AF522424

HYGIENE AND HEALTH

HYGIENE AND HEALTH

M.N. Ahmed

ANMOL PUBLICATIONS PVT. LTD.
NEW DELHI - 110 002 (INDIA)

ANMOL PUBLICATIONS PVT. LTD.
4374/4B, Ansari Road, Daryaganj
New Delhi - 110 002
Ph.: 23261597, 23278000
Visit us at: www.anmolpublications.com

Hygiene and Health

First Published, 2005

ISBN 81-261-2316-8

PRINTED IN INDIA

Published by J.L. Kumar for Anmol Publications Pvt. Ltd., New Delhi - 110 002 and Printed at Mehra Offset Press, Delhi.

Contents

Preface ix

1. **Introduction** 1
Food Quality • Various Products

2. **Correcting the Wrong** 8
Food Adulteration • Legal Aspects • Fake Brands • The Standards

3. **Role of Food** 20
Food Values • Adequate Nutrition • Novel Foods • Processed Foods • Food for Infants

4. **Ideal Diet** 28
Nutritional Requirements • Balanced Diet • Human Needs • Health and Diseases • International Units • Adequate Diet • Milk and Milk Products • Vegetables and Fruits • Cereals and Cereal Products • Energy and Oxidation • Chemical Analysis • Family Food Budget

5. **Diseases of Kidney** 71
Nephrotic Syndrome • Renal Failure

6. **Defects in Cardiovascular System** 80
Hypertension • Atherosclerosis

7. **The Diabetes** 90
Pancreatitis • The Causes • Symptoms • The Treatment

8. **Diseases of Liver** 103
Viral Hepatitis • Hepatic Percoma and Coma • Cirrhosis of Liver

9. **Peptic Ulcer** 110
Aetiology • Dietetic Management • Ulcerative Colitis

10. **Stomach Diseases** 115
Gastro-intestinal Problems • Dyspepsia • Diarrhoea and Dysentery • Malabsorption Syndrome • Constipation • Nutrition in Allergies

11. **Problem of Obesity** 125
The Causes • The Treatment

12. **Diet Therapy** 133
Therapeutic Modifications • Liquid Diets • Soft Diet • Bland Diet • Acidic and Alkaline Foods • Items at Work • Biotin • Pantothenic Acid • Folacin • Folacin Deficiency • Fat-soluble Vitamins • Recommended Allowances • Vitamin K • Vitamin P

13. **Special Diet** 170
During Nervous Disturbances • Epilepsy • In Alcoholism • In Gout and Osteoarthritis • In Fevers • During Deficiency Diseases • The Treatment • Underweight

14. **Specific Nutrition** 193
During Pregnancy • The Complications • During Lactation • During Old Age • During Adolescence • For School Children • For Pre-school Children • The Requirements • During Infancy

15. **Value of Food** **224**
Quality of Food • Consciousness about Health

16. **Desirable Food** **234**
Judging the Quality • The Evolution
• Adulteration of Food • Check and Control

17. **Food Preparation** **254**
Cooking Food • Various Methods • Media of Cooking • Microwave Cooking • New Trends • Art of Cooking • Various Methods • Processing of Food

18. **Safety from Deterioration** **291**
Preservation • Processing • Concentration
• Fermentation

19. **Preserving Agents** **334**
Food Additives • The Requirement • Role of Additives • Unintentional Additives

20. **Aspects and Prospects** **360**
Great Source • Value of Food • Various Patterns
• Effect of Population • Future Prospects

Bibliography 375

Preface

Tourism and Hotel Industry are the two significant sectors of modern day economy and are complimentary to each other. The new world order has turned the whole mankind into one family or society. Today's world is a global village, where distances have no meaning. Although, tourism and travelling are the two phenomena, as old as the civilized world, yet, tourism evolved into a regular and well-organised industry, during the last century only.

Hotel industry is part and parcel of tourism sector. The tourists are honoured guests and the hotels offer them the demanded hospitality. Hence, the two form a correlated industrial sector, which is growing and flourishing fast, with promises for future.

Extension of education and expansion of knowledge have created a new anxiety, among the members of the new generation, regarding the above said two areas. In fact, the two sectors offer high profile career avenues and good opportunities for aspirants and job-seekers. However, like other disciplines, Tourism and Hotel Management also require proper training for professionals. Hence, a large room for exhaustive and exclusive books on the subject, is there.

This series of comprehensive books has been outlined within the parameters of the syllabi of various universities and institutes, in a broad-based manner, in order to cover all streams of the discipline and for the benefit of students at graduate and post-graduate levels.

The undersigned is confident of a due recognition and proper acknowledgement from concerned circles. Further expectation is that this series of useful books would prove to be practically helpful to the professionals and students equally.

— **Editor**

1

Introduction

The concept of hygiene is a new concept. Along with sanitation, it gives a broad based meaning. The word 'sanitation' is derived from the Latin word 'Sanus' meaning 'sound and healthy' or clean and whole. The modern interpretation of the term is broad, including knowledge of health and sanitary conditions as well as full acceptance and effective application of sanitary measures. The National Sanitation Foundation, a non-project, non-commercial organisation with headquarters in the School of Public Health at the University of Michigan, proclaims that sanitation is more than religious sanctions or a code of laws in these words:

> Sanitation is a way of life. It is the quality of living that is expressed in the clean home, the clean farm, the clean business and industry, the clean neighbourhood, the clean community. Being a way of life, it must come from within the people, it is nourished by knowledge and grows as an obligation and an ideal in human relations.

So, people need to be protected against food which has been contaminated by bacteria which are harmful. People also need to be protected against the sale of adulterated food, foods of inferior quality and false advertising. Some of these problems require government help; others depend upon individual understanding and vigilance.

Food is frequently subjected to chemical and biological contamination in a number of ways and this has a direct extensive and important bearing on public health. There is clear evidence now that a vast amount of human diseases and suffering is directly due to the consumption of infected and contaminated food.

Food hygiene means all measures necessary for ensuring the safety wholesomeness and soundness of food at all stages from its growth, production, manufacture until its final consumption.

Diseases transmitted by contaminated foods are classifed as foodborne infections and intoxications. Foodborne infections are usually gastro-intestinal disturbances caused by living organisms, while intoxications are diseases caused by chemical poisons in foods. Poisons may be microbial or non-microbial in origin. Some poisons are even naturally present in foods. Deliberate adulteration of foodstuffs and the use of an ever increasing number of chemicals in agriculture, dairy: farming, storage and processing of foods is currently introducing a number of highly toxic substances into present day foods. A knowledge of the variety of toxicants found in foods due to lack of food sanitation and hygiene, faulty methods of cultivation, harvesting, transport, storage, processing, distribution and cooking, is therefore necessary for every consumer.

Food Quality

The importance of an intelligent selection of fruits and vegetables for use in the home must not be ignored. This necessitates a knowledge of the characteristics which denote good quality in the various products.

Fruits : Fruits such as apples, pears, peaches, plums and tomatoes should have! full colour, a reasonable degree of firmness and an absence of surface defects such as scars and bruises.

Berries : Berries of all sorts and grapes should have full colour, should be firm and have a plump, fresh appearance. They should be dry, clean and free from foreign material, including sand and leaves.

Citrus : Citrus fruits should be well coloured and heavy for their size. They should have a fine-textured bright skin, russetting of the skin, if extensive, need not adversely affect interior quality. Grapefruit should be flat rather than pointed at the stem end. Oranges should have rough and loose skins which are characteristic of this variety of fruit.

Salad Plants : Salad plants and greens which include spinach, should be of green colour, fresh, crisp, and tender. They should be free from wilted yellow leaves. Headed types of salad plants like some varieties lettuce should be fairly firm. Carrots and other root vegetables she be firm, of good shape, clean and fresh looking. The pods of lima beans peas and all vegetables of similar type should be of a good green colour and well filled with seeds. They should be clean and bright in appearance and crisp and firm in texture. Snap beans should be of a healthy green or yellow colour according to the variety. The pods should be clean and fresh in appearance and firm, tender and crisp in texture. The enclosed beans should be small. Cauliflowers should be either white or creamy-white in colour. The head should be firm and compact, not open and loose, a condition which is indicative of growth of the flower clusters. Broccoli should be of a good dark green colour. The clusters of buds should be compact and should not show any of the purple or yellow colour of the flower. The stems should be tender, firm and crisp. Potatoes should be smooth, shallow-eyed and free from any green coloration. The colour of skin and the size and shape of this vegetable vary with variety. Onions should be dry, hard, bright and well developed.

Selection of Eggs : The shell of an egg may be either off-white or white in colour depending upon the breed of the hen producing it. But irrespective of colour, the shell of a fresh egg always has a delicate velvety appearance called "bloom" that is due to the protective mucous coating with which the shell is supplied when the egg is laid. The inner air cell of fresh egg is small. The egg contents, when broken out from the shell show an upstanding, well coloured yolk covered with a clinging layer of thick egg-white which, in turn, is surrounded by a relatively smaller amount of thin egg-white. The yolk may be either golden or light yellow in colour depending upon the amount of carotenoid pigments contained in it, and the white is practically colourless or possibly slightly opalescent. There is no odour other than that characteristic of an egg and upon being put to food use the flavour will be excellent

Meat : Good quality requirements are as follows: The flesh must be firm, the fasciculi should be small, contributing thereby a fine grain and velvety texture to the lean part of the cut. The colour of the flesh must be characteristic of the animal origin—a bright cherry-red for beef, pinkish red for lamb, and greyish pink for veal and pork. The bone must be relatively small and when cut, must be red and spongy in appearance, denoting youth; this is in contrast to white, hard and flint-like bone which denotes age. The fat must be white and firm and there must be plenty of marbling. Finally there must be a relatively small proportion of connective tissues.

Fish : Fish is a food that deteriorates quickly unless handled with great care. When buying fish from the market the purchaser should be able to recognise the characteristics that indicate freshness of the product. Some of these are: Vertebrate fish: the gills should be bright red, the eyes clean, bright and slightly bulging. The flesh should be firm and, when pressed with a finger, sufficiently elastic to spring back into place. Shell-fish: those such as lobsters and crabs should be alive when purchased, shrimps should have firm not flabby bodies, oysters, clams and the like should be alive and their shells tightly closed or if relaxed they should be closed when the fish is handled. Always the odour of fish should be fresh with no suggestion of putrefaction.

Milk : The quality of milk is determined by the grades given to it. The criteria for grading milk as laid down by the Milk Ordinance and Code are on the basis of (1) the bacterial count per given volume of the milk as determined by laboratory investigation, and (2) whether the milk comes from daily farms which meets with designated requirements.

Certified Milk is milk which conforms to the requirements of the Medical Milk Commission and is produced under the supervision of the state or local board of health. It may either be raw or pasteurised. Such milk is the highest quality of milk obtainable and is often used for infant feeding.

Grade A Raw Milk must not exceed the limit of bacterial count permitted and it must meet the highest standards of sanitary production.

Grade A Pasteurised Milk must be of similar quality with these differences: before pasteurisation the bacterial count may be higher than for raw milk of this grade; but after pasteurisation, it must be lower for grade A pasteurised than for grade A raw milk.

Grade B Milks, raw and pasteurised fall below the standards set for raw and pasteurised milk of grade A quality, but they must none the less meet specified criteria, both the limit of bacterial load and sanitary conditions of production that are permitted for raw milks of these grades.

Grade C Milks Raw and Pasteurised are products which violate the requirements for grade B products raw or pasteurised. Such milk should be used only for cookery purposes. This is especially true of the grade C raw milk.

Fats : Fats and oils may have one or more of five principal uses in the average institution food service. The uses may be as a spread on breads and toasts; flavouring or it may be an ingredient of a sauce or dressing for raw or cooked foods such as white sauce, mayonnaise, French dressing and tartar sauce. Another use is in frying, basting and other methods of cooking food. Lastly, for shortening, as in the making of doughs and batters. In each case, flavour, form and other physical and chemical characteristics, as well as food habits to which we are accustomed, influence the choice of fat and its use.

Colour, flavour, odour, consistency, keeping quality and nutritive value are important factors to keep in mind when selecting fat for the purpose of spreading or seasoning. Added to the above would be the emulsifying property and stability under heat for fats to be included in sauces and cooked foods. Oils are used in salad dressings and in browning and frying.

Fat for frying or shortening should be bland and should impart no flavour of its own to the fried food. It should resist rancidity and have a high smoking point, long frying life and low turnover or absorption by the food.

Various Products

These include wheat, rice and corn in their various forms. The kinds of cereal grains are the dried fruits of grasses and although the seed structure varies characteristically with each kind, there are basic similarities among all of them. The first is the likeness of the kernel to a well-wrapped sealed parcel. If the package is broken, the possibilities of rancidity increase. Early measures taken to prevent rancidity in milled products include removal of the germ in the process of refining the cereal which reduces the national nutritive value of the cereal. Regarding rice, brown rice has a higher fat content and a high nutritive value.

Food Poisoning : Bacteria enter the body through either food or water from a contaminated source and cause poisoning which, in the majority of cases, turns out to be fatal. Practices to prevent food poisoning are:

1. Observe the rules of food hygiene at every stage in the handling of food. People known to be harbouring infections should not be allowed to handle foodstuffs in the critical stages of preparation and distribution.
2. Keep perishable foods under deep-freeze or refrigeration immediately after purchase to prevent multiplication of bacteria already present. The refrigerator should be kept clean and foodstuffs must be placed in it in such a way that cold air can freely circulate around different items.

This is to make sure that the foodstuffs kept in the fridge are cooled rapidly and kept cold. No spoiled food should be placed in a refrigerator.

3. Cook foods for a sufficient length of time and at temperatures high enough to destroy the bacteria. Meat should be cut into small pieces to ensure thorough penetration of heat. If required in large chunks meat should be roasted or pressure cooked.

4. Do not keep foods exposed, especially after cooking. If the food is to be consumed later, it should be promptly cooled and put in the refrigerator.

5. If the food has been refrigerated for a long time, it should be reheated before consumption.

6. Foodstuffs such as custard-filled bakery products should be reheated in an oven at 200° C for 20 to 30 minutes before consumption.

7. Keep storage, cooking and service areas clean and free from insects and rodents.

Thus, careful selection of foodstuffs and observing certain food sanitation measures prevent all the food-borne infections and other diseases which are hazardous to health.

2

Correcting the Wrong

Food Adulteration

The practice of adulteration of foodstuffs and marketing of substandard or materials of poor quality is widely prevalent in our country. It has been roughly estimated that over 50 per cent of marketed foodstuffs available today are adulterated in one way or another. The percentage varies from region to region. It is an unpalatable fact for a nation to admit, but there is little doubt that the Indian consumer, unlike his Western counterpart, cannot take the purity of foodstuffs for granted. Despite the existence of legislation to prevent adulteration of foodstuffs, a very large number offered to the consumer today are injurious to health.

One of the causes of adulteration is that there is a wide gap between production and supply of food articles. The temptation for quick gain and easy profits amongst most merchants, slow action by the authorities, the poor enforcement of Prevention of Food Adulteration Act and leniency shown to traders in regard to the enforcement of the laws on food safety, lengthy procedural wrangles and delays, due to various loopholes in our legal system, contribute to the rampant adulteration of foodstuffs. The gullibility of the predominantly illiterate masses coupled with ignorance, apathy and indifference make for easy adulteration. In a developing country, the cost factor is the most crucial point for a large segment of the population, the cheapest product is preferred to the best. There are a large number of mushroom industries to cater to this section.

Almost all foods, milk, cereals, dais, spices, ghee, oils and beverages are adulterated. The adulterant used generally mixes well with the major food article in colour, shape, size and appearance. The more highly priced foods and those foods which are in great demand are the ones more often widely adulterated. By adulterating the foodstuffs, the merchant is benefited in many ways. First more weight is added to the commodity. Secondly, addition of colour improves the appearance of the product and hence substandard product can fetch higher price. Thirdly, new product when combined with the old one, lowers the quality and at the same time substandard commodity is sold at a higher rate. The ingenuity, imagination and initiative shown in adulteration make it difficult for an average buyer to detect it at first sight. Sometimes, it can be detected only in well-equipped laboratories. Besides the relatively harmless forms of adulteration like addition of water to milk, moisture to butter, mixing of edible oils with cheaper edible oils, many types of adulteration are positively injurious to health.

Rice and pulses are often polished with talc, a silicate containing asbestos fibre, which is not removed even after washing, cleaning and cooking. The Japanese have traced cases of stomach cancer to this practice. The other common adulterants used in cereals such as rice and wheat are clay particles, grit, soap stone and weed seeds. Most yellow pulses are adulterated either with kesari dal or by polishing with metanil yellow, a cheap soluble coal tar dye that makes the pulses deceptively brighter and cleaner looking. Metanil yellow is a highly toxic substance with accumulative tendencies, which over the years build up enough toxicity in the body to cause testicular degeneration in the male. When khesari dal is consumed continuously for a few months, it results in the development of lathyrism, a permanent paralysis of the lower limbs.

Spices, particularly because of their high cost, are the most adulterated item in food commodities. Turmeric is coated with lead chromate or metanil yellow to give a lustrous yellow colour. Black pepper is sometimes mixed with papaya berries. Foodgrains and pulses are often indiscriminately sprayed with insecticides to prevent infestation or to destroy pests; chillies are soaked in soluble coal tar dyes to give them a deeper hue, while sawdust, blackgram husk, and used tea leaves are utilised for adulterating tea dust/leaves. These are a few of the many common practices that are used today. Many cheap sweets, sherbets in variety of colours and ice fruits are adulterated with many non-permitted coal tar dyes. These undesirable colours can impair the liver and can be the cause of cancers. Similarly, lead chromate when added to turmeric powder can cause lead poisoning resulting in stiffness of limbs and paralysis. Mineral oils and other non-edible oils when mixed with edible oils can induce nausea, purging, impaired liver functions and cancer. Continuous use of mustard oil with more than 11 per cent argemone seed oil causes the disease 'epidemic dropsy' in people. Further, many mould-infested grains and oil seeds are further processed into flours and oils. Here the main danger is due to the mould growth which produces many hidden toxic substances called mycotoxins. These can cause various diseases and they act as nervous and neurotoxins impairing the general health. Some also have been found to be carcinogenic.

The menace of food adulteration exists all over the world. In developed countries, due to the implementation of food laws for the last few decades, there has been a significant improvement in the quality of food. But due to tremendous improvement in food industry and technology, various chemical substances like artificial colours, preservatives, antioxidants, emulsifiers, flavour and taste improvers are increasingly being used. Some of these pose a great threat to the health of the people. As against this, in developing countries adulteration is found to be rampant even in primary articles of food like milk, ghee, edible oils and foodgrains. Shortage of food and spiralling prices have aggravated the problem. Thus all countries in the world have to grapple in their own way with problems raised by food adulteration.

Legal Aspects

In India, as early as in 1860, adulteration of food was dealt with in certain sections of the Indian Penal Code (Sec. 272,273). Later it was included under the provisions of the Municipal Act. But as a comprehensive act, it was first promulgated in Bombay State in 1899. Subsequently similar acts were enacted by other states also. In the erstwhile Travancore State an Act—The Travancore Prevention of Adulteration Act—was enacted in 1931. Besides food adulteration, adulteration of other articles was also made an offence under this act But then acts were not comprehensive in many ways. The punishment prescribed was not deterrent enough to prevent adulteration of food efficiently. There was no uniformity of standards prescribed for various food articles. The necessity of a comprehensive act applicable to all the states was felt. In 1938 the Central Advisory Board of Health was established. This Board in its report stressed the necessity for efficiently tackling the problem by all states. When the Constitution of India was framed the topic of prevention of adulteration of food was brought under the concurrent list and the P.F.A. Act was formulated in 1954. It was enacted on June 1,1955. After about ten years of implementation of the Act, the position was reviewed and some amendments were made in the Act in 1964 to plug loopholes and to give more protection to the honest traders. Again in 1976 some other important amendments were made to the present act to make it more effective and purposeful. These amendments came into force from April 1,1976.

Object of the Act : What the consumer wants is genuine, wholesome food, of nutritive value, free from any health hazard. He also expects that labelling must be truthful and there shall not be fraudulent claims of any kind by any statement, device or design. The interest of the trader is not only to sell the food articles to the consumers but also to make the maximum profit out of it. This conflicting interest of the consumer on the one hand and the traders on the other, lead to unhealthy practices in trade. It is to prevent such practices that the Act has been made. Though the consumer's interest is the foremost in the P.FA. Act, that of the traders have also been accommodated reasonably as far as scientific grounds and consumers' interest permit.

***Important Provisions of the Act*:** Food has been defined under the Act as articles other than drugs and water, which are ordinarily used as food ondrink and all articles which enter into and are used in the preparation of human food. Another definition of 'primary food' has also been introduced by the amendment act of 1976. Primary foods are products of agriculture or horticulture in its natural form.

The term adulterated has been defined under Section 2 of the Act: An article of food will be deemed to be adulterated if it is not of the nature, substance or quality demanded by the purchaser and is to his prejudice or not of the nature, substance or quality which it purports to be; if an article is partly or wholly substituted by the cheaper substance; if any constituent of the article is extracted from it, if it is prepared or exposed for sale under insanitary and unhygienic surrounding; if it contains prohibited colouring matter or preservative or permitted colouring matters and preservatives in excess of the permissible limits; if it does not conform to the standards under all these conditions it will be deemed to be adulterated. There is a provision that a primary food will not be deemed to be adulterated if it does not conform to standards due to natural causes beyond the control of human agency. In short, anything which lowers the quality of a food article has been brought wider the definition of adulteration.

Fake Brands

Sale of food articles without proper labelling, imitation of other food articles and coating food articles to give improved appearance are brought wider the definition 'misbranding'.

Prohibitory Section : Section 7 of the P.F.A. Act prohibits the sale of (a) any adulterated food, (b) any misbranded food, (c) any article of food for the sale of which a licence is prescribed except in accordance with the conditions of the licence, (d) any article of food and sale of which has been prohibited by the Food (Health) Authority in the interest of public health, (e) any article of food in contravention of the provision of the Act and Rules, and (f) any adulterant.

Crime and Punishment : Infringement of the provision of Section 7 is punishable under Section 16. Various offences and punishments for each have been detailed under mese sections. This section has been amended by the amendment act of 1976. Non-graded punishment, depending on the nature of the offence has been laid down. For the sale of adulterated food the minimum punishment is six month's imprisonment and a fine of rupees one thousand. If the adulterant is of such a nature as to cause death or grievous hurt when consumed by a person, the punishment is imprisonment for a term of three years which may extend to life imprisonment and a fine which shall not be less than rupees live thousand. Punishment has been prescribed for sale of misbranded food and the sale of adulterant. Preventing a Food Inspector from exercising his powers and duties under the Act, using a report of the Public Analyst of Director of Central Food Laboratory for advertising purposes, not issuing warranty, issuing false warranty, tampering of seized food articles are all punishable under the law.

Protection of the Traders : Section 7 of the Act prohibits the sale of adulterated food or any consumable article, by any person either by himself or by any person on his behalf. Prima facie it may seem that an innocent person who buys a food article from a wholesaler or manufacturer and sells it without knowing that it is adulterated is punishable under the Act. Sections 14, 14 A, 19(2) and 20A are meant to protect honest vendors of food articles. Section 14 lays down that no manufacturer, distributor or dealer of any article of food shall sell such article to any vendor unless he also gives a warranty in writing about the nature of substance and quality of such food to the vendor. Insistence of warranty at the time of sale by the manufacturer, distributor or dealer would make it easy to pin down the responsibility with the offender. The amendment of 1976 makes this easier by incorporating a provision that a cash bill can also be considered as a warranty. According to Section 14A, the vendor has to disclose to the Food Inspector the name, address and other particulars of the person from whom he purchased the food article. This helps the Food Inspector to proceed against the warrantor also. According to Section 19(2) of die Act, a vendor shall not be deemed to have committed an offence if he proves that he purchased the food article with a proper warranty, that he stored the article properly and that he sold it in the same condition in which it was purchased. Section 19(3) confers a right on the warrantor to appear in court and give evidence. The law thus protects the warrantor also against spurious warranties. When warranty is proved, the vendor can be exonerated and the warrantor can be proceeded against. As per Section 20A during the trial, when warranty is proved the court can proceed against the warrantor as though a prosecution has been launched against him.

The Standards

There are two standards set up by the government to help the manufacturers, the traders and the consumers to ensure quality. They are 'Agmark' standard and 'Indian Standards Institution mark.

Agmark Standard : The Directorate of Marketing and Inspection of the Government of India have set up this standard. This grades goods into (1) Special (Grade I), (2) Good (Grade ft), (3) Fair (Grade m) and Ordinary (Grade IV). These standards also specify the type of packaging to be used for different rent products. An Agmark certificate is issued to traders and the mark on commodities provides assurance of the quality to the consumer.

Indian Standards Institution (IS1) : The ISI mark on food is a guarantee of good quality. This institution prescribes standards for various food items and issues certificates, to traders.

Common Food Adulterants

Foodstuffs	***Common Adulterants***
Milk and milk products	Water, removal of butter and addition of refined oil.
Milk, liquid	Fat addition of skimmed milk reconstituted from skimmed milk powder.
Milk powder	Staich, dextrins.
Cream	Other fats.
Ice-cream	Non-permitted colour, artificial sweetness, other fats and gelling agents.
Butter	Other fats.
Ghee	Hydrogenated fat.
Vegetables oils and fats	
Vanaspati	Animal fat and other high melting fats.
Vegetable oil	Argemone oil, mineral oil, orthotricresyl phosphate, cheap non-edible oils.
Spices and condiments	
Whole turmeric	Coating of lead chromaie or coal-tar dyes.
Turmeric powder	Coal-tar colour, yellow earth, starch or talc coloured yellow by coal-tar dye.
Curry powder	Starch coloured red by coal-tar dye.
Coriander seeds	Other seeds coloured green.
Coriander seed powder	Powdered bran or sawdust coloured green with dye.
Chilli powder	Starch coloured brown by coal-tar dyes.
Mustard	Argemone seeds.
Cumin	Artificial jeera like product.
Black pepper	Dried papaya seeds.
Asafoetida	Resins and other plant gums.

Foodstuffs	Common Adulterants
Cereals	
Wheat and rice	Stones.
Wheat flour	Tapioca flour, talc
Semolina	Tapioca semolina.
Pulses	
Bengal gram dal	Khesari dal (Lathynis sativus)
Red gram dal	Coloured yellow with coal-tar dye.
Bengal gram flour	Tapioca flour or starch coloured yellow with dye.
Sweetening agents and soft drinks	
Honey	Coloured canesugar syrup.
Soft drinks	Artificial sweeteners (Saccharin).
Beverages	
Coffee powder	Exhausted coffee powder, roasted husk or date seed or tamarind seed powder.
Tea	Other leaves with added colour, exhausted tea leaves.
Miscellaneous	
Processed arecanut (Supari)	other seeds or nuts broken and coloured.

Consumer Protection

For consumer protection there are a number of laboratories in central and state level. They are set up to collect samples and to analyse it. Some of the Government agencies are:

(1) Municipal Laboratories in big cities.

(2) Food and Drug Administration Laboratories of States.

(3) Central Food Testing Laboratory of the Government of India, and

(4) Laboratories of the Export Inspection Council.

Municipal Laboratories

In municipalities of big cities like Mumbai, Delhi, Chennai and Kolkata they have set up their own testing laboratories. According to the Prevention of Food Adulteration Act the Municipal analyst qualification must be scrutinised. Chemical and microbiological analysis of all kinds of foods are essential in the laboratory. Nutrient analysis like fat content of milk, contamination of water or pesticide residue in parts per million in foods etc. are some examples of the test conducted there.

These laboratories are under the Health Officer of the state. Health inspectors under him make periodical rounds of the various wards and collect samples of food suspected to be adulterated. Samples are sealed in the presence of the vendor and witness and sent to the municipal laboratory for analysis. The Health Officer can take action against the manufacturer of the food if he is found to be guilty. The manufacturer can defend himself in the court of law. Depending on the severity of crime he can be punished by a fine or imprisonment or both.

Food and Drug Administration : Some state Governments have laboratories throughout states. The Director of the Administration is empowered through his staff to collect samples which are suspected to be adulterated and have them analysed by the Health Officer of a municipality. The Food and Drug Administration has jurisdiction all over the state as compared to municipal laboratories which work only within city limits.

The Central Food Testing Laboratory : The Government of India has established a Central Food Testing Laboratory in Kolkata for carrying out analysis of all foods. These laboratories are very well equipped and carry out even sophisticated and sensitive analyses. These laboratories are the ultimate authority in determining whether a food sample is adulterated or not in cases of conflicting reports of analyses from two laboratories, the authorities concerned usually refer the case to this laboratory. Usually analysis carried out by these laboratories are accepted as the last word in analysis of food.

Export Inspection Council Laboratory : The Government of India has made it mandatory for all exporters to have their products analysed so as to ensure the quality of foods exported. Frozen food items like seafood, canned fruits and vegetables are also analysed before export. It also sees to it that all the foods exported conform to the minimum requirements as laid down by the council. The council has laboratories in all the major parts and the samples analysed. Without the council's certificate no food can be exported.

Quality Checking Agencies

Quality Control Laboratories of Companies : Most of the companies which manufacture food products have well equipped quality control laboratories to check the quality of their products. The ingredients used for manufacturing and the products are examined physically, chemically and microbiologically. The taste, weight, volume, colour, keeping quality, packaging all these factors are checked.

In the dairy industry microbiological centre of the milk, are taken and the fat content determined, the former gives an idea of the sanitary condition under which the milk was collected, the latter whether any cream had been removed. Proper pasteurisation is also checked before supply.

In canning fruits and vegetables the fresh materials are visually inspected and all the bruised and spoiled ones removed. Oxidity of fruits like mangoes, cherries, tenderness of vegetables like green peas are determined to estimate duration of processing time, accelerated storage tests at higher temperature one conducted to ensure the keeping quality of the canned food.

In freezing, quality control checks at various stages of

processing are carried out to see that the final frozen product conforms to the prescribed microbiological standards, weights after thawing and drying are taken to make sure that the customer gets the right weight. Biscuit, dairy, fruit and vegetable canning industries set up their quality.

Quality Control Laboratories of Consumer Cooperation : Apna Bazar in Mumbai, Super Bazar in Delhi, Chinthamani in Coimbatore have criteria for selection of food items which they sell in their shop. If the qualities are not fulfilled they will not accept materials.

Testing Laboratories : There are a number of private testing laboratories which carry out tests of all food materials on payment. Government has recognised certain private laboratories and certificates given by them are valid for legal purposes.

Consumer Guidance Society : A consumer guidance society has been formed in India with Bombay as its headquarters and with branches in major cities. They create consumer awareness of the various forms of adulteration and develop consumer resistance to such adulterated food products through various communications and mass media.

3

Role of Food

Food is essential for human existence just like the air we breathe or the water we drink. The food that we eat is utilised in the body and the assimilated substances are used for the growth and maintenance of tissues. A living organism is the product of nutrition. The human being requires more than 45 different nutrients for its well-being. Food materials ingested by the body are digested, absorbed and metabolised. Useful chemical substances derived from food by the body are called nutrients. A number of foodstuffs have to be selected to get all the nutrients. The health of a person depends on the type and quantity of foodstuff he chooses to make his diet For sustaining healthy and vigorous life, diet should be planned according to the principles of nutrition. Extensive research work carried out on human beings and on experimental animals throughout the world has provided us with sufficient knowledge on nutrition and health. World Health Organisation defines health as "the state of complete physical, mental and social well being and not merely the absence of disease or infirmity".

Food Values

Nutrition is the science of food values. It is relatively a new science which was evolved from chemistry and physiology.

Nutrition is often mentioned as a branch of chemical science or biochemistry. The effect of food on our body is explained in nutrition. In other words, nutrition is defined as food at work in the body. In a broader sense nutrition is defined as the combination of process by which the living organism receives and utilises the materials necessary for the maintenance of its functions and for the growth and renewal of its components. Nutrients are defined as the constituents of food which help us to maintain our body functions, to grow and to protect our organs. There are six major nutrients in our body. They are carbohydrates, proteins, lipids, vitamins and minerals. The human body requires 17 vitamins and 24 mineral elements for various day-to-day activities. The composition of human body is 60-62 per cent water, 17 per cent proteins, 14 per cent fat, 6 per cent minerals and 1 per cent carbohydrates. In infants the percentage of water is more as compared to an adult. In women water content is slightly lower whereas fat content is more than in men. Fat deposition in the body increases with age.

Percentage Composition of Human Body

Nutrients	*Man*	*Woman*
Water	60-62	54
Protein	17	15
Fat	14	25
Minerals	6	5
Carbohydrates	1	1

Vitamins are present in negligible amounts.

Relationships of food to health have been made from the research conducted by chemists, microbiologists, pathologists and nutritionist from the past two centuries.

Human nutrition is governed by many factors like food habits and behaviour, food beliefs, ethnic influences, geographic influences, religious and sociological factors, psychological factors, food and production, income, national and international food policies, food technology, processing, fisheries, transportation, marketing, educational status and other mass media facilities.

The benefits of good nutrition are health, happiness, efficiency and longevity.

Adequate Nutrition

When all the essential nutrients are present in a correct proportion as required by our body, it is called optimum nutrition or adequate nutrition. Optimum nutrition is required to maintain good health.

There are certain signs of good nutrition. They are height and weight for the age, clear complexion, fresh and lively skin and hair, healthy pink nails, correct posture and gait, inquisitive and alert eyes, good appetite and bowel evacuation, emotional maturity and confident deeds and pleasing personality and optimism in life and overall health.

Undernourishment : When almost all nutritions are below the requirement, the condition is known as undernourishment Under nourishment may be defined as a state of partial starvation. An undernourished person manifests symptoms of deficiencies and feels unwell. Poor body weight, poor resistance to infection, weakness, apathy and general ill-health are symptoms of undernourishment.

Malnutrition : Malnutrition is an impairment of health either from a deficiency or excess or imbalance of nutrients. Malnutrition is a condition when one or two nutrients are less or are in excess in the body. This again manifests in disorders and discomforts. Severe malnutrition in certain phases of life can do irreparable damage to the body. Physical, mental and intellectual well-being in a person is affected due to malnourishment. Emotional upset and intellectual dwarfism create personality problems in later life. Impaired functional ability and deficient structural integrity result from malnutrition. Marasmus, kwashiorkor, xerophthalmia, scurvy, rickets, osteomalacia, beri-beri, pellagra and anaemia result from the deficiencies of protein, calories, vitamin A, vitamin C, vitamin D, B-complex vitamins and minerals, respectively. Malnutrition creates lasting effect on the growth and development of a person. Permanent retardation of the central nervous system occurs due to protein calorie malnutrition in early life. Thus nutrients from food sources enable one to keep fit and maintain health. These substances include energy which gives the capacity to work, proteins which form our body muscles, bones, blood, body fluids, enzymes, hormones, antibodies, organs, skin, hair and nervous tissues. Food also supplies minerals and vitamins which protect our organs and regulate their functions and other physiological processes.

Classification of Foods : Based on these functions, foods are grouped into energy-yielding foods, body-building foods and protective foods. Nutrients which engage in these activities are known as energy-yielding nutrients, body-building nutrients and protective nutrients. Carbohydrase, fats and proteins release energy on metabolism in our body.

1 gm of carbohydrates provides	- 4 kcals
1 gm of proteins provides	- 4 kcals
1 gm of fat provides	- 9 kcals

Cereal grains like rice, wheat, ragi and maize, roots and tubers like potato, sweet potato and tapioca are good sources of carbohydrates. Fats are considered the concentrated source of energy as they supply more than double the quantity of carlories compared to carbohydrates and proteins. Though proteins yield energy, normally they are considered body-building foods. Nutrients like proteins, mineral salts like calcium, phosphorus, iron and water are body-building nutrients. Their sources are body-building foods. Just like a house is built from wood, brick, cement, sand, iron rods, nails and other materials our organs in the body are built from the substances derived from food.

Protein foods like milk, meat, fish, eggs, pulses, grams and nuts are essential to build our tissues and to form blood.

Our body functions are regulated by water, certain minerals and vitamins. They are essential for the well-being and working of the body. They are called protective foods. Foods rich in protein, minerals, vitamins and water are termed as protective foods. Water is necessary for various body processes.

Minerals like calcium help in controlling blood clotting, muscular contraction and for the efficiency of heart muscles. Iron is essential for blood formation and iodine is necessary for regulating body function through the thyroid gland.

Vitamins are essential for regulating the body process such as growth, muscular coordination of various organs and functions of several organs like eyes, ears, nose and skin.

Thus foods play a prominent role in providing physical, mental and social well-being which is otherwise known as health to the people. Health is reflected in a person's nutritional status. Nutritional status is the condition of the individual as influenced by the utilisation of the nutrients. Dietary history, physical examination and laboratory examinations reveal it

Novel Foods

Food industry has brought out some novel protein-rich foods which can be used for combating malnutrition. Some of them are from unusual food sources which were never considered as consumable by our forefathers. Leaf and grass proteins, food yeast, algae and microbial synthesis of proteins from hydrocarbons are some of the novel food sources now available.

Leaf Protein Concentrates : Proteins from fibrous materials of leaf are separated and leaf protein concentrates with 30 to 35 per cent of the original nitrogen can be extracted from leaves. Outstanding work in this field has come from Pine et al in 1961. Leaf protein concentrates can be incorporated with milk or in common flours or dal powders for children's foods.

Food Yeast : Yeast is capable of converting carbohydrate to protein. About 16 to 33 per cent of this type of conversion is possible by yeast. Thus it can be incorporated at 5 to 10 per cent level in children's foods. Food yeast is a pale yellow product. It has a characteristic nut-like taste. This can be incorporated in low cost foods for infants, it can also be used for overcoming protein malnutrition among children.

Algae : A unicellular green algae chlorella contains a protein content of about 50 to 60 per cent. This can be incorporated with soups, noodles and in baked items. Even though it is nutritionally good, its acceptability is very poor.

Microbial Synthesis of Proteins from Hydrocarbons : Certain petroleum hydrocarbons can be converted to proteins through microbial use. Its utilisation for human beings is not established even though as an animal feed it is used.

Processed Foods

Modern technology has made many food sources into processed items. Food industry is developing in accordance with modern living. Almost all food groups are now processed into readymade or ready for table items. Pre-cooked or half cooked items are also available. Examples of some of these items are given below.

Cereals: Starch is a polysaccharide and it is used in cookery. It is manufactured from corn, potato, sweet potato and tapioca. In the market it is available as tapioca starch, arrowroot starch and starch products like sago or custard powder where cornstarch is flavoured with vanilla and edible colour and corn syrup.

Rice is available in processed form as instant rice or quick cooking rice. It is prepared by cooking rice and dehydrating the cooked rice so as to retain a porous structure.

Puffed rice from paddy and from parboiled rice is available in the market.

Cornflakes from corn can be used as a breakfast item.

Barley is processed into barley flour and pearl barley. Malted barley is breakfast item.

Oats is available as oatflakes in processed forms.

Breakfast cereals and infant foods are often prepared from cereals. Flaked items from all cereals, puffed wheat, rice, barley and corn are available in the market. Shredded breakfast cereals like shredded wheat is a pre-cooked item.

Food for Infants

Most of the infant foods contain both cereals and milk and these pre-cooked cereals are eaten as gruels with water or milk. Rice noodles are popular in some of the Far East countries. Sago or sabudana is made from rice, or other cereals. Biscuits and breads are also processed cereal products.

Pulses are processed into puffed grams. Now commercial instant mixes of cereal, dal, fermented products are also available. Ready mixes of South Indian dishes like idli and dosa are prepared by using baker's yeast or baking soda and acidifying agents like citric acid.

Puffed chickpeas and peas and canned dry peas are available as processed items.

Roasted groundnut and protein isolates from soyabean or peanut can be used in the production of toned milk and protein-rich biscuits or bread. Soyabean milk powder and butter are available in the market.

Milk powders, malted milk powders, various weaning foods, ice-cream mix, cream and condensed milk, cheese, khoa-based sweets, channa or paneer-based sweets like rasogulla and sandesh are some of the processed milk products. New milk-derived products like Miltone and Chai-sathi are available, especially in North India.

Fruits are processed into fruit juices. Today even bananas and guavas are used to prepare juice. Fruit juice concntrates and fruit juice powders are made from juices along with syrups or squashes. Cordials, ketchups, sauces, jellies, jams, marmalades, artificial syrups, dried fruit and salad, preserves, candies, glaced and crystallised fruits and fruit-cereal flakes are available in the market as processed foods.

Vegetables are processed into soups, purees, canned or frozen and dehydrated forms.

Egg powder, egg albumin powder, custard or caramelised custard powder and readymade puddings are some of the processed forms of egg available in the market.

Meat is processed into canned meat, cured meat, smoked meat, sausages, cutlets, soup powder and as dehydrated meat.

Strained baby foods with meat are being manufactured in some places.

Fish is processed into frozen, canned and dried forms. Fish protein concentrates and fishmeal and strained baby foods with fish are also available as processed items in developed countries.

All food items are processed in very many ways and they are marketed in various forms. Pickled and fermented items of innumerable sources are also available in the market.

4

Ideal Diet

Everyone knows that good diet is needed to sustain good health. By health we mean the well-being of an individual in physical, emotional and social conditions. Just the presence or absence of a disease cannot label a person as healthy. Sound emotional and mental condition of an individual is contributed by good nutrition. A healthy person will have a positive attitude towards life. A good natured person full of life reflects his better health standards. A good or adequate diet is known as 'balanced diet'. A balanced diet yields daily nutrients in the proper amounts and proportion required by the body.

Nutritional Requirements

Nutritional requirements vary according to age, sex, physical activities and other physiological conditions. The National Institute of Nutrition is engaged in research work on the dietary pattern of Indians and their requirements of various nutrients. The Nutrition Advisory Committee of the Indian Council of Medical Research made recommendations in 1944 for all nutrients. They were revised in 1958 and 1968. In 1980 further recommendations were made by the Nutrition Advisory Committee and the latest requirements are available now for formulating balanced diets for various groups. A balanced diet must supply enough food to the body for deriving energy. Energy is simply expressed as the capacity to do work. For basic activities like heart beat, breathing and excretion energy is required. Energy is stored as carbohydrate in foods. Cereals like rice, wheat, millets like ragi or bajra contain much carbohydrates in the form of starch. Starchyuits like banana and roots like tapioca, potato, yam, colocasia and sweet potato are rich in carbohydrates. Energy requirements for various age groups are given elsewhere and for an adult sedentary man 2,400 kcals are required and for a sedentary woman 1,900 kcals are recommended. In a balanced diet energy from cereals should not exceed more than 75 per cent of total requirements. Energy derived from fat or oil should not exceed 15 per cent of the total calories and from refined carbohydrates (sugar and jaggery) has been recommended around 5 per cent of the total calories.

A balanced diet must supply enough protien for building up our tissues in various parts of our body. When some tissurs get worn out or used up proteins repair and replace them. Proteins are essential for the secretion of digestive juices and synthesis of enzymes and hormone production. Dietary proteins are used again for the synthesis of body ins. Protein requirements must be met by dietary proteins. Usually in requirement is in terms of body weight, that is, 1 gm of protein to body weight is the recommendation. Even though animal ins are of superior quality it is not a practical suggestion to depend on them for dietary proteins. In an average Indian diet pulses are a very important source of proteins. When nutritional scores are given to jus proteins egg has a high score of 90 per cent whereas vegetable proteins score only 45 to 50 per cent in the case of pulses and 45 per cent to cereals. But it can be improved by incorporating pulse and cereal proteins; 40 to 60 gms of pulses and 150 to 250 ml of milk can provide enough proteins in a vegetarian diet For non-vegetarians 20 to 30 gms of pulses and one egg or 30 gms of meat or fish and 100 to 150 ml of k provide the protein requirement If no pulse is used non-elarians can take two eggs or 50 gms of meat or fish or 30 gms of fish neat and one egg.

Fats and oils are other major nutrients in a balanced diet. Fats are icentrated forms of energy. Fat soluble vitamins are utilised only in presence of fat For males 40 to 65 gms of fat and for females 20 to gms of fat must be included in a balanced diet. Vitamins are essential the proper functioning of our body. Small quantities of vitamins own dramatic effect on our body. Organs like eyes, alimentary canal, in and mucous membraneous structures depend on vitamins for their formal structure and functions. Leafy vegetables, other vegetables, yellow vegetables and roots and tubers provide almost all the vitamins required by our body. About a quarter kilogramme of vegetables is required in our daily diet to ensure vitamin supply. Raw vegetables or sprouted grams or fruits are essential to supply vitamin C. Minerals like calcium, phosphorus, iron and trace elements and salts are essential to laintain good health. Sodium chloride is essential to regulate water metabolism in our body. A balanced diet provides enough vitamins and minerals from natural sources. Tonics or supplements are not required or people who consume balanced diets. The Indian Council of Medical Research has designed Recommended Dietary Allowances for various nutrients. They have also formulated composition of balanced diet for various groups. These allowances are designed to serve as a guideline for planning diets. Suggestions are given for substituting foods for-non-vegetarians and additional allowances during special conditions.

To include the above nutrients in daily diet certain guidelines are suggested by the ICMR. Food items which contribute the same nutrients are grouped together and certain food groups are evolved. Foods are grouped into 11 groups based on their nutritive value. They are cereals and millets, pulses, nuts and oilseeds, vegetables, fruits, milk and milk products, meat, fish, eggs and poultry, fats and oils, sugar and jaggery and spices and condiments.

Cereals and millets constitute 70 to 80 per cent of calories and proteins of low income group. Except ragi all cereals are poor in calcium. Dried pulses are rich in proteins and a cereal-pulse combination is an excellent substitute for animal proteins—pulses are also good sources of many B vitamins and sprouting enhances the vitamin C content of pulses. Nuts and oilseeds are good sources of proteins, certain B vitamins, vitamin E and minerals like phosphorus andiron.

Vegetables are the storehouse of carotene, riboflavin, folic acid, vitamin C and calcium. Vegetables also supply water and roughage to the body. Leafy vegetables, other vegetables and roots and tubers are the different types of vegetables. Fruits in general are a good source of vitamin C. Milk is nature's best food as it is almost complete except for iron and vitamin 'C. Like milk, egg also contains proteins of high biological value. Egg is a rich source of vitamin A and some B vitamins. Animal foods like meat, fish and poultry are rich sources of proteins and B vitamins. Fatty fish are good in fat, vitamin A and D and small fish with bones are good sources of calcium. Liver and other organ meats are good sources of proteins, vitamin A, B complex, B12 and iron.

Sugar and jaggery are good sources of energy and honey and jaggery contain minerals like iron. Condiments and spices are mainly used to enhance palatability.

For non-vegetarians pulses can be reduced to 50 per cent and instead of that, one egg or 30 gms of meat or fish can be included. If no pulse is taken two eggs or 50 gms of meat or fish can be included.

Balanced Diet

For planning a balanced diet for labourers, low cost nutritious foods must be included. Ragi, tapioca, sweet potato, clusterbeans, bittergourd, soyabeans, drumstick leaves, various types of leafy vegetables, cowgram, horsegram, groundnut, Indian gooseberry, guava, papaya, mango, cashew fruit and other seasonal fruits can be used liberally to make a low-cost balanced diet Sprouted pulses and cheap vegetables that can be used as raw salads also must be included to meet the vitamin C requirement.

The ICMR Advisory Committee (1981) recommended the composition of balanced diet and it is given below:

Food Item	*Adult Man*			*Adult Woman*		
	Seden-tary	*Moderate Work*	*Heavy Work*	*Seden-tary*	*Moderate Work*	*Heavy Work*
Cereals	460 gm	520 gm	670 gm	410 gm	440 gm	575 gm
Pulses	40 gm	50 gm	60 gm	40 gm	45 gm	50 gm
leafy vegetables	40 gm	40 gm	40 gm	100 gm	100 gm	100 gm
Other vegetables	60 gm	70 gm	80Lgrn	40 gm	40 gm	100 gm
Roots and tubers	50 gm	60 gm	80 gm	50 gm	50 gm	100 gm
Milk and milk products	150 ml	200 ml	250 ml	100 ml	150 ml	200 ml
Oil and fat	40 gm	45 gm	65 gm	20 gm	25gm	40 gm
Fruits	60 gm	60 gm	60 gm	60 gm	60 gm	60 gm
Sugar and jaggery	30 gm	35 gm	55 gm	20 gm	20 gm	40 gm

For non-vegetarians pulses 5O per cent less + one egg or 30 gms fish or meat, if no pulse, 2 eggs or 50 gm fish or meat

A Sample Diet for a Sedentary Woman

Time	*Meal*	*Menu*
6.30 a.m. -	Bed coffee	
8 a.m. -	Breakfast -	Chapathi, Groundnuts-Tomato curry, Coffee
12.30 Noon -	Lunch -	Rice or Chapathi, Brinjal and horsegram curry Amaranth or spinach pugath, Lassi, Carrot salad.
4 p.m. -	Tea -	Vegetable vermicelli uppuma, Mint leaf chutney, Tea.
8 p.m. -	Dinner -	Wheat dosa or phulkas, Sprouted greem gram curry, Fruit cup.

Quantities of various food groups can be distributed according to te composition given by ICMR. This above diet provides:

Calories	-	2420kcals
Proteins	-	53 gms

The idea that the body's needs are definite and can be measured is a very recent one. We are so accustomed to eating to satisfy hunger that for centuries this criterion accepted by most people without question. Plenty was, in general, associated with health and want with starvation.

And yet, throughout the ages there have been those few who have seen a little further into the meaning of nutrition. We know from the book of Daniel of how he asked that he and his companions might eat a simple diet of pulses and water and how, after ten days during which this was permitted, 'their countenances appeared fairer and fatter in flesh than all the children which did eat the portion of the king's meat.' This was probably the first dietary experiment ever to be recorded.

We also know how, in the Middle Ages, illness and loss of life from scurvy led to the recognition that food could prevent and cure certain diseases but the connection between man's daily food and his health was only dimly acknowledged and in a very limited field.

Fortunately, the pleasures of a mixed diet led those who could afford it to eat a variety of foods. The greater the variety, the greater chance there was that all the vital and necessary factors would be included. Hence disease was most prevalent in institutions where the food was restricted and monotonous and among the poor who could not afford variety.

It was Sanctorius (1561-1636) who showed, by sitting on a chair suspended from the arm of a balance while he ate a meal, that afterwards the increase in weight which had taken place was gradually lost again. He described the loss as due to 'insensible perspiration.'

This proved the first basic fact that body-weight was connected with food eaten and that living, even without any conscious exertion, causes loss of weight.

This led in time to the acknowledgment that all the activities of the body derived their energy from the slow combustion of the foods eaten or (in starvation) of the body itself.

An adequate diet is one of that provides all the essential nutrients in sufficient quantities to meet the needs of the body. Thus far, the energy and nutrient needs, including carbohydrates, fats, proteins, minerals, vitamins, and water. The information concerning each of the nutrients in terms of the day's food is now brought together. Easy rule-of-thumb methods for knowing which foods and how much of each one are needed to provide an adequate diet have been developed on the basis of *food groups;* for this purpose, foods similar in nutritive value are considered together as a group. The pattern for the adequate diet is developed by recommending sufficient food servings from the various groups.

Human Needs

The food shortages during and after the 1914-18 war and the resulting ill-health of children, especially in Eastern Europe, made the general public realize for the first time that starvation was not the only consequence of a poor diet. Enough food to satisfy hunger sometimes failed to protect from diseases of malnutrition. Food had to be of the right and, to be fully protective, had to contain the essential vitamins as well as the basic nutrients : protiens, fats, carbohydrates and mineral salts.

Information to have extracted from old records about diets known to have been associated with deficiency diseases. Beriberi had occurred most commonly in countries where rice formed the bulk of the food eaten and had been known to disappear when some of the rice was replaced by vegetables. A diet provided for the U.S.A. garrison of Porto Rico consisted of rice, beans, potatoes, onions and meat with some extra fruit and vegetables, and on this, cases of beriberi occurred. Using recent values for the vitamins B_1 content of these foods, we find that the daily diet contained about 0.5 mg. of vitamin B_1 per man. This represents an average intake, and implies the some men ate less and some more, the former being without doubt those who succumbed to beriberi. The rations were later improved. Less rice and onions were given and more beans, potatoes and meat, and with the change, beriberi disappeared from the camp. The vitamin B_1 of the improved ration calculated by modern methods was just over 0.8 mg. per man — an increase of only 0.3 mg. but it made the difference between beriberi and protection. This difference is about two-millions of the total weight of a man's daily food, so it is not surprising that vitamins, active in such minute amounts, remained undiscovered for so long.

During the 19th century, scurvy was common in prisons and in other institutions, not to be punitive. In 1822 the meals in Millbank Penitentiary are described as:

For females — morning	9 oz. bread
	¾ pint gruel (made with barley)
noon	9 oz. bread ¾ pint soup evening ¾ pint soup.

The bread would have been made from stone-ground flour and would contain plenty of vitamin B_1, so as we should expect, there is a history of beriberi in such a prison, but any vegetables used in the preparation of the soup would be unlikely to retain any vitamin C during the cooking and it recorded that 448 prisoners did in fact show signs of scurvy in one year.

During the war of 1914-18, both scurvy and beriberi occurred. Soldiers of the Indian Army who ate few vegetables and little if any meat, suffered from scurvy. The British on the other hand, who ate vegetables, but while in India had rice or refined cereals, went down with beriberi. In 1916, special hospitals for the admission of cases of scurvy were operated in Baghdad and other parts of the Middle East.

A valuable study was made between 1920 and 1930 on the effect of increasing the quantities of protective foods in the meals of schoolboys. Records were kept of the heights and weights of boys between the ages of 10 and 18 at a large public school. Conditions of housing, the amount of physical exercise taken and other possibly influential factors remained relatively constant during period and the boys were, by accepted standards of nutrition, well fed. However as a result of an increasing awareness of the importance of vitamin-containing food the authorities altered the diet, so that the boys ate less bread and more milk, vegetables and butter. The results of these changes as seen in records kept over a long period were published by the medical officer (Friend, 1935).

At all ages there was an increase in both height and weight, this being greatest, as one would expect, during the years of most rapid growth.

It may be argued that increase in size does not necessarily mean better health and we are all familiar with overweight children who are abnormally fat but, in general, and where large numbers are concerned, the rate of growth of children can be taken as one indication of physical progress.

This study as important a being the first of its kind undertaken on an adequate scale and over a long enough period to give reliable results.

With the increasing consumption of vegetables and fruits in Great Britain, scurvy, at one time described as the 'English disease,' became rare and the introduction of cod liver oil as a supplement for infants reduced the incidence of rickets, but the new knowledge of the importance of vitamins as protective factors roused great interest in nutrition and people began to wonder how present-day diets would stand up tests of adequacy.

The first report of a large-scale investigation into modern diets was published by J. Boyd Orr in 1937. He divided the community into six sections according to income and estimated the amounts of money spent on food and also the consumption of protective foods in the different income groups. He found that with rise of income, more protective foods were eaten and that in three lowest groups, the amounts of Vitamins A and C eaten were very low.

Investigations on similar lines were made in the United States and from all the data collected, it became possible to make a fairly good estimate of the amounts of the more common vitamins contained in the daily food of normal healthy people and also the amounts below which deficiency diseases were liable to occur.

Tables setting out probable human requirements were published by a Technical Commission of the League of Nations in 1937 and by the Government Bureau of Home Economics, U.S.A. (Stiebeling, 1933). This was before the adoption in the United States of international units, so the results are not comparable but the attempt to express human needs in terms of quantities of vitamins was in itself a great advance.

Later, tables using international units were prepared by the National Research Council of the U.S.A. and these gave (except for vitamin C) figures surprisingly close to the League of Nations recommendations. The most recent publication is that the British Medical Association, 1950.

	League of Nations 1937	*National Research Council 1945*	*British Medical Assoc, 1950*
Vitamin A	2,000-4,000 i.u.	5,000 (optimum)	i.u. 3,000 i.u.
Vitamin B_1	1 mg. approx.	1.5 mg.	1.4 mg.
Vitamin C	30 mg	75 mg.	20 mg.
Vitamin D	—	—	400 i.u.

During the war of 1939-45 there were many cases of dietary deficiency including beriberi in the Japanese prison camps. Some of the doctors who were among the prisoners kept record of the occurrence of beriberi and also of the vitamin B_1 of the diet and the history of the Porto Rico garrison was repeated. When the intake fell blow 0.5 mg. vitamin B_1 (or about 0.2 mg. per 1,000 nonfat Calories) men succumbed to beriberi; when it rose above these levels, the men's health improved (Smith and others, 1951).

The Register-General's Statistical Review which is published every year gives details of the number of deaths from different diseases. Although the causes of scurvy and rickets were known in the 1920s, and the foods effective for prevention were available, the diseases did not disappear immediately. There was, however, a steady drop in incidence. This demonstrates that not only must protective foods be available, but the public must be educated to use them properly. Free supplements for the provision of vitamins A, C and D were made available for infants during the war years but all mothers did not avail themselves of the opportunity to have them. The number taking them has increased considerably in the last few years with a corresponding drop in rickets almost to the point of disappearance (Registrar-General, 1949, 1950 and 1952) and the health of children in this country has steadily improved.

Health and Diseases

Most of the vitamins, being growth-promoting substances in the sense that they are needed for full structural and functional development are needed greater amounts during childhood when growth is taking place and during pregnancy and lactation for the same reason.

Vitamin A : Vitamin A is stored in the liver and during adult life the daily needs can be supplied to a considerable extent from these reserves. Volunteers who deliberately consumed diets very low in vitamin A were able to continue doing so for several months without developing any gross signs of deficiency. But in spite of this there is general agreement that it is better to consume enough to guard against any chances of deficiency and, in the table, the recommended levels of vitamin A vary very little.

Whether taken as vitamin A itself or in the plant form carotene, this factor is always converted into vitamin A used as such in the animal body. But the two forms are not of equal physiological value, unit for unit. It is usually reckoned that the number of international units needed in the form of carotene is about twice the number needed as vitamin A itself. Even this ratio is not the same for all foods. The carotene of green vegetables supplies to the body about half as many units of vitamin A as the number obtained by chemical estimation, but yellow vegetables like carrots supply only about one-fifth or one-quarter (Graves, 1942).

Increased Needs for the Vitamin A : Vitamin A being used by the body to maintain the health of the skin, teeth and mucous linings of the respiratory organs is needed especially in illness in which these are involved. To guard against them, supplies in the daily diet should be kept up to the standards given. In treatment higher doses are available in pharmaceutical preparations can be prescribed. Dases up to 100,000 or 200,000 i.u. are sometimes given daily.

The B Vitamins : The need for vitamin B_1 varies according to the amount of food eaten and the energy expended in movements in all kinds.

As muscular activity, which depends on the oxidation of carbohydrates, continues throughout life, vitamin B_1 must be continuously supplied. Moreover, this vitamin differs from vitamin A is not being stored for long periods. In general, the fat-soluble vitamins tend to be stored in the body, but the water-soluble vitamins, i.e. those of the B group and vitamin C, are not stored If more is eaten than needed it is rapidly excreted again in the urine.

Because vitamin B_1 is used day by day, as it is consumed, it has been much easier to find out exactly what the daily needs are in fact, as early as 1934, Cowgill was able to suggest a mathematical formula to express the daily needs in terms of body weight and calorific intake.

Increased Needs for Vitamin B : As vitamin B_1 is concerned with carbohydrate metabolism, any conditions which involve a higher calorific intake, e.g heavy manual work, climbing, Article exploration, naturally call for higher intake.

In those diseases, too, in which the rate of metabolism is increased, more vitamin B_1 is needed.

Riboflavin and nicotinic acid also take part with vitamin B_1 in energy relations and the amounts needed are related to the amount of vitamin B_1 In foods, these vitamins of the B complex occur together and a shortage of one usually implies a shortage of the others. It is only when the staple cereal happens to be grossly short of a particular factor as, for example, polished rice and vitamin B_1 or maize and nicotinic acid, that well-defined deficiency diseases such as beriberi and pellagra occur. In countries where mixed diets are customary, deficiencies are usually less severe but of a mixed type. For example, a mild shortage of riboflavin will produce, in some individuals, roughness and redness of the skin over the nose and some cracking of the lips, easily cured by the consumption of extra quantities of one or two foods rich in riboflavin such as eggs or liver.

Similarly a shortage of nicotinic acid, not enough to cause pellagra, may produce digestive disturbances, a reddening of the skin of the face and hands and feelings of depression.

Nicotinic acid is concerned in healthy people with the control of movements of precision and if its supply is limited subjects may find themselves unusually clumsy.

The varying responses of individuals to diets deficient in the B vitamins was puzzling until, as a result of a long series of observations, it was learnt that these factors are also synthesized within the body of man and the higher animals though not by it. The intestinal tract contains warm semifluid material rich in nutrients and is, as we know, a medium in which there is normally an expensive bacterial flora. These organisms are not disease-producing. They merely live in and with man. Their power of synthesizing vitamins is a relatively recent discovery. They seem to specialize in the factors of the B group but some can also synthesize vitamin K (Najjar and Barrett, 1945).

Ruminants, whose large rumen in the first part of the digestive tract is the site of vitamin formation, obtain so much riboflavin and nicotinic acid from bacterial activity that they fail to develop rigns of deficiency even on diets lacking these vitamins. But in man the bacteria carry on their synthetic activities much further down the digestive tract and, although undoubtedly some of the B vitamins produced in this way are available for human use, enough of each is not formed to satisfy all human needs.

It is, however easy to see that in conditions such as diarrhoea in which the contents of the alimentary tract move along quickly, less than the normal amounts may be absorbed and symptoms of deficiency may occur if the condition is not checked. The recent use of some of the new drugs, sulphonamides and antibiotics has also revealed that these, too, affect the activities of the vitamin-B-producing bacteria. The drugs inhibit not only the growth of disease-producing organisms but also the synthesis of the B vitamins in the intestine. This interference with production may be great enough to cause true secondary deficiencies in patients who may not have been very well supplied with vitamins before. Cases have been observed with signs of peripheral neuritis, enlarged heart and swelling of the limbs, indistinguishable from true beriberi. Other patients develop a sore mouth and red scaling of the skin recalling deficiencies of nicotinic acid and riboflavin.

In the treatment of these secondary deficiencies very large doses have to be given — a hundred or more times the amount needed for normal health.

Vitamin C : Vitamin C, also water-soluble, is another vitamin which should be taken daily, although the body stores are not exhausted as rapidly as those of vitamin B_1

There is difference of opinion about the amount of vitamin C needed to maintain health. The American in which estimate is higher than the British. An experiment in which volunteers did without any vitamin C for months showed that they could do so without developing any gross signs of scurvy, and the quantity needed for health has consequently been placed at a lower level than formerly. But, as the signs of deficiency develop in such an insidious manner, it is probable that minor degrees of vitamin C deficiency are fairly common though not always recognized as such.

It is known now that vitamin C is concerned not only in protection against scurvy but in the healing of wounds, in the prevention of shock from injury, in the tolerance of high atmospheric temperature and in the control of body fluids. These processes are common in everyday life and probably account for the daily use by the body of vitamin C.

Increased Needs for Vitamin C : When any of these, conditions are actually present or exaggerated the need is correspondingly increased. Very large doses (up to 1 g.) are given before operation to prevent shock and in the treatment of severe injuries and larger than normal doses are given to man doing heavy work in an excessively hot humid atmosphere

Large amounts of vitamin C are available in fruits and vegetables and some reason or other an individual does not eat or can not eat these foods, then tablets of the synthetic vitamin or some other pharmaceutical preparation must be taken. The massive doses are, of course, always given by means of a pharmaceutical preparation.

Vitamin D : It will be noticed that the table gives the same figure for the human requirement for vitamin D except in the case of infants under one year and for expectant and nursing mothers. This uniform level is an fact a confession that very little is known about varying needs.

At one time it was assumed that vitamin D was needed only during the period of active growth. This view is no longer held and it is thought that the fragile nature of the bones people of older may be related to their low consumption of vitamin D foods.

The figures for human needs given in the B.M.A. table have been obtained by studies of dietary surveys, of individual diets, of diets associated with deficiency diseases and so on. The first estimates were made by the Health Committee of the League of Nations; these were followed by American estimates and finally the table quoted here was produced. Considering the magnitude and difficulty of the task, it is astonishing how closely the various estimates agree and it is probable that these recently published figures are as near the truth as we are likely to get.

The question has to be asked : to what extent do individuals eat diets which satisfy these needs? How easy or difficult is it to obtain an adequate diet?

There are several ways of approaching this problem. We can see whether there is any evidence that people are better fed now than formerly or we can study foods which are normally eaten in ordinary homes and see if they supply the needs.

Reference has been made to the effect of adding protective foods to the diet of schoolboys and to the increases in height and weight produced as a result. Data on the height and weights of London school children during the first half of this century have recently been published and these show the same kind of increase. It may not be totally due to nutrition, but it is not unreasonable to conclude that improved feeding due to increased knowledge of nutrition has also played a part in producing these effects.

If we approach the problem from the dietary angle, we can analyse representative diets and estimate their vitamin content. This is a useful exercise and a comparison between the foods eaten on several different days or by different individuals shows how wide the variation in vitamin content can be.

Following examples of meals will illustrate this point. These show that the value of a diet depends on the *choice* of foods, and that likes and dislikes are of themselves not reliable guides; there must be knowledge also.

Amount *Oz.*	*Vit. A or equiv. in carotene* *i.u.*	*Vit.* B_1 *μg.*	*Ribo-flavin* *μg.*	*Niacin* *μg.*	*Vit C* *mg.*	*Vit D* *i.u.*	
Meal 1							
Roast beef	3	42	33	195	3,900	—	
Yorkshire pudding							
3 oz. = flour	1	_	34	23	450	-	-
milk	1½	45	18	54	-	-	0.45
egg	½	125	19	85	-	-	8.5
cooking fat	1/8	-	-	-	-	-	-
Roast potatoes	6	-	180	26	1,200	15	-

Contd...

	Amount Oz.	*Vit. A or equiv. in carotene i.u.*	*Vit. B_1 µg.*	*Ribo-flavin µg.*	*Niacin µg.*	*Vit C mg.*	*Vit D i.u.*
Cabbage	4	288*	4	28	320	28	-
Apple pie= flour	½	-	17t	11	225	-	
cooking fat	¼	-	-	-	-	-	
apple	2	4	6	-	50	1.6	-
sugar	¼	-	-	-	-	-	-
Custard= milk	2	60	24	72	-	-	0.6
powder	neg	-	-	-	-	-	-
		564	335	564	6,145	44.6	9.55
		i.u.	µg.=	µg.=	µg.	= mg	i.u.
			.335	.564	6.145		
			mg.	mg.	mg.		
Proportion of day's need approx.		1/8	¼	1/3	½	All	1/40
Meal 2							
Cheese	1	369	9	140	100	-	4
Lettuce	2	727*	34	40	200	6	-
Tomato	3	540*	60	30	300	21	-
Wholemeal bread	3	-	270	150	1,800	-	-
Butter	½	568	-		-	-	8.5
Orange	3	48	60	30	300	48	-
Coffee= milk and sugar	5	150	60	180	-	1	1.5
		2,402	493	570	2,700	76	14
		i.u.	µg.=	µg.=	µg.=	mg.	i .u.
			.493	.57	2.7		
			mg.	mg.	mg.		
Proportion of day's need approx		¾	1/3	1/3	1/5	All	1/90

Meal 3							
Fried white fish	4	-	40	160	2,400	-	-
Fried potatoes	6	-	180	60	1,200	12	-
Rice pudding							
4 oz.							
= rice	1/3	-	5	6	100	-	-
milk	2½	75	30	90	-	-	.75
sugar	1/6	-	-	-	-	-	-
Stewed apple, 4							
=raw	3	7	9	-	75	2.4	-
		82	264	316	3,775	14.4	.75
		i.u.	μg.=	μg.=	μg.=	mg.=	i.u.
			.264	.316	3.775		
			mg.	mg.	mg.		
Proportion of day's need approx		1/40	1/5	1/6	1/4	1/2	negligible

Meal 4							
Sausages, pork	3	-	210	150	1,500	-	-
Baked beans	3	35	60	30	600	-	-
Mashed potatoes	6	-	144	96	1,350	12	-
Prunes	4	103	32	68	-	-	-
Custard= milk							
powder	3	90	36	108	-	-	.9
		228	482	452	3,450	12	.9
		i.u.	μg.=	μg.=	μg.	= mg.	i.u.
			.482	4.52	3.45		
			mg.	mg.	mg.		
Proportion of day's need approx		1/13	1/3	1/4	1/4	3/5	negligible

For green vegetables : Carotene =40 per cent as vitamin A

Yellow veg. =25 per cent

Half the value of uncooked flour.

Where no value is available for vitamin B_1 in cooked food, the figure for the uncooked food is halved.

International Units

Vitamins A and D are usually expressed in international units (i.u.)- Human or animal requirements for other vitamins are usually given in milligrammes, but the value in foods is often expressed in microgrammes (1/1000s of miligramme) so as to avoid the use of decimals.

In the tables, the value of *individual* foods are given in microgrammes for the same reason but the *total* values and the requirements are given in milligrammes for comparison with other published figures.

Conversions —Weight and Household Measures

5 oz. milk	= 1 teacupful
1 oz. cheese is the same size as	1 oz. butter (1/4 of 1/4- 1b. pack)
1 oz. bread	= ¼ in. slice from square loaf
1 oz. cake	= portion 3 x 1 x 1 /2 in.
1 oz. Castle pudding is the same size as 1 oz. cake	
1 oz. biscuits	= 2 biscuits (2 1 /4 in. in diameter)
1 oz. flour, rice, oatmeal, custard, powder, sugar, etc.	= 1 well heaped tablespoonful
½ oz.	= 1 level tablespoonful or 1 well heaped teaspoonful
1 oz. jam	= 1 dessertspoonful
2 oz. potato (mashed), green vegetables, root vegetables or peas	= 1 heaped tablespoonful
2 oz. tomato	= 1 egg-size tomato

4 oz. stewed fruit	= 5 small plumps (with juice) or 4 tablespoonfuls of soft fruit
3 oz. meat	= 4 thin slices (approx. 3 x 4 in.)
1 oz. bacon	= 1 rasher (approx. 1/8 x 7 x 2 in.)
4 oz. fish	= portion approx. 3 x 3 x 1/2 in.
2 oz. herring	= 1 small herring (approx.5 in. long)

Adequate Diet

A plan for selecting an adequate diet developed around 4 *food groups* will now be discussed. There are other plans, developed on the same principle as the 4-group plan, differing only in number of groups. All of the plans are developed in accordance with food habits of the people and the foods available to them. In case the habits of eating and the food supply are different, the food patterns are of necessity also different.

The 4-group plan is flexible, permitting for a wide choice of foods within most of the groups. Meals planned in one home are likely to differ from those in another, even though the meals in each home follow the same food pattern. Foods selected by persons eating out may vary widely, and still at the same time each is in complete accordance with the recommendations of the same food pattern.

Four-Food Group Plan : The 4-group plan (milk, meat, vegetable-fruit, cereal) was developed in 1958 and is a simplified version of the 7-group plan that originated during wartime 1943. In this 4-group plan the citrus fruits, green and yellow vegetables, and other vegetables and fruits are combined into one group, and the butter fortified margarine group omitted. The daily quantities of each group of recommended to provide the *foundation* of an adequate diet and the main nutritive contribution of each group are given. Calories are the least well supplied by this pattern. However, as a usual practice, facts and sugars, which are not listed, are eaten as such or combined in baked goods and desserts, with a result that the energy intake is increased. Also to satisfy the appetite, additional servings from the food groups may be experted, which will contribute both to the energy and nutrient intake.

The 7 food groups	*Daily amounts*	*Min nutritive contributions*
Green and yellow vegetables	1 or more servings	Vitamin A value Ascorbic acid Iron
Oranges, grapefruit, tomatoes or raw cabbage or salad greens	1 serving	Ascorbic acid
Potatoes, other vegetables and fruits	2 or more servings	Vitamins and minerals in general Cellulose

The 7 food groups	*Daily amounts*	*Min nutritive contributions*
Milk and milk products	Children ¾ to 1 quart Adults 1 pint	Calcium Riboflavin Protein Phosphorus
Meat, poultry, fish and eggs	1 serving meat, fish or poultry 1 egg(at least 4 a week)	Protien Phosphorus Iron B- Vitamins
Bread, flour and cereal (whole grain enriched or restored)	3 or more servings	Thiamine Niacin Riboflavin Iron Carbohydrate Cellulose
Butter or fortified margarine	2-3 tbsp.	Vitamin A Fat

The basic 7 food groups.

The 4 food groups contributions	*Daily amounts*	*Main nutritive*
Milk group:	Children 3-4 cups	
Milk, cheese, rice	Teen agers 4 or more cups	Calcium
cream (cheese and ice cream can replace	Adults 2 or more cups	Riboflavin
part of the milk)	Pregnant 4 or more cups Women	Protein
	Nursing 6 or more cups Mothers	Phosphorus
Meal group	Protein	
Beef veal pork, lamon,		Phosphorus
Poultry, fish, eggs	2 or more serving	Iron
dry beans and peas as alternates		B-vitamins
	4 or more serving, including a dark green or deep yellow vegetable at least every other day.	

Contd...

The 4 food groups contributions	*Daily amounts*	*Main nutritive*
Vegetable-fruit group	A citrus fruit or other fruits or vegetable rich in ascorbic acid- daily Other fruits and vegetables including potatoes	Vitamins Minerals Cellulose
Bread-cereals group (Whole grain) ebrichesd restored)	4 or more servings	Thiamine Niacin Riboflavin Iron Carbohydrates Cellulose

The 4-food group plan.

The percentage of the Daily Recommended Allowances provided by the foundation pattern will vary with individual needs. The person with a greater requirement will have those needs less well satisfied, of course, than the person with a lesser daily·need. A day's dietary planned with the use of the 4-food group is illustrated in table . This menu contains more than the minimum number of servings in three of the four groups of plan (see Fig.). The nutrients contributed by foods in the four foundations groups in this dietary are shown in Table. Butter, jelly, mayonnaise, lemon pie, and sugar are not included in the calculations. A comparison of the percentage of the Daily Recommended Allowances provided by foods in the 4-group plan is made (Fig.). Young men obtained a lower percentage of their allowance from the foundation groups simply because the recommendations for men are higher for some nutritents than for women. However, the young man, in satisfying his energy need and promoted by a natural urge to eat, selects more of all food groups. The result is that in actual practice the diets of young men are, as a rule, more nearly adequate than those of young women.

The 4-group plan is useful as an education tool to show the foundation for an adequate diet. Because it is such a simple plan, some may not realize its importance. For the most efficient use of the 4-group plan, one should know the main nutrients contributed by the various foods in each group.

The Nutritive Value of Food Commodities : Each food group, and each food within the group, makes a particular contribution to the nutrient content of the diet.

Comparison of the Nutrients Sulphide by the 4-Food Groups from the Above Menu to the NRC Recommended Daily Allowances for Young Women and Men

Young women (18-35 years)

Young men (18-35 Years)

Some foods supply many more of the nutrients and in much greater concentration then do athors. The nutritional contribution of the major food commodities, milk and milk products; meat, fish, and poultry vegetables and fruits; and cereal and cereal products, will be discussed in the following paragraphs.

Menu with the Four-Group Plan as a Guide

Breakfast		*Lunch*		*Dinner*	
Orange juice	4 oz	Swedish meat balls	3 oz	Veal cutlet	3 oz
Egg. soft-cooked	1	Green beans	½ c	Baked potato	1 med
w.w. toast	2 sl	Waldorf salad	2/3 c	Brocciol	2/3 c
Butter	1 pat	Pan roll	1	Hard roll	1
Jelly	1 tbsp	Cup custard	6 oz	Butter	1 pat
Milk, whole	8 oz	Iced tea	8 oz	Lemon pie	1 sl
		Snack -1 milk shake	Iced	tea	8 oz

Milk and Milk Products

Milk is considered as nature's "most nearly perfect food." Most of the known essential nutrients are found in milk, but it is a much better source of some than others. Milk and milk products are excellent sources of calcium, protein and riboflavin. Vitamin A, phosphorus, and thiamine are also supplied in good amounts. Milk and milk products are poor sources of iron and of ascorbic acid.

The importance of including milk or milk products in the diet so as to obtain sufficient calcium is well known. For students, or anyone for that matter, drinking milk is one of best ways of assuming an adequate calcium intake. Each gram of milk contains about 1 mg of calcium, with a glass of milk supplying about one-third of the recommended calcium intake for the college student.

Milk contains protein of high biological value; and so complements the incomplete proteins of cereal products, fruits, and vegetables. Since milk can very well be served as a beverage at each meal of the day, a source of complete protein can therefore be assured. The protein value of milk is that each ounce contains about 1 gm of protein.

Evaporated milk contains the same nutrients as whole milk. The process of evaporation, and pasteurization also, reduces the thiamine and ascorbic acid content by about one-fifth to one-fourth. Evaporated milk is convenient to use and economical.

The fortification of milk with vitamin D is a god public health measure. By adding vitamin D to milk the essential nutrients for bone formation, calcium, phosphorus, protein, and vitamin D, are brought together in one food.

The popularity of non-fat milk solids is increasing because of the lower cost, ease of storage, and lower Calorie intake. With the removal of cream from the milk, which is done prior to drying, the caloric value is reduced by about one-half. In addition, vitamin A and other fat-soluble vitamins are removed. If nonfat milk solids are used to replace the whole milk, care must be taken to provide for additional vitamin A value from other sources such as green and yellow vegetables and liver because milk is depended on to provide some of the vitamin A need.

An ounce of Cheddar-type cheese provides about the same nutritive value as a glass of milk. In the manufacture of cheese some of the whey is removed, taking with it some of the water-soluble nutrients including lactose, the water-soluble vitamins (B-group), and minerals. Cottage cheese made with rennet has a higher calcium content than that made entirely by the souring of the milk (acid coagulation). In this process calcium, which is soluble in an acid medium, is carried into the whey.

Food	Measure	Energy, Cal.	Protein, gm.	Calcium, mg.	Iron mg.	Vit. A IU	Thiamin, mg.	Riboflavin, mg.	Ascorbic Acid mg.
Milk group									
Milk (beverage, custard, milk shake)	2½ C	400	22.5	720	0.3	875	0.2	1.05	5
Ice cream (shake)	1/8qt	145	3	87	0.1	370	0.03	0.13	1
	Total	*545*	*25.5*	*807*	*0.4*	*1245*	*0.23*	*1.18*	*6*
Meat group									
Egg, soft, ck,	1	80	6	27	1.1	590	0.05	0.15	—
Egg (custard)	1	80	6	27	1.1	590	0.05	0.15	—
Meat balls	3 oz	245	21	9	2.7	30	0.07	0.18	—
Veal cutlet	3 oz	185	23	9	2.7	—	0.06	0.21	—
	Total	*590*	*56*	*72*	*7.6*	*1210*	*0.23*	*0.69*	—
Vegetable-fruit group									
Orange juice	4 oz	50	.5	13	0.3	245	0.11	0.03	64
Green beans	1/2c	15	1.0	31	0.4	340	0.04	0.06	8
Apples	1/2c	35	tr	4	0.2	25	0.02	0.01	1
Celery	1/4c	4	tr	10	0.1	60	0.01	0.01	2
Potato, baked	1 med	90	3	9	0.7	tr	0.10	0.04	20
Broccoli	1/2c	20	2.5	66	0.6	1875	0.07	0.15	68
	Total	*219*	*7.0*	*124*	*2.1*	*2435*	*0.32*	*0.28*	*150*
Bread-cereal group									
Bread,w.w.	*2sl*	*110*	*4*	*44*	*1.0*	*tr*	*0.10*	*0.06*	*tr*
Roll,pan	*1*	*115*	*3*	*28*	*0.7*	*tr*	*0.11*	*0.07*	*tr*
Roll, hard	*1*	*160*	*5*	*24*	*0.4*	*tr*	*0.03*	*0.05*	*tr*
	Total	*385*	*12*	*96*	*2.1*	*tr*	*0.24*	*0.18*	*tr*
Grad total		*1734*	*100.5*	*1108*	*12.4*	*5000*	*1.05*	*2.35*	*169*

Table Nutritive Value of Milk and Some Milk Products

Milk and Milk Products	*Energy Cal.*	*Protein, gm.*	*Calcium, mg.*	*Irons mg.*	*Vit. A. IU*	*Thiamine, mg.*	*Riboflavin mg.*	*Ascorbic Acid, mg.*
Milk, whole (I c)	160	9.0	288	0.1	350	0.08	0.42	2
Buttermilk, cultured, skim (Ic)	90	9.0	298	0.1	10	0.09	0.44	2
Evaporated, water added (I c)	173	9.0	318	0.2	410	0.05	0.42	1
Cheese, process (I oz) 105	7.0	219	0.3	350	trace	0.12	0	
Chesse, cottage, creamed, skim milk (1/2 c)	120	15.5	106	0.3	190	0.03	0.28	0
Ice cream (1/8 qt)	145	3.0	87	0.1	370	0.03	0.13	1

Table Nutritive Value of Some Meat, Fish, Poultry, and Egg

Food	*Energy Cal.*	*Protein, gm.*	*Calcium. mg.*	*Irons mg.*	*Vit. A. IU*	*Thiamine, mg.*	*Riboflavin mg.*	*Ascorbic Acid, mg.*
Beef, round (3 oz)	165	25.0	11	3.2	10	0.06	0.19	0
Beef, liver, fried (3 oz) 195	22.5	9	7.5	45,200	0.22	3.55	23	
Pork, lean and fat, loin roast (2 oz)	310	21.0	9	2.7	—	0.78	0.22	0
Chicken (3 oz)	170	18.0	18	1.3	200	0.03	0.11	3
Salmon (3 oz)	120	17.0	—	0.7	60	0.03	0.16	0
Egg (1)	80	6.0	27	1.1	590	0.05	0.15	0

Value depends on amount of bone consumed.

value. They provide protein and iron, with some phosphorus, thiamine, riboflavin, and niacin.

Meat, Fish, Poultry, and Eggs : Meat, fish and poultry are very similar in their nutritive.

The protein in this group of foods, as in milk, is of high biological value. A 3-oz serving of meat supplies approximately 20 gm of protein, which is about one-third the Recommended Allowances for young adult women and over one-fourth for young adult men.

Iron is present in relatively high concentration in the organ meats, particularly liver and kidney, and in to a lesser amounts in muscle tissues. Meat is poor source of calcium . Some fish products, mainly shell fish and canned salmon, in which a portion of the bone is edible, are somewhat better than meat as a source of calcium.

Pork muscle is high in thiamine content whether other muscle meats contain only moderate amounts. The glandular organs, liver, kidney, heart, and tongue are higher than muscle meats in riboflavin content. Liver, the storage place for vitamin A, is only edible animal tissue containing any appreciable amount of this vitamin.

Eggs provide protein, iron, phosphorus, vitamin A, and riboflavin to the diet. The protein in egg, which is located both in the yolk and the white, is of good biological value. One egg contains about 6 gm of protein, approximately two-thirds the amount in one glass of milk. Phosphorus is distributed in both the white and the yolk. Iron and vitamin A are contained only in the yolk. Table. gives the nutritive value of some kinds of meat, fish, poultry, and eggs.

Vegetables and Fruits

As a group, vegetables and fruits are the source of minerals, vitamins, and cellulose to the diet. Not to be disregarded is the interest they add because of their variety in colour, flavor, and texture. The great number of fruits and vegetables available for use differ markedly in nutrient content. For the sake of clarity they are grouped according to their contribution of nutrients to the diet.

Mostly the green and yellow vegetables and fruits are outstanding in their vitamin A values. One serving of sweet potatoes, carrots, kale or cantaloup furnishes sufficient vitamin A to meet the Recommended Allowance for vitamin A for persons of all ages. In addition leafy-green vegetables provide more calcium, iron , ascorbic acid, and the B-vitamins than other vegetables. Some of the green vegetables, spinach, chard, sorrel, and beet greens contain oxalic acid, which combines with calcium during digestion forming an insoluble salt that cannot be absorbed, and makes the calcium in those vegetables of no use to the body. However, these green vegetables, even though not supplying calcium, are invaluable in the diet for the generous amounts or iron, ascorbic acid, and vitamin A value they provide. The ascorbic acid content of broccoli, Brussels sprouts, kale, and similar vegetables is quite high.

Head lettuce, celery, cabbage, and other light green vegetables are important source for cellulose. Raw cabbage is a good source of ascorbic acid. The light green vegetables are low in vitamin A value.

Citrus fruits and tomatoes are good sources of ascorbic acid. Tomato juice contains about one-third as much as the citrus fruits. Since they are available the year round and are well liked, it is customary to include citrus fruits in most dietary plans. Other foods like strawberries, cantaloups, kale, and green peppers are also rich in ascorbic acid as citrus fruits, but due to cost, unavailability, or lack of acceptance, do not fit into the diet as a routine item as well as citrus fruits. Ascorbic acid is easily destroyed during storage, freezing, and cooking. Citrus retain their ascorbic acid content better than other foods due to the preserving action of the acids they contain.

Vegetables of the seed, root and tuber classes, like Lima beans, corn green peas, sweet potatoes, and white potatoes are higher in carbohydrate content than other varieties. Starch is stored in these areas of the plant's structure.

Vegetables and fruits as a rule provide lesser protien, fat, and total Calories. Table shows the contribution of some fruits and vegetables to the diet.

Cereals and Cereal Products

Cereals are seeds of the grass family—wheat, corn, rice, oats, rye, and barley. From these cereal grains flours (whole wheat, white rye, barley etc.) are manufactured for the preparation of the many varieties of breads, cakes, pastries, breakfasts cereals, macaroni products, hominy corn sirup, corn meal, and other products. Whole wheat has the following composition in terms of grams of the constituent per 100 gm of whole wheat: 72 carbohydrate, 2 fiber, 12 protein, 2 fat, 2 ash, and 10 moisture.

In many countries cereals are the main food of the diet, furnishing 50 to 90 per cent of the total calories; in the United States about one-third of calories is from cereal or cereal products. More wheat and corn is grown in U.S.A. than other cereals; most of the wheat and corn is used for human consumption, a large part of the corn fed to livestock.

The cereal grains are easy to grow, easy to store, and have good keeping qualities. Whole grain cereals contribute calories (mainly in the form of carbohydrate), thiamine, iron, riboflavin, and partially in complete protien. Cereals are easy to digest, have a blend flavor, and supply roughage or cellulose.

In the preparation of cereal products for the market, parts of the cereal grain are removed. In the case of brown rice only the outer husk is removed whereas in the preparation of white rice all of the outer coats are wheat flour is made from the entire grain except for the husk; white flour is just the endosperm portion. Most of the cellulose, minerals and B vitamins are in the outer layers or coats of the grain. The endosperm portion contains the carbohydrate and incomplete protein. The germ contains most of the fat of the grain and some of the thiamine. Because the fat tends to become rancid during storage and also seems to hold a great attraction for insects, the germ is usually removed in milling. Furthermore, the public prefers the refined product for mouses.

Nutritive Value of Some Fruits and Vegetables

Food	*Energy Cal.*	*Protein, gm.*	*Calcium, mg.*	*Irons mg.*	*Vit. A. IU*	*Thiamine, mg.*	*Riboflavin mg.*	*Ascorbic Acid, mg.*
Apple (1 med)	70	tr	8	0.4	50	0.04	0.02	3
Banana(1 med)	85	1.0	8	0.7	190	0.05	0.06	10
Broccoli, ck (1/2 c)	20	2.5	66	0.6	1875	0.07	0.15	68
Cabbage, ck (1/2 c)	18	1.0	38	0.3	110	0.04	0.04	28
Carrots, ck (1/2 c)	23	0.5	24	0.5	7610	0.04	0.04	5
Green beans, ck (1/2 c)	15	1.0	31	0.4	340	0.04	0.06	8
Kale, ck (1/2 c)	15	2.0	74	0.7	4070	—	—	34
Lettuce, Iceberg, (50 gm)	7	0.4	10	0.2	167	0.03	0.03	3
Lima beans, ck (½ c)	90	6.0	38	2.0	225	0.15	0.08	14
Orange juice, fresh (1/2 c)	50	0.5	13	0.3	245	0.11	0.03	64
Peaches, cn (1/2 c)	100	0.5	5	0.4	550	0.01	0.03	4
Potato, white, baked (1 med)	90	3.0	9	0.7	tr	0.10	0.04	20
Tomato juice (1/2 c)	23	1.0	9	1.1	970	0.07	0.04	20

Cereal and Cereal Products	*Energy Cal.*	*Protein, gm.*	*Calcium, mg.*	*Irons mg.*	*Vit. A. IU*	*Thiamine, mg.*	*Riboflavin mg.*	*Ascorbic Acid, mg.*
Otameal, ck (1 c)	130	5.0	21	1.4	0	0.19	.0.05	0.3 0
Rice, white, enriched ck (1 c)	185	3.0	17	1.5	0	0.19	0.12	1.6 0
Macaroni, unenriched ck (1 c)	155	5.0	11	0.6	0	0.02	0.02	0.4 0
Macaroni, enriched ck (1 c)	155	5.0	11	1.3	0	0.19	0.11	1.5 0
Cake, plain (3 x 2 x ½)	200	2.0	35	0.2	90	0.01	0.05	0.1 0
Bread, white, unenriched (1 sl)	60	2.0	16	0.2	0	0.2	0.02	0.3 0
Bread, whole wheat (1 sl)	55	2.0	23	0.5	0	0.06	0.03	0.7 0
Muffin, enriched (1)	140	4.0	46	0.8	50	0.08	0.11	0.7 0
Biscuit, enriched (2 1/2" diam)	140	3.0	46	0.6	0	0.08	0.08	0.7 0
Pan roll, enriched (12 per Ib)	115	3.0	28	0.7	0	0.11	0.07	0.8 0

The protein in cereal products varies in biological efficiency but as a whole is classified as partially incomplete. However, with supplementation or protein from milk or meat or eggs, the cereal protiens make a significant contribution to the diet. About 20 per cent of the protein in diet is from cereal sources; on low-cost dietaries the percentage is relatively higher. Milk and cereal make a good nutritional team, cereal supplying iron, thiamine, and partially complete protein, and milk providing calcium, vitamin A, and complete protein. The use of the milk solids (dried milk) in bread improves the nutritive contributions of this product.

It is important that whole grain, restored or enriched cereals, and cereal products be selected for the diet in order to benefit from their greater nutritive contributions. Table gives the nutritive contributions of some cereal products to the diet.

Energy and Oxidation

Energy for physiological activity is ultimately obtained from the sun. The sun gives out energy in the form of visible light waves and invisible ultravoilet rays. When these impinge on green plants, the latter are able to absorb the energy and build-up compounds and such as sugar and starch from the carbon dioxide of the air and the water of soil. The compounds become storehouses of energy within the green plants.

By the action of oxygen on these carbon compounds, they can again be broken down through a series of stages into carbon dioxide and water and, in the process, the stored energy is once more liberated. This breakdown happens in the plants themselves when they respire and is the source of energy used by them for growth, development and reproduction.

But far more energy is stored in starch and sugar than is used by the plants and, when animals eat the plant products, this energy becomes available to them.

Animals, too obtain oxygen from the air in breathing. This is transferred in the lungs to the blood and is carried to all parts of the body. Food which is eaten, digested and absorbed is also taken in the circulation to organs where it can be temporarily stored. Most of the starch and sugar eaten is stored in the form of another carbohydrate, glycogen, in either the liver or the muscles, and as we have seen, is broken down to provide energy.

The recognition of these facts led to a great deal of work on the quantities of food needed to produce the energy for certain tasks and it was found that the energy value of a food could be expressed in terms of a heat-unit or calorie. A calorie is the amount of heat-energy required to raise the temperature of 1 g. of water through 1 °C. This was found too small a unit to be convenient for expressing the energy values of foods, so a unit was chosen of 1,000 calories or 1 large Calorie (spelt with a capital C).

The next step was to find out how many calories were required by individuals of different weights, both resting and carrying out tasks with different energy requirements.

The following are average values:

	Calories
Metabolism of sleep (8 hours)	518
Basal metabolism while awake (16 hours)	1,152
Allowance for light work	1,200
Total	2,870

(Best and Taylor, 1950).

Daily Calorin Allowances for Adults

Requirment	*Description*	*Calorie requirement*
0	No work, almost basal (e.g. lying in bed).	1,750
1	Sedentary work (30 Cals/hr.) and little travelling (65 Cals.)	2,250
2	Light work (70 Cals. /hr.) and travelling (130 Cals.)	2,750

Contd...

Requirment	*Description*	*Calorie requirement*
3	Medium work (100 Cals./hr.) and travelling (130 Cals.	3,000
4	Heavy work (200CaIs. / hr.) and travelling	(130 Cals.)
	Extremely heavy work (450 Cals./hr.) and travelling (130 Cals.)	5,000
0	No work, almost basal (e.g lying in bed)	1,500
1	Sendentay work (30 Cals./hr.) and little travelling (50 Cals.)	2,000
2	Light work (70 Cals./hr.) and travelling (100 cals.)	2,250
3	Medium work (100 Clas./hr.) and travelling (100 Cals.).	2,500
4	Heavy work (200 Cals./hr.))	
5	Very heay work work(200 Cals./hr.) and travelling (100 Cals.)	3,750

The recognition that the quantity of food required could be exactly measured so captured the imagination that for many years no thought was given to the quality of the food supplied. Calories were all important and the neat way in which a man's energy needs could be expressed numerically no doubt delayed the recognition of the more subtle needs for particular factors in foods.

This is doubtless one reason why vitamins were not discovered until the present century, and why are still ignorant about certain aspects of nutritional requirements.

It is, however, established that the basal needs for calories, are best met by a balance between protiens, fats and carbohydrates: other needs are adequate amounts of fluid, certain mineral salts and vitamins.

Although this book is mainly concerned with vitamins, it is not possible to study them without reference to other nutrients.

The Table shows present-day views of human requirements of vitamins and calories.

The figures given in the table are, of course, averages. As with all physiological functions, there are great individual variations but these can be discovered only by experience. However, an example will serve to illustrate the point. Mr. A, a lean, bony man, has a hearty appetite and seems able to eat as much as he likes without showing any tendency to grow fat. By contrast Mr. B, who is also physically active, puts on weight without apparently eating to excess. These two seem to have different basal mechanisms for the use of food, one making his calories go futher, as it were, than the other.

The same seems to be true, to some extent for vitamin needs. Among people in a group living on a diet deficient in one or other of the vitamins, some will show signs of disease, others, whose needs are evidently less, will escape.

Both nicotinic acid and nicitinatmide are physiologically active as what was originally the P-P factor. To avoid confusion with nicotine (which has no vitamin activity) the term Niacin was introduced in the U.S.A. and has been used in the table compiled by the B.M.A. Committee on Nutrition.

In planning diets, however, the table given can safely be used as a guide. Any individual idiosyncrasies in the nature of special needs must be allowed for separately.

Methods of Assessing the Adequacy of Diets : How can you assess that a diet which has been planned or eaten is adequate in nutrient content? There are various procedures for assessing the nutritive value of the diet. The most simple of these is the use of a "score card." The use of a food pattern as a guide in planning an adequate diet has already been discussed, and score cards have been developed for determining how well diet meets the suggested pattern. A more precise method of evaluating the

Vitamins in Nutrition and Health

Report of the Committee on Nutrition- B.M.A. 1950. p. 22 and p. 23 (extract)

Age and sex	Requirement class	Calories	Vit. A &- carotene i.u. daily	Vit. D i.u. daily	Thia min mg. daily	Niacint mg. daily	Ribo flavin mg. daily	Vit. C mg. daily
Both								
0-1		1,000	3,000	800	0.4	4	0.6	10
2-6		1,500	3,000	400	0.6	6	0.9	15
7-10		2,000	3,000	400	0.8	8	1.2	20
Males								
11-14		2,750	3,000	400	1.1	11	1.6	30
15-19		3,500	5,000	400	1.4	14	2.1	30
	sedentary work	2,250	5,000		0.9	9	1.4	20
	medium work	3,000	5,000		1.2	12	1.8	20
	heavy work	4,250	5,000		1.7	17	2.6	20
Females								
11-14		2,750	3,000	400	1.1	11	1.6	30
15-19		2,500	5,000	400	1.0	10	1.5	30
	sedentary work	2,000	5,000		0.8	8	1.2	20
	medium work	2,500	5,000		1.0	10	1.5	20
	very heavy work	3,750	5,000		1.5	15	2.2	20
Pregnancy								
1st half		2,500	6,000	400	1.0	10	1.5	40
2nd half		2,750	6,000	600	1.1	11	1.6	40
Lactation		3,000	8,000	800	1.4	14	2.1	50

Vitamin B_1, aneurin and thiamine are synonymous but the most recent recommendation is that Thiamine should be adopted as the chemical name of vitamin B_1.

nutritive adequacy of diets is computing the nutrient content of each food using a food composition table. The most precise method of all is actual laboratory determination of the energy, protein, mineral, and vitamin content. The choice of the procedure for evaluating the energy and nutrient content of a diet depends on the use to be made of the findings and the accuracy with which the food consumption data were collected.

Use of Dietary Score Cards : Dietary score cards set up for evaluating the diet on the basis of food groups are used mainly as a basis for nutrition education programs (Tables). A limitation of each score card is its failure to give the complete nutritive contribution of each food. On the other hand, it is a commendable educational tool in that it encourages a varied diet and provides a good "rule of thumb" for the selection of an adequate diet.

Use of Food Composition Tables : By far the most common method of determining the nutrient content of the diet is the use of food composition tables. In various chapters of the book of the food tables have been used in the study of the energy value and content of the different nutrients of various foods. The values are obtained by laboratory analysis with each representing many determinations.

The composition of the same food varies widely, specially in fruits and vegetables. Growing conditions, variety, fertilizer treatment, care in handling, all make a difference. Preparation of the food for the table preservation, and storage also have an influence on the composition of most foods.

A Dietary Score Card

Foods	*Each Day You Need*	*Score for Your One Day Score*
Green and yellow vegetables (raw or cooked in small amount of water)	1 serving	10
Oranges, grapefruit, tomatoes, or other vitamin-C-rich food	1 serving	10

Contd...

Foods	*Each Day You Need*	*Score for Your One Day Score*
Potatoes and other vegetables and fruits	3 servings	5
Milk and milk products	Children, 3-4 cups Adolescents, 3-4 cups Adults, 2 cups	20
Meat, poultry, or fish	1 serving	15
Meat, poultry, fish, or meat alternates (dried beans, peas, peanut butter)	1 serving	10
Eggs	1 daily (at least 4 a week)	5
Cereal, whole grain or enriched	1 serving or 2 slices bread	
Bread, whole grain or enriched	1 or 2 slices at every meal	5
Butter or other fats	2 to 3 level tbsp butter or enriched margarine	5
A good breakfast, including some form of protein, as milk or egg		10
	Total	100

Those who have compiled food tables have had to decide on the values that they considered most representative for inclusion in the table. The necessity of exercising judgment in preparing a food table accounts for some of the differences that exist among the compilations of food composition values. As a rule the most food table includes new data add to the accuracy.

Short Methods Using a Food Composition Table : Short method for dietary calculation have been developed in which foods similar in composition are grouped, together, a representative value for each of the nutrients is calculated, and the values listed in a table. Totalling the amount of foods of like composition in a diet and computing the nutritive contribution of the group is shorter, of course, than computing each food separately. That is the manner in which the short methods save time in calculation.

The short methods are found to agree with the long or usual method if applied to a varied diet, and if the food habits do not differ widely from the usual pattern of the dietary habits of the people of a country as a whole. In regions where there is a relatively higher intake of certain foods, such as corn meal in the southern region, a revision in the cereal and bread portion of the table becomes necessary to obtain an accuracy approaching that of calculating each food individually. For survey studies the shorter method of dietary calculation has been found satisfactory. Time required for computation can be reduced without great sacrifice to accuracy.

Chemical Analysis

In research studies designed to determine quantitatively the nutrient intake as part of a metabolic balance study, the composition of a food is determined by laboratory analysis rather than by use of a food composition table Laboratory Analysis is the most accurate of any procedure for determining the nutritive value of food, since the nutrient content of some foods varies widely. To illustrate, the ascorbic acid content the thirteen different varieties of potatoes ranged from 8.2 to 17.4 mg. per 100 gm. of fresh weight, and for thirty-five varieties of cabbage from 32.4 to 100.7 mg. per 100 gm. of fresh weight. It should be recognized, however, that the fruits and vegetables vary more in composition than most other foods.

The differences between computed and analyzed values for given diets have been studied. It is generally concluded that agreement is sufficiently close to warrant the use of food tables in dietary surveys, reserving laboratory analyses for controlled studies.

Family Food Budget

Ultimately, daily menus, a market list, and a plan for purchasing food must be made by families who maintain households and by agencies who make allowances for families in need of assistance. The Consumer and Food Economics Research Division of the U.S. Department of Agriculture prepares materials that are of genuine assistance as guides in planning food budgets. The quantities and kinds of foods needed to adequately nourish different individuals are estimated at low-cost, moderate-cost, and more expensive diet. The Research Division has prepared plans for twenty age-sex groups and for eleven food commodity groups. These groups include milk and milk products; meat, poultry, and fish, eggs, dry beans, peas, and nuts; grain products; potatoes; citrus fruits and tomatoes; dark green and dark yellow vegetables; other vegetables and fruits; fats and oils; sugars and sweets.

To plan a food budget for a family of a certain size it is necessary to add together the estimated quantities needed for each family member. For example, a week's food plan for a family of a man and a woman both 33 years of age, a girl 8, and a boy 11 would be as summarized in Table.

The student of nutrition is aware that merely planning for kinds and amounts of food is not enough; the planning is made best with knowledge of the food preferences of the family and the availability and price of these foods. The budget plan allows for choice of foods within the commodity groups. Further adjustment can be made even between the groups with a knowledge of food values. For instance, potatoes could not substitute for eggs nutritionally, but another serving of meat would substitute very well.

The estimated cost of one week's food supply for a four-member family (a girl 8, a boy 11, man and woman each 33 years of age) as of January 1963 was $32.80 for the moderate-cost plan (Table).

It is gratifying that an adequate diet can be provided at different cost levels. The low-cost plan contains substantially more potatoes and grain products. The lower-cost meat cuts can be used in the limited-expense plan with the assurance that the nutritive value is equal to that of the higher-priced cuts. The moderate-cost and liberal plans include more milk, eggs, meat, fruits and vegetables. More expensive items such as foods out of season and the more highly processed foods are allowed in the moderate-cost and liberal plans.

Quantity of Food for a Family of Four for One Week

Food Groups	*Unit*	*Low-Cost Plan*	*Moderate Cost-Plan*	*Liberal Plan*
Milk, milk products	qt	16.5	17.5	19.0
Meal, poultry, fish	lb	11.5	17.2	20.8
Eggs	no.	25.0	29.0	29.0
Dry beans, peas, nuts	lb	1.4	.9	0.9
Grain products	lb	12.5	11.5	10.9
Potatoes	lb	10.0	8.5	7.8
Citrus fruit, tomatoes	lb	7.5	9.0	11.5
Dark green, deep yellow vegetables	lb	3.5	3.5	3.5
Other vegetables, fruits	lb	19.8	22.5	25.2
Fats, oils	lb	3.1	2.8	2.8
Sugars, sweets	lb	3.0	3.9	4.6

Cost of one Week's Food at Home[1] Estimated for Foods Plans at Three Cost Levels, June 1964, U.S.A. Average

Sex-Age Groups[2]	*Low-Cost Plan, Dollars*	*Moderate Cost Plan, Dollars*	*Liberal Plan, Dollars*
Families			
Family of two 20-35 years[3]	14.60	19.60	22.70
Family of two, 55-75 years[3]	12.20	16.50	18.70

Contd...

Sex-Age Groups[2]	*Low-Cost Plan, Dollars*	*Moderate Cost Plan, Dollars*	*Liberal Plan, Dollars*
Family of four, preschool children[4]	21.40	28.40	32.80
Family of four, school children[5]	24.60	33.00	38.30
Individuals[6]			
Children under 1 year	2.90	3.80	4.10
1-3 years	3.70	4.80	5.50
3-6 years	4.40	5.80	6.70
6-9 years	5.20	7.00	8.30
Girls, 9-12 years	6.00	8.00	8.90
12-15 years	6.60	8.80	10.20
15-20 years	6.90	9.00	10.20
Boys 9-12 years	6.10	8.20	9.40
12-15 years	7.10	9.70	11.00
15-20 years	8.30	10.90	12.60
Women, 20-35 years	6.20	8.30	9.40
35-55 years	6.00	7.90	9.10
55-75 years	4.70	6.90	7.80
75 years and over	4.70	6.20	7.20
Pregnant	7.50	9.60	10.80
Nursing	8.60	11.10	12.30
Men 20-35 years	7.00	9.50	11.20
35-55 years	6.60	8.80	10.20
55-75 years	6.00	8.10	9.20
75 years and over	5.60	7.80	8.90

Food Values and Food Costs : The buying of food is the largest single expense in the budget for most families. An average of 19 per cent capita of disposable personal income is spent for food in the United States. With increasing income, the per cent going food diminishes.

Economical purchase of food makes it possible to provide adequate diets at lower cost. Some nutrients are provided at less expense by one food or group of foods than by others. The approximate percentage of the food dollar spent for milk and milk products; meat, fish, poultry, eggs, dry beans, and nuts; vegetables; fruits; and grain products is shown in Fig. Other foods not included in Fig. are fats, sugar, and sweets, and miscellaneous items, which account for about 20 per cent of the total food expenditure. The protein group of foods is the most expensial, amounting to 37 cents of the food dollar or 37 per cent of the food expenditure. Milk and milk products account for 15 cents of the food dollar, vegetables 12 cents, grain products 11 cents, and fruits 8 cents.

Foods differ in the economy with which they provide the nutrients of the diet. Protein, calcium, vitamin A value, and thiamine were selected to illustrate this point. Using Fig. as a guide, in each food group if the nutrient bar exceeds the cost bar in length, that food group is a good buy for providing that nutrient, because the per cent of the expenditure for that group of foods is less than per cent of the nutrient obtained. The relative lengths of the bars will vary, of course, with price. It can be clearly seen that the milk group of foods is an excellent buy for calcium but only fair for supplying thiamine; the meat, fish, poultry, eggs, dry beans, and nuts group is a good buy for protein but a poor buy for calcium; vegetables are excellent for vitamin A, poor for protein; fruits are not a good buy for the nutrients listed, but had ascorbic acid been selected as one of the nutrietns in the illustration, fruits would appear as good buy for that nutrient. Grain products are a good buy for protein and thiamine, and it may be surprising to note, for calcium, accounted for in part by the use of bread containing non-fat milk solids. Of course, little if any vitamin A value is furnished by grain products. The protein of cereals is economical to purchase and becomes of the good nutritional quality when supplemented with milk or other sources of complete protien. Grain products are a good buy for protein because, as shown in the cost bar is shorter than the protein bar.

5

Diseases of Kidney

Kidneys are the major excretory organs in our body. They are also called as the guardians of the nutritional wealth of our body. All useful substances and nutrients are reabsorbed by the proximal convoluted tubules of nephrons. In renal failure excessive loss of water, electrolytes, calcium and phosphorus and proteins take place.

The kidneys which weigh only 0.3 per cent of body weight perform very important functions. Formation and expulsion of urine, maintenance of normal nutrition, acid-base and electrolyte balance and secretion of certain hormones like renin and erythroprotein are the major functions of the kidneys.

The waste products of the body, especially the end products of protein, metabolism, are excreted by the kidneys. Urea is the major component of urine which is about 30 gms in urine. Urea is derived from ingested food and from the breakdown of body tissues. If urea is more than 4 per cent of urine, complications occur in the body. In renal disorders urine formation is affected. A healthy person's kidney filters about 170 litres of fluid and 1 to 2 litres of urine is produced. Acid and basic mineral salts and other nitrogenous products of protein metabolism such as uric acid and creatinine are eliminated by the kidney. Ammonia is synthesised by the kidney and excreted through urine.

Nephritic syndrome, nephrotic syndrome and chronic renal failure are the common disorders of the kidney.

Acute Glomerulonephritis : This disease is also known as Bright's disease. In this condition inflammation or degeneration of the kidney takes place.

Nephritis is characterised by oliguria, hematuria, nitrogen retention, hypertension, oedema and proteinuria. Glomeruli, tubules and intestinal tissues are affected. Usually it occurs in children due to streptococcic infections like scarlet fever, tonsillitis, pneumonia and other respiratory infections. If children are affected 85 to 95 per cent make a complete recovery whereas if adults are affected only 50 per cent gain complete recovery. Carelessness in treatment and dietetic control leads to chronic renal failure. Renal infarction, acute polyonephritis and metallic poisoning also cause acute glomerulonephritis.

Dietary modification includes a low protein, low sodium, low potassium, high carbohydrate diet with moderate fluid content. In the acute state of illness nausea and vomiting occur and normal food consumption is impossible. At the end of the second week normal diet can be given.

Carbohydrate is included liberally to supply 1,700 kcals per day. Cereals in all forms are allowed, but no cooking salt is added.

A low protein diet is recommended so as to give rest to the kidney. Complete proteins are better to ensure maximum utilisation.

If anuria develops protein should be stopped. When urine formation is about 500 to 700 ml, about 0.5 gm protein per kg body weight is allowed.

Vitamins, especially vitamins C and B complex, are recommended in very high quantities. More than 100 mgs of vitamin C is recommended.

In acute nephritis kidney is unable to do proper filtration, therefore, sodium and potassium are not excreted and electrolyte balance and water balance are disturbed. If oedema is present, sodium is restricted. When urine formation is reduced potassium is also restricted.

Fluid intake is regulated based on urine formation. Intake and output of fluid and urine must be checked; 1,000 ml plus output of urine is the best method of calculation of fluids.

A soft, low protein, low sodium must be suggested to the patient. Animal proteins like meat, fish, eggs, liver and other flesh foods, milk in excess, excess peas, beans, pulses and all nuts are restricted in nephritis diet Papad, chutney or pickles are avoided.

Bread, chapathis of wheat, rice, millets, breakfast cereals, 3 cups of milk and milk products, all vegetables, roots and tubers, sugar and jaggery, boiled sweets, fresh fruits, arrowroot, cornflour and plain biscuits are allowed.

A Sample Diet for an Actue Glomerulonephritis Patient

Time	*Meal*
6 a.m.	Coffee
8 a.m.	Bread, Butter (2 slices), Jam, Grape juice.
11 a.m.	Orange juice.
12.30 p.m.	Tomato rice or soft chapathi (2 nos.) Tomato curry, Steamed cabbage raita, Fruit juice.
4 p.m.	Rava ladoo (2 nos.), Tea
7 p.m.	Sago pudding (1 cup)
8 p.m.	Soft chapathi (2) or uppuma (1-2 cup), Tomato-dal mashed, Fruit salad.
10 p.m.	Milk (skimmed milk)

The diet supplies 1,850 kcals, proteins-36 gms, fat - 32 gms.

Nephrotic Syndrome

Albuminuria, haematuria, oedema and proteinuria, hypertension and diminished renal functions are the common symptoms of nephrotic syndrome. Serum cholesterol levels are raised, nitrogenous waste products are retained and gradually uraemia or renal failure occurs. Renal excretory capacity is maintained even if only 10 per cent of kidney tissues are in working condition. After that excretory and regulatory functions of the kidneys are affected and the waste products are accumulated in the blood. This condition is known as uraemia. Chronic glomerulonephritis, vascular kidney diseases like malignant hypertension, hypertensive, arteriosclerosis, atherosclerotic nephrosclerosis and vascular lesions produce degenerative destruction of nephrosis. Diabetes develops nephropathy which gradually destroys nephrons. Neglected gout and congenital abnormalities like polycystic diseases present since birth eventually lead to renal failure.

Dietetic management includes enough calories, fat and a high protein and high vitamin C content in the diet; 2,000 kcals, 1.5 to 2 gms of protein and 1 gm fat/kg body weight are recommended. A high protein diet is required to meet the heavy loss of albumin and protein depletion of the tissues. Since proteins are lost, resistance power is reduced and the patient becomes susceptible to infection. So a high protein diet is essential.

Sodium is restricted to prevent oedema. Cooking salt is restricted and readymade foods where salt is added are also avoided. But severe sodium restriction may lead to body depletion of sodium. For a nephrotic patient 500 mgs to 800 mgs of sodium is recommended. Substitutes for sodium must be carefully selected as it may affect the potassium elimination. Fluid is restricted only when the kidney is affected in its functions accompanied by oedema.

Cereals in all forms are allowed for a nephrotic patient. Pulses, beans, fleshy foods like meat, fish, eggs are allowed. Milk is not allowed but skimmed milk can be used. Soups are excluded but vegetables, roots and tubers, cooking fat, sugar and jaggery, pastries, dessert, sweets and fruits are allowed. Condiments and spices, papads, pickles and chutney are not permitted.

Sample Diet for Nephrotic Syndrome

Time	*Meal*
6 a.m.	Coffee
8 a.m.	Rava porridge, Toast, Poached egg, Coffee.
10 a.m.	Lime juice, Banana
12.30 p.m.	Rice or soft chapathi, Pumpkin dal curry, Meat cutlet, Vegetable salad, curd
4 p.m.	Coffee, Pancake.
8 p.m.	Chappati, Tomato-dal curry, Fish molee, Spinach or amaranth saute.
10 p.m.	Milk (skimmed milk)

This diet supplies 82 gms, proteins 3,200 kcals fat, 80 gms.

Since calcium and potassium deficiency may accompany severe proteinuria, bone rarefaction and hypokalemia are common in nephrosis, low sodium milk with potassium supplements is essential in the treatment of this condition. A soft bland diet is suggested. Vitamin supplements, especially vitamin C, are essential. Thus a high protein, high carbohydrate, salt free, moderate fat with restricted fluid are recommended for a nephrotic patient.

Renal Failure

Diminished renal function leads to renal failure. It can be acute or chronic in nature. Waste products are accumulated in the blood and tissues and anuria occurs in acute renal failure. Headaches, nausea, drowsiness, lethargy and coma are the symptoms. In chronic renal failure, functioning nephrons are few. Nephrons are hypertrophied. Infection or trauma creates new catabolic loads to the damaged nephrons and blood urea may rise only 10 to 15 mgs per 100 ml daily. Cardiovascular oedema, neurological changes, skin and skeletal changes are common.

Dietetic treatment aims to minimise protein catabolism, to avoid dehydration and overhydration, to control electrolytes and fluid loss through vomiting and diarrhoea, to arrest acidosis and to minimise complications. A minimum of 600 to 1,000 kcals mainly from carbohydrate and fats is recommended. Protein foods are restricted except in the case of peritoreal dialysis or haemodialysis. In this condition 40 gms of protein is recommended. Usually the protein content of the diet varies depending upon the urea content of the blood. Fluid content is calculated based on urine formation. Total loss plus 500 ml is the allotment. Sodium restriction is also judged by the physician based on sodium loss in the urine. Hyperkalaemia or potassium intoxication produce deleterious effects and potassium sources like tomato juice, coffee or tea, cocoa, and molasses are avoided. Since normal food is not given, other sources of potassium-rich vegetables or beans are not included in the diets. A planned diet is not possible because of the severe complications in uraemia. If the condition improves liberal amounts of protein can be included with a high carbohydrate content. A bland, easily digested diet with sodium restriction, if there is oedema, is recommended for uraemia.

Urinary Calculi : In urinary calculi stones are developed anywhere mong the urinary tract, in the kidneys, ureters, bladder and urethra. Small foci are formed and supersaturated urinary salts are precipitated around the foci of mucoid structures. Mucopolysaccharides and mucoprotein combine with chemicals bound to form the foci. The end products of protein metabolism leaves uric acid, phosphate and oxalates, sodium, calcium and magnesium. A urine concentrated with calcium phosphate and ammonium phosphate predisposes stone formation. Abnormal colloids in the urine cements precipitated crystals around the foci, and concentration of urine due to low fluid intake helps the calculus formation.

Aetiological factors are heredity, climate, fluids, vitamin B complex deficiency, vitamin A deficiency and excessive vitamin D and calcium content, hyperthyroidism and frequent infections. People residing in hot climates are more prone to develop renal calculi compared to people of other areas. During summer calculi occurs more often as compared to in cold weather.

Due to high perspiration in tropical areas urine becomes concentrated if large quantities of fluids are not ingested daily. A high fluid intake of more than 8 to 10 glasses enables the urine to be in dilute state. This prevents stone formation. Urinary oxalate excretion is more if tryptophan content in the diet is more. B complex vitamins, especially B6, decreases the urinary oxalate excretion. Vitamin A deficiency causes roughening of the epithelial tissues in our body, thereby helping the precipitation of stones in the renal system. Vitamin D is essential for proper bone calcification and if excess vitamin D with calcium is administered as supplements it can produce urinary calculi in later course. In hyperparathyroidism the breakdown of bone matrix is more which leads to inorganic calcium and phosphorus deposits in the urinary tract. Prolonged bed rest and congenital malformation in renal pelvis, ureter or bladder, prostate enlargement and urinary infection can also produce calculi.

Renal calculi are with calcium combined to oxalates, urates, or phosphates and high oxalate content in the diet. Excessive uric acid releases high inorganic phosphates in the diet; low urinary magnesium and high calcium excretion are the direct causes for urinary calculi.

Dietary Modifications : The role of diet in the formation of stones is not clearly known. Even though formation of stones is a metabolic defect where certain chemicals are either excreted more or retained more in the urine, foods rich in such chemicals are restricted as a dietary modification for urinary calculi. Two commonest types of stones in the adult population are those made of uric acid and of calcium oxalate. In a stone-forming person, especially in oxalate stones, the patient absorbs and re-excretes a greater proportion of calcium from a normal diet compared to a non-stone-forming person. In magnesium deficiency excessive oxalate is excreted. Uric acid calculi are common in adults. Increased uric acid content in urine makes the calcium oxalate in the urine less soluble and develops stones with calcium oxalate and traces of urates. Acidification of the urine is dangerous in such patients because of the high solubility of free uric acid in acid medium. In alkaline medium uric acid combines with alkali and forms alkaline urates.

Protein is the main source of uric acid in our body. In starvation body proteins are depleted and breakdown of protein and fat helps the liberation of uric acid. If excessive fluid is ingested this can be minimised. A high fluid intake is recommended for all three types of urinary calculi. A dilute urine prevents precipitate formation around the matrix. Acidity of the urine must be regulated. Purine content in the diet has to be reduced in low uric acid diets. Organ meats like kidney, liver, brain, heart and sardines. Fish, fish roe, herrings are rich in purine content. These foods are strictly prohibited in urinary calculi and in gout. Beans, peas, cauliflower, spinach, amaranthus, meat, seafoods, yeast and wholegrain cereals are moderate in its purine content. All other vegetables, fruits, milk, eggs, refined cereals and cereal products, sugar and sweets are poor in purine content

If the stone is a calcium oxalate stone, high fluid intake reduces the concentration of calcium and oxalate iron in the urine. Acidification of the urine by taking acidifying agents keep the calcium and oxalate in solution. Calcium and oxalate intake must be avoided. Calcium-rich foods are milk and milk products, small fish with bones, canned sardines, beans, prawns, crabs, cauliflower, egg yolk, molasses, potatoes, tapioca, colocasia, ragi, gingerale, cane sugar and onion. Foods rich in oxalates are beef, coffee, cola drinks, tea, cashewnuts, chocolates, grapes, plum, leafy vegetables, beetroot, yam, gooseberries.

Even though dietary oxalates are controlled endogenous production of oxalates takes place independent of exogenous dietary supply. Often calcium phosphate stones are formed and to avoid this along with calcium, dietary phosphates also must be restricted. Milk, cheese, milk products, wholegrain, cereals, bran, oatmeal, eggs, organ meats, nuts, soyabean, meats, banana, carrot, cherry and soft drink are rich in phosphorus content. A high fluid intake, about 3 litres, is essential to prevent stone formation. Urinary infection produces complications and care must be taken to prevent it.

High intake of calcium, hypervitaminosis D, prolonged skeletal immobilisation, prolonged acidosis, postmenopausal osteoporosis and hyperparathyroidism produce hypercalcinuria. If any of these cause hypercalcinuria it must be treated first. Vegetarian diets are more appreciated for urinary calculi.

6

Defects in Cardiovascular System

A healthy human heart is an extremely efficient muscular organ contracting and relaxing 1,00,000 times per day. A person is said to be as old as his arteries because once the arteries of the heart, kidneys or brain show degenerative changes these organs suffer. The heart pumps the blood and pushes it through the body.

The arteries branch into smaller capillaries and supply nourishment and oxygen to each and every cell in our body. The veins collect the impurities and impure blood from the cells and bring it back to the heart. This is how complete circulation takes place in our body. The force exerted by the heart as it pumps the blood into the large arteries creates a pressure within the arteries. The pressure depends on various factors and the most important of them is the size and nature of the arterial walls. They have high elasticity so as to dilate and constrict on pumping of the heart. The more constricted the arteries the higher the pressure tends to be. Thus it is the amount of constriction which determines the level of blood pressure rather than the force of the heart's pumping. Indirectly this affects the force of pumping. Narrowing, hardening and degeneration of arterial walls produce high blood pressure and coronary heart diseases. Atherosclerosis, a progressive vascular disease, reduces the elasticity of arterial walls and causes degenerative changes. Ninety five per cent of coronary heart diseases are due to coronary aheroma and arteriosclerosis. No doubt cardiac diseases are a menace to health because kidneys, brain, lungs and extremities are affected due to cardiac upset. The diseases of the heart may be classified as functional or organic. The pericardium, endocardium or the myocardium are the different parts of the heart. Any of these can be affected and at times blood vessels within the heart or leaving the heart or the valves can be diseased. Enlargement of the organ also brings disorder. When the heart is not able to maintain the normal function heart failure occurs. Weakness, pain in the chest, dyspnoea on exertion, loss of appetite and digestive disorders manifest as the first symptoms of heart diseases. Atherosclerosis and hypertensions are the common heart diseases.

Hypertension

High blood pressure, commonly known as hypertension, is not a disease but only a symptom indicating that some underlying disease is progressing. Cardiovascular diseases, renal diseases like glomeulonephritis, polycystic renal disease, pyelonephritis, tumours of the brain, or adrenal glands, hyperthyroidism or diseases of ovaries and pituitary may cause hypertension. However, the majority of patients with high blood pressure arc grouped as patients with "essential hypertension" for which the cause is unknown.

Predisposing factors of hypertension are heredity, stress, obesity, smoking, high viscosity of the blood due to too many red blood cells in the circulating blood, narrowing of the main blood vessels near the heart or aorta due to congenital malformation and excessive hormone secretions especially cortisone, aldosterone, adrenaline and non-adrenaline.

Studies conducted on parents and their children and siblings showed that there is a strong tendency for hypertension to run in families. Hypertension is often mentioned as a disease of modern living because city dwellers are more prone to it compared to rural people. Usually a villager leads a quiet life whereas a city dweller leads a mechanical life with various stresses and strains. People who are usually tense show high blood pressure as compared to a normal person. Overwork, unhappy home, marital disharmony, financial worries, and generation problems can create continuous stress. If the cause of stress is isolated half the problem is over. People who cope with their problems quickly, worry less and produce less pressure compared with a person who always broods over a problem.

Obesity has a tendency to increase blood pressure. When the weight is brought down pressure usually falls. People with sedentary work suffer more from hypertension in contrast to a moderate or a hard worker.

Smoking of cigarettes causes rise in blood pressure. Nicotine in the tobacco causes the release of adrenaline and non-adrenaline from the adrenal glands which increases blood pressure. Atheroma, a condition where deposits of fatty materials line the blood vessels which later break up causing blood clots, is more common among smokers. Coronary thrombosis occurs more among hypertensive patients who smoke.

Symptoms of Hypertension : Mild and moderate hypertensions usually produce no symptoms. The first symptom may be, if any, headache towards the back of the head and neck on walking. All headaches need not be related to hypertension. Giddiness, unexplained tiredness, change in eyesight, especially a blind spot when they look in one or another direction and shortness of breath, are signals of rise in blood pressure. Acute attacks of breathlessness in the night are very harmful. Reduced blood supply due to constriction of arteries, especially coronary arteries, makes the heart work hard and this may cause angina pectoris, a discomfort of pain usually felt in the centre of the chest. If a coronary artery is completely blocked the condition is known as thrombosis. And it is often referred to as 'heart attack'.

Hypertension patients are more prone to coronary and cerebral thrombosis. Cerebral thrombosis is one of the causes of a 'stroke'. Depending upon the site and position of the blockage in the artery the patient may become unconscious and go into a coma. Cerebral haemorrhage also causes a stroke. In this condition, an artery may rupture and the blood flow thus destroys a part of the brain. This stage is mentioned as 'apoplexy'. Therefore, hypertension can produce such complications if neglected.

Dietary Treatment : 'Kempner's rice-fruit-sugar diet' is very effective in severe cases. It provides about 2,000 kcals, 5 gms fat, 20 gms protein, 150 mgs sodium and 200 mgs chloride. It consists of boiled or steamed rice, 250 to 350 gms (dry) in weight. Rice is cooked in water or in fruit juice. No salt is added. Fruits may be eaten raw or stewed with sugar or as fruit juices. Free fluid should be limited to 700 to 1,000 ml only as fruit juice. Vitamin supplements other than vitamin C are essential; 5,000 I.U. of vitamin A and 1,000 I.U. of vitamin D, 5 mgms of the amino chloride, 5 mgs of riboflavin and 25 mgs of niacinamide are essential. Calcium pentothenate 2 mgs is also recommended in this diet. Hospitalisation is essential and it provides rest to the patient.

The normal diet prescription of a hypertension patient is a low calorie, low fat, low sodium diet with normal protein in it. Since obesity is common among those patients with essential hypertension, weight reduction is essential. A moderate amount of protein, that is, 1 gm of protein per kg (ideal weight) body weight is recommended. If kidney diseases cause hypertension, low protein diets of 20 to 30 gms are recommended. As a general rule 1,000 to 1,200 kcals and 50 gms of protein are recommended. Though animal protein has no direct relation in increasing the pressure, their cholesterol content and saturated fatty acid content have harmful effects in a hypertension patient.

Since atherosclerosis accompanies hypertension high intake of fat, especially animal fat and vanaspati, and coconut oil are restricted. About 30 gms of vegetable oil is recommended.

Low sodium diet is generally prescribed for a hypertension patient; 2 gms and 5 gms sodium restriction is introduced in cardiovascular renal diseases and in hypertension, respectively. Low sodium foodstuffs are to be selected for a hypertension patient. Animal foods are rich in sodium content and seafoods and canned foods are better avoided in a low sodium diet. Foods rich in sodium are beef, kidney, liver, beetroots, enriched breads and cereals, salted butter, items where baking powder is used, cereal brans, kidney, liver, beetroots, cornflakes, salted butter, baking powder, riceflakes, cream, soda, egg, sardines, tuna, skimmed milk, onion, legumes and vegetables like cabbage. Cooking salt, salted preserves, and snack items and chips are not allowed in a low sodium diet.

Foods allowed in a low sodium diet are bread, chapathi, breakfast cereals or wheat, rice, millets or oats without salt, pulses, vegetable soups, vegetable salads from selected vegetables like tomato, sprouted green gram, vegetables like potato, yam, drumstick, beans, vegetable oils, sugar, jaggery, honey, desserts, dried fruits except raisins, and fresh fruits. Beverages except milk drinks are allowed.

Animal foods like meat, fish, chicken, eggs, beetroot, carrots, leafy vegetables, sweets and pastry, readymade food items where salt is used, papad, chutney, pickles and canned foods are excluded. Also milk is minimised in sodium restricted diet

Fluid content of a hypertension diet depends on oedema in the body.

A Low Sodium Diet

Time	*Meal*
6 a.m.	Coffee
8 a.m.	Sweet potato stuffed chapathi Pineapple, Coffee.
11 a.m.	Grape juice
12.30 p.m.	Rice or chapathi, Fish curry, Carrot kheer, Cucumber raita.

Time	*Meal*
4 p.m.	Banana, Toast, Mango, Coffee
8 p.m.	Rice gruel or soft chapathi, Green gram curry, Meat cutlet, Fruit juice.
9 p.m.	Milk

This diet provides 62.5 gms protein, 516.6 mgms sodium, 38 gms fat and 2015 kcals.

A Sample Diet for a Hypertension Patient

(No Salt is added)

Time	*Meal*
6. a.m.	Coffee
8. a.m.	Soft chapathi (2 in nos), Egg curry (less oil), Plantain, Coffee.
10. a.m.	Lime juice
12.30. p.m.	Potato-tomato soup, Rice or chapathi (50 gms), Bittergourd with tamarind juice, Tomato curry, Drumstick pugath, Curds, Guava.
4. p.m.	Tea, Vermicelli savoury
6. p.m.	Buttermilk
8. p.m.	Chapathi, Tomato-dal mashed, Orange.
10. p.m.	Milk (skimmed milk)

This diet provides 50 gms protein, 1,800 kcals and 750 mgs sodium.

Atherosclerosis

Atherosclerosis is a chronic vascular disease characterised by thickening, hardening and loss of elasticity of the arterial walls. Lipids infiltrate the arterial wall of an atherosclerosis patient which is followed by degenerative changes. One of the major causes of heart attacks is atherosclerosis. Coronary arteries, which supply blood to the heart muscles, are affected because of the deposits of plaques containing fat, especially cholesterol. Sometimes the plaque becomes very thick and the inner lining of the arteries bursts which leads to clot formation or thrombosis. This blocks the blood supply within the heart and the heart muscles suffer from lack of oxygen causing myocardial infarction. If the damage is severe the heart fails to function and death may occur immediately. Atherosclerosis of the cerebral arteries causes paralysis or stroke and in the renal arteries it leads to high blood pressure.

The raised plasma lipid level is due to heredity, age, hormones, high calorie intake, cholesterol content in the diet, triglycerides in the diet, plasma lipo protein content, total fat content, saturated and unsaturated fat content in the diet, protein content of the diet, vitamin and mineral content in the diet, and smoking and emotional stress in the person. Longstanding hypertension and diabetes predispose to atherosclerosis. This disease is common among males and among obese people.

Heredity plays an important role in coronary heart disease. Short, stock, short-necked persons are more exposed to this disease compared to tall, thin people. Dietary habits and living pattern of the family may also contribute to it.

The onset usually takes place during early adult life but symptoms are manifested only at the age of 50 or above. Myocardial infarction and ischaemic heart diseases are observed in infants and children but atherosclerosis occurs in an adult age.

Sex hormones have some influence in the occurrence of atherosclerosis. Atherosclerosis is common among male members and it occurs among women after menopause, at the same rate as in males.

Oestrogen administered to males reduces the plasma cholesterol level in coronary artery disease even though it is not practical. In hypothyroidism total blood lipid and cholesterol level are high.

The serum lipids rise with an increase in total calorie intake. Obese people are more prone to atherosclerosis and obesity is the result of high calorie intake. Studies have shown that in communities where calories and fats are consumed in large quantities the incidence of atherosclerosis is more.

The cholesterol content in the diet has high relationship with the development of adieromatous patches in the arterial walls. An excess of cholesterol and saturated fat-laden foods in the body can lead to the hardening of the arteries.

Among the Bantus in Uganda where fat consumption is very low the incidence of coronary heart disease is not seen.

Fats in food materials are mainly saturated (hard) fats which are solid at room temperature, mono-unsaturated fats and poly-unsaturated fats are soft. Saturated fats are rich in cholesterol. Egg yolk, organ meats like heart, brain, liver, kidney, shellfish like oysters, crabs, prawns, shrimps, lobsters, dairy products like butter, cream and milk and all animal products are rich in cholesterol content- Pork, mutton fat, hydrogenated oils and coconut oil and palmoil are also rich in cholesterol. Low consumption of saturated fats reduces coronary infection, sudden death and cerebral infarction. As a whole vegetarians have a low plasma cholesterol but it is elevated if animal foods are included. Plasma cholesterol is elevated in pregnancy, diabetes, nephrosis, obstructive jaundice, cirrhosis, hypothyroidism and in cholecystitis. Low plasma cholesterol level is seen in hyperthyroidism, anaemia and in acute infection.

Cholesterol is synthesised in the liver and in the intestine. Dietary Cholesterol content regulates the endogenous production. But even in a cholesterol-free diet endogenous production continues. Fasting, low cholesterol diet and increased bile flow reduces the synthesis by the liver. A small quantity of cholesterol is essential as it forms an insulating sheath for nerves and raw materials for hormones. In all tissues some amount of cholesterol are present and form some chemical agents which determine our growth, energy and sexual characteristics. Bile contains cholesterol. But excess cholesterol in the blood causes artery blockage. High cholesterol or saturated fat content in the diet produces excess cholesterol in the blood. To limit the fat content in the diet poly-unsaturated fats like sunflower oil, saffola oil, corn oil, soyabean oil, groundnut oil, sesame oil, rice bran oil and other vegetable oils can be used.

Sistosterol, a vegetable sterol of cholesterol family, interferes with cholesterol absorption. If five to ten grams of this is given to a person sistosterol combines with the cholesterol of food and bile to form unabsorbable compounds. Soyabean and cottonseeds are rich in sistosterol.

Lipo proteins are compounds of lipids attached to proteins of different densities. This makes insoluble lipids soluble for transport. Parts of cholesterol, neutral fat and phospholipids attach themselves with protein to form proteins. Alpha, beta and prebeta lipo proteins are in our blood. In coronary heart disease the pre-beta and beta lipo proteins are increased.

Dietary advice is the first thing required in the management of patients with high cholesterol and triglyceride level. Total calories should be reduced to bring down body weight to ideal weight. Latest studies have shown that ingestion of large quantises of sucrose causes an elevation of blood triglycerides because sucrose increases the intestinal synthesis of cholesterol in the body. So a moderate to low calorie diet according to weight is recommended for an atherosclerosis patient. Protein allowance of 1 gm per kg of body weight is permitted but animal proteins are not recommended for an atherosclerosis patient. Low fat, low cholesterol diet is prescribed for an atherosclerosis patient. Animal fats, organ meats, eggs and seafoods are restricted and so vitamin deficiency, especially vitamin A deficiency, may occur. Supplement of vitamin A is essential. Leafy and other vegetables can be used liberally, but since they are not palatable without salt and seasoning the patient has to develop a habit to consume it.

Foods allowed are skimmed milk, coffee and tea in limited amounts, soft drinks, non-fat cereal foods like rice, wheat, biscuits, breads, roots like potatoes, pulses, lean meat, small fish, fowl, vegetable oils, all fruits and vegetables, sugar, honey and desserts and fruit preparations where fat is not used.

Foods avoided are whole milk, cream, cereal preparations and snack items where baking soda is used, fried and baked items where cream or fats are used, bakery items, animal foods, like meat, only fish, animal fats like butter, ghee, hydrogenated fats like vanaspati fats like vanaspati, pickles, nuts, papads and preserves where fats are used.

Three or four smaller meals are suggested instead of two big meals. The evening meals must be two hours before retiring to bed. Regular exercise and relaxed mental attitude help to reduce pressure. Aggressiveness, tensions and worries increase the pressure. Dietary fibre reduces the food consumption and so a high fibre diet is recommended. Since vegetable proteins have a tendency to reduce blood cholesterol, a vegetarian diet is more appreciated for an atherosclerosis patient. The pectin in fruits also reduces the cholesterol content of blood. Heavy smokers and uncontrolled diabetics and alcoholics have a higher death rate from heart attacks.

A Sample Menu for Atherosclerosis

Time	*Meal*
6 a.m.	Coffee
8 a.m.	Dry chapathi, Red gram dal curry, Coffee.
10 a.m.	Lime juice
12.30 Noon	Steamed vegetable pulao or chapathi, Tomato-peas salad.
4 p.m.	Ragi porridge Pury plantain
6 p.m.	Buttermilk (non-fat)
8 p.m.	Chapathi, Fish curry, Potato-spinach

This diet provides 44 gms protein, 24 gms fat and 1,384 kcals.

7

The Diabetes

Diabetes is a chronic metabolic disorder that prevents the body from using energy from carbohydrate. This inefficiency of the body to utilise glucose may be partial or complete in a diabetic. When we eat carbohydrate, it is digested and absorbed as glucose. Glucose is stored in the form of glycogen which is otherwise known as 'metabolic fuel'. Glycogen supplies glucose to the cell when energy is required in excess or in fasting. Thus, excess glucose is converted to glycogen and glycogen is converted to glucose in a normal person's body. Insulin, a hormone secreted by islets of langerhans, which are spread out in the pancreas, regulates the chemical changes for the energy balance. Lack of insulin causes diabetes mellitus. In young diabetics, deficiency of insulin and in adult obese diabetics the overweight and in senile diabetics fibrosis in pancreas are the causes.

Diabetes, the Latin word, means 'flow through' and mellitus means "honey" and clinically it is manifested by the overflow of sugar or glucose in blood and urine instead of getting converted into glycogen.

Pancreatitis

Pancreatic disease may be due to congenital or inflammatory diseases, tumour or tracoma.

In pancreatitis the enzyme production is inadequate and this interferes with normal digestion. In pancreatitis undigested protein and fats are found in the stools. Some starch also may be present often.

These are two types of pancreatitis: Acute Pancreatitis and Chronic Pancreatitis.

Acute Pancreatitis : Inflammation of the pancreas takes place in this condition. The blood supply to the pancreas is poor and so the outflow of pancreatic juice is also less. Haemorrhagic necrosis of the pancreas and peritonitis are the other complications.

Aetiological factors are alcoholism, biliary tract disease, tracoma, virus infections, tumours, nutritional deficiency, certain vascular diseases, metabolic diseases or gallstone.

Symptoms : Sudden onset of severe upper-abdominal pain radiating to the back is the first sign of pancreatitis. Epogastric tenderness, distension, constipation, nausea and vomiting occur. Moderate fever, jaundice, high serum amylase and lipase, hyperlipermia, hypocalcemia are the other symptoms.

Treatment : Medical treatment for the control of pain and vomiting and to reduce pancreatic secretion and replacement of fluids are essential.

Dietary treatment consists of parenteral administration of 2,000-2,500 ml of glucose (10%) depending upon the blood sugar level. A diet of clear liquids or some synthetic fibre to a soft or bland diet depends on the condition of the patient.

Chronic Pancreatitis : This disease may be described as progressive fibrosis of the pancreas due to recurrent occurrence of pancreatitis. Periodic pain, recurrent attacks of burning, epigastric pain, especially after meals with fat, flatulence, anorexia, weight loss, nausea, vomiting, defective digestion of protein and fats are the major symptoms. Liver and gall bladder enlargement and jaundice may present chronic changes of pancreatitis, often lead to destruction of the islets of langerhans, fibrosis and pseudocyst and pancreatic calcification.

Dietary Treatment : A low fat, high carbohydrate, high protein diet is required. Alcohol should be completely prohibited. From carbohydrate and protein a diet has to be built. Skimmed milk can be included. Small helpings of low fat, lean meat, broiler chicken, small fish, fruit juices, semi-synthetic fibre-free diet are suggested. Pancreatic secretions are greatly affected and so easily digestible carbohydrate sources are recommended.

A Sample Menu for a Chronic Pancreatitis Patient

Time	*Meal*	*Menu*
6 a.m.	-	Milk (skimmed milk)
8 a.m.	Break fast	Bread or idli with jam or sugar, Orange juice.
10 a.m.	Mid-time	Lime juice with glucose.
12 p.m.	Lunch	Double boiled rice or soft chapathi, Vegetable puree, Baked chicken cutlet, buttermilk, Fruit juice.
2 p.m.	Mid-time	Water melon
4 p.m.	Tea	Tea, Biscuits, Plantain
6 p.m.	Mid-time	Tender coconut water
8 p.m.	Dinner	Bread and jam or rice, Vegetable puree, Buttermilk, Lemon pudding (skimmed milk)
	Bed time	Rava gruel

The Causes

At least two per cent of the world's population suffer from diabetes and the main causes are genetic, endocrine and others.

Age, sex, heredity, obesity, virus infections, emotional stress and glandular disorders also cause diabetes.

Age is a factor because half of all cases occur in the age group of 50 to 60 and only five per cent of diabetics are under ten years of age.

Though the disease affects both the sexes, in younger group more boys develop diabetes and in the mature group more women develop it. On the whole men are more prone to diabetes.

Genetic factors contribute if the patient is below 40 years. But all children of diabetic parents are not affected. If both parents are diabetic one child out of four may be a diabetic. But others may have a tendency to develop it as they become old. If one diabetic marries a diabetic carrier half of their children will be potential diabetics. If a diabetic marries one who is neither diabetic nor a diabetic carrier none of the children will have diabetes.

Obesity is a strong predisposing factor in middle-aged diabetes. The percentage of obese people developing diabetes is greater than a normal person. Eighty per cent of the diabetics are obese. Middle-aged diabetes is due to increase in the size of fat cells and not the number. The insulin secreted by the body is not enough to convert it into glycogen. Normal amount of insulin is secreted in an obese diabetic patient also. In a juvenile diabetic body weight is often less and insulin secretion is also less. In adults diabetes commonly occurs among sedentary workers compared to labourers.

Latest researches have shown that virus infection may be a reason for diabetes because virus infections even could put strain on the body. But no clear evidence is yet found even though researches are diverted on this line.

Various emotional setbacks like worry, strain, rundown feeling, listlessness contribute to the physiological upsets in the body. In emotional disorders more adrenaline and cortisone are released which can lead to diabetes.

Glands like pituitary secrete growth hormones and over-secretion of growth hormone may overstretch the pancreas's ability to cope with the rapidly increasing size in the body.

Damage or tumours in pancreas, pancreatitis, and hemochromatosis and disorders of glands like acromegaly, Cushing's syndrome cause diabetes.

Symptoms

Disturbed metabolism of carbohydrates, protein and fat brings about many symptoms. Polyuria or frequent and large outflow of urine occurs because of the large amount of glucose content in the kidneys. Polydipsia or excessive thirst is another cause because of great loss of body fluids in the urine. Dehydration may occur if fluid is not taken in polyphagia or increased appetite results from the inefficiency of the body to utilise carbohydrate foods. General weakness and loss of body weight take place because of the depletion of body fat to energy purposes. Decreased resistance to infection especially staphylococcal infection, and tuberculosis, occur in poorly regulated cases of diabetes. Delayed wound healing occurs because of high blood sugar and oedema. Degenerative changes like peripheral neuritis, retinitis, diseases of coronary arteries and arteriosclerosis are symptoms of advanced cases or poorly adjusted diabetes. Ketosis or acidosis is another symptom because of high depletion of fat from the body.

Urine changes show certain biochemical indices. Glycosuria and ketoneuria are common. In glucose urea sugar is found in the urine. Glucose tolerance test, a test used to diagnose diabetes, must be done before confirming diabetes by glycosuria because sugar occurs in urine due to other causes also. Pentose uria takes place in the inefficiency of body to use pentose and lactose uria in lactating mothers. In ketoneuria ketones like aceto acetic acid are present in urine. Hyperglycaemia is another symptom when blood sugar level is above 120 mg per 100 cc of blood.

In a national survey it was found that only in 30 per cent of those diagnosed as diabetics had hyperglycaemia. So the confirmation of diagnosis of diabetes depends on urine test and blood examination in the fasting state. Glucose tolerance test is used to detect diabetes.

Glucose Tolerance Test : The test is performed after a fast of 12 hours or more. Dissolve 100 gms of glucose in 250 ml of water. Take a blood sample of the patient before giving the known sample of glucose. Again blood samples are taken to test content at the end of 1/2,1,2 and 3 hours after giving the glucose.

The blood sugar rises 1/2 to 1 hour after taking glucose even in normal persons. After one hour it falls down. By the end of the second hour, normal sugar level is obtained in a normal person. In a diabetic person maximum sugar concentration reaches by the second hour and falls down very slowly. Elevated blood sugar level is accompanied by glycosuria.

Metabolism in Diabetes : Diabetes is also known as a disease of metabolism because normal metabolism of carbohydrate, proteins and fats is affected in this condition.

Carbohydrate Metabolism : The body converts the ingested food into carbohydrates and fats. Glucose is formed not only from carbohydrates but from proteins and fats also. Amino acids from protein foods are used mainly for tissue building and maintenance. The amino acids remaining in the amino acid pool are deaminised by the liver. Some portion of this deaminised molecule of amino acid is left out which is oxidised to glucose and fatty acids. Thus, on a low carbohydrate diet glycerol function of the fat molecule and amino acids are used for energy.

In a diabetic patient, due to deficiency of insulin, the metabolism of carbohydrates is disturbed. Decreased oxidation of glucose in the tissue results in high blood sugar level and glycosuria. Sorbitol, a hydrogenated sugar, is less sweet and is absorbed slowly by the intestinal tract. This is due to its conversion into fructose by the liver before converting it into glucose.

Protein Metabolism : The breakdown of protein is more in a diabetic patient due to reduced carbohydrate utilisation. Nitrogen excretion is more and negative nitrogen balance is common. So protein requirement is high in a diabetic to ensure essential amino acid supply.

Fat Metabolism : In a diabetic patient glycogen is not synthesised and so fatty acids are metabolised by the liver for energy purposes. End products of fat metabolism are released by the liver into the bloodstream. Acetone, acetic acid and beta-hydroxybutyric acid are the end products of fat metabolism and together they are known as ketone bodies. Due to excessive release of ketone bodies in the blood the acid base equilibrium is disturbed and gradually acidosis develops. This condition can lead to dehydration and coma. Acetone is a volatile substance which is excreted through lungs and so it gives out a characteristic odour to breath.

Clinical Types of Diabetes : Dietary modification suggests three categories of diabetics: juvenile diabetics, adult diabetics and senile diabetics.

Juvenile Diabetes : This occurs in children below the age of 15 years. Acute symptoms occur. Insulin production is minimal with the tendency to develop ketosis. Most of the juvenile diabetics lose weight because of abnormal carbohydrate metabolism. Dietary habits of the child and at times of the family have to be changed. Information regarding selection of food and substitutes should be known to the child because complications are more in this age group.

Adult Diabetes : Usually obese people are diabetic. Middle-aged diabetics, show increase in the size of fat cells and glucose deposition is not possible in cells as there is no space there. Insulin secretion in an obese diabetic may be normal but because of lack of available space for conversion of glucose to glycogen, its storage is affected and hyperglycaemia and glycosuria occur. Insulin therapy is not necessary for an obese diabetic. Weight reduction often corrects the disease in them.

Senile Diabetes : This occurs among elderly people. This is mainly due to diminished insulin production by the pancreas in fibrosis or in tumours. These subjects require more insulin to bring their blood sugar to normal.

The Treatment

Dietetic treatment aims at bringing the blood sugar level to normal along with proper health of the patient Intake of calories are an important yardstick in bringing the normal blood sugar level. Body weight has to be watched carefully. Weight check-up and urine examinations are indispensable in the treatment of a diabetic. Calorie distribution in various common food items must be made clear to a diabetic, so that they can adjust their intake by themselves in course of time. The ideal body weight of the patient must be calculated and known to the patient

The calorie content of the diet must be calculated to the ideal weight. If the actual weight is more, calories must be reduced to bring down the body weight by breaking the body fat. Calorie intake also varies depending upon the type of activities the patient is engaged in. A sedentary worker requires 30 kcals per kilogramme of body weight whereas a moderate worker needs 40 kcals and a heavy worker 50 kcals per, kilogramme of body weight, respectively. Once the weight is reduced by an obese person enough calories must be supplied to keep the body in normal condition.

Dietary instructions given to a diabetic must be simple. The National Institute of Nutrition has classified all foodstuffs into exchange groups for the benefit of a diabetic's selection. With careful selection from this exchange group a diabetic can consume any item within the limits. The aim is to select a low carlorie diet and items rich in carbohydrate are better restricted for wide choice.

Having gained an elementary knowledge of the calorie content of various foodstuffs from the exchange list one can select a low calorie diet. In our country 60 to 75 per cent of the total calorie intake is from carbohydrates and so in a reducing diet or in a low calorie diet the amount of carbohydrate has to be reduced. Places where roots like tapioca (cassava) are used as the major source of carbohydrate, incidence of diabetes is more. In South India, especially in Kerala, pancreatitis or pancreatic diabetes is very common.

There is no other disease in which diet takes on a greater role as in diabetes. The patient must actively cooperate for the management of dietary treatment. Even though there are many complications of diabetes like paralysis, coronary thrombosis, blindness and coma, diabetes is no more a dreaded disease. A well managed diabetic with diet control, insulin therapy or oral drugs, weight check-up, urine and blood examination has a good expectancy of life. On the contrary negligence of the condition causes irreparable damage to the arteries, gangrene, kidney diseases or other complications of diabetes. Success or failure in the treatment of a diabetic patient depends on dietary regimen. Optimum nutrition is essential to lead a healthy life but it must be judiciously selected. Normal nutrition, normal weight, normal blood sugar level and minimum complications are the objectives for the treatment of diabetes.

Distribution of calories in terms of carbohydrates, proteins and fats is the first step. The total calorie requirement for the ideal weight has to be calculated in terms of activity. In an obese diabetic 10 kcals per kilogramme of body weight is reduced, as also for a sedentary and moderate worker, and 5 kcals per kilogramme for a labourer. In an underweight diabetic 5 kcals per kilogramme of body weight is increased for all three groups.

Caloric distribution for the total diet is 60 to 70 per cent from carbohydrate, 15 to 25 per cent from fats and 15 to 20 per cent from proteins. These calories are distributed as 1/5th of the total for breakfast, 2/5th for lunch and 2/5th for dinner.

Calorie distribution can be calculated by another method. Total calories for ideal weight of a normal, obese or underweight person can be calculated based on their activities. For example, for a normal sedentary man with an ideal weight of 65 kilogrammes the total calorie requirement is 65 x 30 kcals = 1950 kcals. Protein requirement for him is 1.2 gm/kg body weight; for 65 kg weight = 65 x 1.25 gm = 81.25 gm. Protein calorie contribution 81.25 x 4 kcals = 324.8 kcals. Non-protein calorie contribution 1950-324.8 = 1625 kcals. Non-protein calories have to be divided between carbohydrate and fat Calories from: carbohydrate 1625/2 = 812.5 kcals. Amount of carbohydrate in diet 812.5/4 = 203 gms Calories from fat 812.5 kcals Amount of fat 812.5/9 = 90.15 gms.

Therefore the ration in grams of carbohydrate, protein and fat in the diet is 203: 81.2: 90.15.

Once the calorie distribution from carbohydrate, protein and fats is calculated, using an exchange list items can be selected for various meals by a diabetic patient. In the exchange list amounts of food groups are given. The availability of local foods and their preparation vary a great deal in each part of our country. Practical suggestions considering locality, availability, economic status and dietary patterns are moire useful. Calorific value of common items must be made clear to them. For example, one cereal exchange of 30 gms contributes 15 gms carbohydrates, 2 gms protein and 70 calories. One thin chapathi requires 20 gms atta, and so 1 chapathi makes 1 cereal exchange. Therefore, 3 tablespoons of cooked rice, one idli, one slice of bread, one medium potato, 3 tablespoons cornflakes, 3/4 cup cooked porridge, 3 Marie biscuits and 1 tablespoon ragi are equivalent in its carbohydrate content with one cereal exchange. For a thin diabetic when 2 chapathis are recommended, for a person with normal weight or an obese diabetic one chapathi is enough.

Among diabetic people there is a wrong notion that wheat products like chapathi or brown bread, millets like bajra or jowar or rava can be eaten in any quantity without harm. They believe that only rice is restricted for them. In fact, all cereals and millets more or less provide the same amount of calories. Since wheat is better in its protein content it is recommended instead of rice to rice-eaters. For a thin or underweight diabetic one exchange of rice can be taken daily. For other groups who prefer rice, two chapathis can be substituted for three tablespoons of cooked rice. For a thin diabetic, if vegetarian, 1 cup thin dal is allowed per meal which supplies 100 kcals per cup. If egg, meat or fish or milk is used for non-vegetarians 200 kcals worth exchange can be included. Leafy vegetables can be included liberally in a diabetic diet. Dates, bananas and dried fruits like raisins are rich in calorie content. Groundnut has high fat content; 100 gms supplies 560 kcals. One cup of coffee with 1 oz milk and sugar supplies 65 kcals, whereas without sugar it has only. One cup of tea with sugar and 1 oz milk has 62 kcals whereas without sugar it has only 22 kcals. Pickles and papads are rich in energy.

Foods to be Avoided and Allowed : In a diabetic diet sugar, pastries, rich sweets, cakes, candy, dry fruits, fats and oils, fruit juices, in-between snacks, coconut, groundnut, fried items like pickles, papads and thick soups are restricted. Salads from raw tomato, cucumber, cabbage, capsicum, green chillies, radish and lemon, sprouted pulses are recommended liberally. Salad dressings are not allowed. Root vegetables are also restricted.

Regular exercises like walking rapidly, running, cycling, household work and light games are good. Exercises helps improve the function of cardiorespiratory organs.

Diabetics with Pregnancy : Complications are common among diabetics with pregnancy. Toxaemia and placental dysfunction can occur. Normal delivery is often difficult and Caesarean operations are necessary. Newborn babies may have congenital malformation and respiratory problems. Jaundice is also common among newborns. A diabetic mother must be under the care of the physician throughout pregnancy. Insulin treatment is preferred to oral drugs. Nutritional requirements are the same as that for a non-diabetic woman. Additional calorie requirements should be evenly distributed to all meals so as to avoid hypo or hyperglycaemia. The insulin intake must be adjusted. All other nutrients recommended for a non-diabetic pregnant mother are advised for the diabetic also. Weight gain of the pregnant mother must be periodically checked because unusual increase in weight during early pregnancy may be due to prematurity of the foetus and excessive weight gain in the third trimester is associated with toxaemia. High calorie items like ghee, nuts, dry fruits, sweets, dal preparations, and coconuts are restricted because they are calorigenic foods. If the dose of insulin is not regulated complications occur in pregnancy and such cases must be hospitalised. Infections during pregnancy in a diabetic mother are a serious complication and emergency treatment is essential. Since diabetes increases the hazards of pregnancy due to dangers of glycogen depletion, hypoglycacmia, acidosis and infection, regular obstetrical supervision is very essential. Early detection of any complaint prevents complications with critical conditions like proliferative retinopathy and nephropathy. Abortion may threaten a diabetic pregnant mother. A diabetic mother may not be able to secrete enough milk and so breast-feeding should not be encouraged in such cases. Often a diabetic pregnant mother is induced even if there is no complication in pregnancy by 36 to 38 weeks of gestation. Usually obstetricians admit their pregnant diabetics three months earlier, to observe the health of the mother and the child.

General Complications : As a rule, even though diabetics are not more prone to infections compared to a normal person, if they fall ill complications are more in them. Cold, pneumonia or vomiting or diarrhoea upset their carefully set balance. Any illness increases the body's need for insulin. Urine and blood tests are necessary to check their sugar level and sometimes two to three times daily checking is necessary. Organs that are mainly affected by diabetes are kidneys, blood vessels, nerves and skin. Often due to excess work the kidney is damaged. Blood pressure may rise because blood vessels, especially arteries, are affected. Arterial walls become thickened and later hardened. Angina and heart pains are more common in diabetics and lead to coronary thrombosis or heart attacks. Blood pressure must be checked periodically. In senile diabetes the circulation of blood in the legs and arms may be reduced. Foot care is very essential in old people because damaged toe nails lead to infection. If abrasions, injuries, cuts, sores or corns occur, they are difficult to heal and may lead to gangrene. Small blood vessels in the eye are damaged and retinopathy in diabetes is common. Blood circulation to nerves suffers due to thickening of small blood vessels in the brain.

Sensitivity and skin's perception capacity are affected and often the skin may become insensitive. Nerve sensation impairment, on and off pains, attacks of "pins and needles" in the legs, feet, arms or hands are common. Warm clothing helps to relieve these conditions. The skin of a diabetic is liable to infection. Sugar content in the urine often causes fungus, skin infections around the genital, especially in women. So personal hygiene is very important in the case of a diabetic.

8

Diseases of Liver

Liver is one of the most important organs of the body. Liver secretes bile and takes part in metabolic processes. It manufactures many important substances. Digested amino acids are received and new proteins are synthesised by the liver. Many metabolic processes of protein take place in the liver. It also plays an important role in carbohydrate metabolism. Liver is the chief storehouse of carbohydrate and it regulates the blood glucose level by converting excess sugar into glycogen.

Liver has a prominent role in lipid metabolism. It converts absorbed fatty acids into circulating phospholipids. It also synthesizes cholesterol and converts it into bile salts. Fats in the liver are oxidized into energy. Again, protein, carbohydrate and fats are interconverted. Bile salts are essential for fat digestion and liver detoxicates poisonous substances from the body. Conversion of beta carotene into vitamin A and storage of vitamins A and D are other functions. Plasma proteins are also synthesised by the liver. Worn out red blood cells are broken down and the liver extracts useful substances. It also stores iron and copper. The intrinsic factor or the anti-anaemic factor is produced by the liver. There is no other organ in our body which takes part in so many vital functions. Thus, a healthy liver is essential for healthy living.

Disorders of liver are jaundice or hepatitis, hepatic percoma and coma, hepatic cirrhosis and fatty liver.

Dietary deficiencies produce liver disorders like fatty liver and cirrhosis of the liver. Protein deficiency, choline deficiency, cystine deficiency, methionine deficiency and B vitamin deficiencies produce either fatty liver or necrosis of liver. Liver injury occurs due to alcoholism. Acute hepatic damage and jaundice occur in malnourished alcoholic patients. Lipid metabolism changes in the alcoholics by enhancing fatty acid synthesis and decreasing its oxidation.

Triglyceride formation is stimulated by alcohol. Cirrhosis of liver occurs among chronic alcoholics.

Jaundice : Jaundice is a symptom which denotes abnormal liver function due to diseases. In jaundice the skin and mucous membranes show a yellow pigmentation due to rise in the serum bilirubin. Jaundice occurs from haemolysis of red blood cells as in yellow fever and pernicious anaemia. Obstruction in bile-flow either through intra or extra hepatic obstruction results in jaundice. A malignant growth, stones or inflammation of the mucous ducts produce obstructive hepatitis. Hepato-cellular jaundice results from damage to the parenchymal cells due to viral infection or due to toxic origins such as poison or drugs.

Viral Hepatitis

Viral hepatitis is otherwise known as infectious hepatitis. This is the common cause of jaundice. Through food or water the virus enters the body. Anorexia, fever, headache, rapid weight loss, loss of muscle tone and abdominal discomforts are the earlier symptoms. These develop into jaundice. The symptoms may continue for 4 to 8 weeks. If proper treatment is not given it leads to permanent liver damage. Living in crowded areas and living on an inadequate diet, especially on low protein diet, and consumption of alcohol while ill, produce complications. Recovery is possible even with restricted diet, rest and supplementation of deficient nutrients, especially vitamins. Prolonged convalescence results in relapse or fatal conditions because of liver cellular collapse. Mortality due to jaundice occurs mainly among malnourished people because an already damaged liver due to malnourishment is further affected by infection. Neglected hepatitis leads to cirrhosis of liver.

Dietetic Management : Modifications in the dietary treatment depend on the liver damage. Since anorexia is an important symptom, normal feeding is difficult in the initial stage. In hospitalised cases intravenous feeding with 10 per cent glucose solution is recommended. As soon as there is appetite simple foods of high nutritional quality can be given.

The objective of dietetic treatment is to avoid further injury and strain to liver, and provide nutrients for regeneration of liver tissues. A high protein, high carbohydrate, moderate fat diet is recommended. Small feeds of attractive meals at regular intervals are better tolerated.

In nasogastric feeding stage about 1,000 kcals are supplied for a person weighing 60 kgs. In severe cases 1,600 kcals to 2,000 kcals are suggested. Once convalescence stage is reached 45 kcals/kg body weight helps to regain normalcy.

Protein requirement varies according to the severity of the disease. With severe jaundice an intake of 40 gms of protein and in mild jaundice 60 to 80 gms of proteins is permitted. If hepatic coma or percoma accompanies it, protein-containing foods are not given as the liver metabolises the end products of intestinal protein. Cereal proteins are better suggested during this condition.

An average consumption of fat along with normal protein intake is recommended. In hepatic percoma and in coma, hepatic cellular failure takes place. Liver cells are not able to metabolise fats, therefore fat is restricted in such cases. In severe jaundice 30 gms of fat is permitted and 50 to 60 gms of fat in moderate jaundice.

High carbohydrate content in the diet is essential to supply enough calories so that tissue proteins are not broken down for energy purpose. For 1,600 kcals diet 300 to 340 gms carbohydrate is recommended.

Vitamins are essential to regenerate liver cells; 500 mgs of vitamin C, 10 mgs of vitamin K and supplements of B complex are essential to meet the daily needs. If anorexia and vomiting after consumption of these supplements are present intravenous administration is essential.

Mineral deficiency occurs if normal food consumption is not possible. Normal serum level of sodium and potassium must be maintained through supplements.

Foods Included : Foods included in viral hepatitis are cereal porridges, soft chapathis, bread, rice, millet preparations, milk, preferably skimmed milk, thin soups from tender vegetables, roots like tapioca, potato, sweet potato, yam, fruits and fruit juices, sugar, jaggery, honey, biscuits, soft custards without butter or cream and light non-stimulant beverages.

Foods Avoided : Foods to be avoided in the diet of a hepatitis patient are pulses, beans, meat, fish, chicken, eggs, soups, sweet preparations where ghee, butter or oil are used, backery products, dried fruits, nuts, spices, papads, chutney, pickles, alcoholic beverages, fried preparations, cooking fats, whole milk, cream, sardines, salmon, fried fish or fish rich in fat. Liberal intake of water is allowed.

The patient needs bedrest but slight movement in the room improves appetite. In moderate jaundice pulses or beans, meat, fish or chicken and eggs are allowed. Though fried foods are restricted cooking fat is permitted. Dried fruits, sweets without much ghee are included. Fruit juices, water and other beverages except alcoholic beverages are allowed.

Hepatitis in infancy and childhood is not complicated if the therapeutic dietary pattern is observed strictly. But hepatitis in pregnancy, especially in the second and third trimester, is harmful to the mother and child.

Hepatic Percoma and Coma

Complications of viral or acute alcoholic hepatitis, accidental damage to the hepatic artery, anaesthetic agents and certain drugs, encephalopathy or surgery of the liver produce hepatic coma and percoma.

Common symptoms of these disorders are confusion, disordered consciousness, tremor of the outstretched hands, psychosis, apathy, and personality changes. Gradually these symptoms lead to death.

The exact cause is that the liver is incapable of detoxicating ammonia from bacterial decomposition of protein foods. In a healthy person's body, the liver converts ammonia into urea and excretes it through kidneys. In liver disorders or in hepatic surgery nitrogenous materials, especially ammonia, get into systemic circulation and reach the central nervous system. The blood ammonium ion level is increased in coma. Along with ammonia, indoles and phenols are also not detoxicated from the body by a damaged liver. There are many toxic products of metabolism in minute quantities which are detoxicated by a healthy liver. All these are accumulated in the body in the coma stage. Again urine is not eliminated properly which affects the concentration of waste products in the urine and in blood. Electrolytic balance is also upset.

Dietetic Management : For a coma patient 1,000 kcals are recommended. A low protein diet is prescribed for a coma patient. The endogenous breakdown of protein can be minimised by a high carbohydrate diet. An improvement in coma suggests 30 to 40 gms protein per day. In acute coma protein in the diet is withheld. As fats are not metabolised they are not given for a coma patient. Carbohydrate rich foods are included liberally as they prevent endogenous breakdown of protein. Glucose is recommended as it is easy to assimilate.

Vitamins and mineral supplementation is essential. Fruit juices, vegetable soups without seasoning, honey and barley water are fed to a coma patient. In most of the cases nasogastric feeding is carried out. The feed consists of :

Orange juice	-	1,000 ml
Glucose	-	200 gms
Water	-	1,000 ml
		2,200 ml

Cirrhosis of Liver

Cirrhosis is a common disease of liver which usually affects alcoholics. Previous occurrence of hepatitis also causes cirrhosis of liver. Undernutrition causes necrosis of liver cells and fatty liver. Fatty liver produces cirrhosis of liver. Toxins of foods like aflatoxins and "bush tea" cause cirrhosis.

In cirrhosis of liver parenchyma is destroyed and it is replaced by fibrous tissues. Gradually all active parenchymal tissues are destroyed and liver function is seriously affected. Morphological changes occur and the liver is contracted and irregularly distorted. In advanced cirrhosis complications arise and one of the common complications is retention of water in the tissues due to hypoalbuminemia. Synthesis of albumin by liver is reduced in cirrhosis which leads to reduced osmotic pressure of the plasma. Due to high portal pressure, fluid is accumulated in the abdominal cavity and ascites occurs.

There are three types of cirrhosis: (1) Diffuse hepatic fibrosis which is also known as alcoholic cirrhosis or portal or Laennec's cirrhosis, (2) Post-necrotic scarring in liver, and (3) Biliary cirrhosis which occurs due to obstruction, infections or toxin. Wasting of tissues, low serum albumin, oedema, ascites and retention of sodium are some of the symptoms. Portal hypertension and lymphatic obstruction cause oedema. In infantile biliary cirrhosis diminished appetite, flatulence, liver enlargement and jaundice occur first. In later stages oedema and ascites occur.

Symptoms : Gastrointestinal disturbances such as anorexia, nausea, vomiting, pain and distension of abdomen are common.

Dietary Regimen : A high calorie, high protein, high

carbohydrate, low fat diet, with vitamins and mineral supplementation is recommended for cirrhosis patients. Calorie content of the diet for a cirrhosis patient is 2,000 to 2,500 kcals. Consumption of food is difficult because of anorexia and ascites. But the patient requires highly nutritious foods because of prolonged undernourishment.

The protein content of the diet varies according to symptoms. If hepatic coma accompanies, protein is restricted. Otherwise a high protein diet of about 2 gms of protein per kilogram of body weight is advisable. Fat is restricted in cirrhosis of liver but 0.5 gm to 1 gm per kilogram of body weight is harmless if enough protein is included in the diet.

Carbohydrate should provide more than 60 per cent of the total carlories so that liver damage is minimised.

Sodium is restricted in oedema and ascites. If there are no ascites very little salt is permitted. Potassium salt is administered for ascites and oedema to prevent hypokalemia. Anaemia is common among cirrhosis patients. So iron supplementation is essential. Vitamin supplementation, especially of B vitamins, is required, to prevent anaemia. Choline and methionine are useful if fatty infiltration is present.

Foods included in a cirrhosis diet are cereals in any soft form, pulses, beans, meat, fish and chicken, soft cooked eggs, vegetables, cooked or pureed sweets, fruits, fruit juices and light beverages. Cooking salt is not added. Papads, chutneys or pickles are excluded in the diet of a cirrhosis patient A smooth or liquid diet is suggested if there is difficulty in swallowing food. Fried items, rich desserts, strongly flavoured vegetables, nuts, milk, salads and seasoned gravies are avoided in a cirrhosis diet.

9

Peptic Ulcer

Peptic ulcer may be defined as an open lesion upon the mucous lining of the stomach or duodenum. Discomfort and burning or gnawing sensation in the abdomen is the first sign of peptic ulcer. When the gastric juice comes in direct contact with the mucous membrane disintegration and necrosis of the tissue occur. Ulcers may occur in the stomach or in the duodenum. In India peptic ulcers are prevalent more in South India Low-protein diet with high spices can be the special reason for their occurrence. Gastric ulcers turn malignant, whereas duodenal ulcers do not become malignant

Aetiology

The exact cause of peptic ulcers remains unknown. Due to unknown reasons the mucosa of the stomach and duodenum become unable to resist the action of digestive juices and part of the tissue is digested and an ulcer develops. Irritation of the mucosa due to alcoholism or dietary irritation from various foods, fasting, mental stress or emotional upset causes peptic ulcers.

Heredity seems to have some influence on the occurrence of

peptic ulcers. Blood group 'O' subjects are more liable to have peptic ulcer. Climatic conditions exert influence on the recurrence of peptic ulcer. Monsoon season records highest admission of peptic ulcer cases.

Normally gastric secretions are more if meet with soups or extractives, condiments like chillies, pepper, ginger or strong tea or coffee or alcohol is ingested. Protein-rich foods as a whole induce secretions of gastric gland. Smoking appears to have an adverse effect. Ulcerogenic drugs such as aspirin and the various salicylates, conticosteroids, phenylbutazone, oxyphenbutaxone and resperine should be avoided. Mental stress in any form increases acidity. Irregular dietary hours and irritating foods aggregate the situation.

Dietetic Management

In no other disease does dictic treatment take such an important role as in peptic ulcers. A soothing diet gives symptomatic relief and an irritating diet produces sensitivity. Dietary habits must be set with a schedule. Persons engaged in certain occupations like busy executives, businessmen and professionals such as doctors are more prone to peptic ulcers and they have to set a time schedule for meals. Rushing before and after a meal should be avoided. Heavy meals should be avoided as distended abdomen causes pain in gastric ulcers and empty stomach causes pain in duodenal ulcer.

The objectives of the diet are to restore and maintain good nutrition to decrease secretion of gastric juices, to neutralise stomach acidity, to decrease gastric motility and to avoid irritation through mechanical movements on the lesion.

To fulfil the above objectives a strict dietetic regimen was set by physicians. The most popular regimen used for peptic ulcers was the Sippy diet. Though it was acclaimed in olden days now it is not practised as it poses problems of deficiency diseases. At present after the initial problems are removed a less restricted or regular diet is recommended.

Sippy's Diet : Every hourly feed consists of milk and cream in equal amounts. Between these feedings neutralising alkaline powders are given. The objective of this diet is to give maximum rest to the stomach. But Sippy's diet is not adequate for longer treatment

Sippy's diet consists of different stages. In the first stage between 7 a.m. and 10 p.m. hourly feeds of milk and cream or olive oil with an antacid are given. In the second stage a milk-based diet with gradual introduction of solid foods is prescribed. In three weeks time the patient is exposed to a bland diet.

After the first stage of Sippy's diet lightly cooked egg, bread and well cooked cereals are recommended. In the third stage the quantity of cereal is increased and strained vegetable soups, purees, vegetables, jam, jelly, strained fruit juices are included. Three regular meals of cereals, steamed fish, minced mutton, chicken along with more milk are recommended in the next stage. A bland diet is suggested after this gradual modification. A bland diet is one which is mechanically, chemically and thermally non-irritating. Smooth consistency, bland taste and moderate temperature are the characteristics of a bland diet.

Foods Allowed : Foods allowed in a bland diet of a peptic ulcer patient are milk and milk products, weak tea, strained bland soup, white bread, soft chapathi of wheat, rice, ragi or maize, other soft breakfast cereal items and pre-cooked infant cereals. Fine cooked cereals, noodles, macaroni, potato, sweet potato or mashed yam, eggs in all forms except fried, baked or ground minced meat or fish, soft cooked mashed vegetables; carrots, peas, beets, strained tomatoes and all other vegetables except coarse fibre or overripe fruits without seeds are allowed. Mashed banana, cooked fruits, desserts, steamed or baked puddings are included.

Foods Avoided : Irritating and solid or hard foods must be avoided. It is better to avoid strong smelling vegetables and meat preparations. Carbonated beverages, cereals and cereal products with bran, fried foods, raw foods, and spiced items are not permitted. Sweets, sweet meats, papad, chutney, dried fruits, vegetable salads, are also avoided.

Strict dietetic regimen is essential to bring satisfactory improvement. The patient must be educated to live with the ulcers. The patient must accept the ulcer rather than resent it. A worrying patient with great mental stress must be admitted in a hospital.

A high calorie, high protein, highly vitaminised soft bland diet is recommended for peptic ulcers. One should suitably modify the work schedule so that there is not much stress or pressure on time. Surgical treatment may become necessary in severe cases. Even after surgery diet control is essential to avoid possible relapse of the condition.

Ulcerative Colitis

Ulcerative colitis is an intestinal disorder which is characterised by inflammation and ulceration of the colon or other parts of the intestine. In severe cases inflammation or ulceration leads to the appearance of blood and mucus in the stools. Intestinal allergy, especially cow's milk allergy, infections and psychogenic factors or nutritional deficiencies of multiple nature cause ulcerative colitis. No specific organism has been isolated for its occurrence.

The onset resembles an attack of dysentery but no organisms can be isolated. In the initial stage constipation, abnormal secretion of mucus or diarrhoea occur. In chronic ulcerative colitis, loss of appetite, nausea, fever, abdominal distention, flatulence, alternating diarrhoea or constipation and bleeding occur.

Dietary Modifications : An adequate diet with high protein and enough fat is recommended. Supplementation of vitamins and minerals, especially iron, is essential. Since significant nitrogen loss through urine makes the serum albumin level low, a high protein intake of 100 to 150 gms/day is required. Sodium and potassium loss is very high and supplementation is essential with a liberal intake of fluid. A bland high protein diet is essential to meet the requirements. If there is milk allergy soyabean milk can be given.

Cereal bran, raw vegetables, dried fruits, nuts, condiments and spices are avoided. If fat is not tolerated, only emulsified fats from egg yolk and butter are included. Small feeds are comfortable for the patient.

Psychological approach to the patient is essential and fatigue or emotional strain must be avoided.

Stomach Diseases

Gastro-intestinal Problems

The relation between nutrition and diseases of the stomach is complex. Modern medicine emphasises the fact that stomach is the seat of all diseases. Diseases of the upper gastro-intestinal cases interfere with the intake of food by reducing appetite, inducing nausea and vomiting, evoking pain or by producing obstruction. The intestinal tract, especially the small intestine, the site of digestion and absorption of nutrients, play an important role in maintaining the general health. Diseases of the intestinal tract impair the functions of intestinal tract and result in poor utilisation of ingested food.

Common disorders of stomach and intestine are:

Gastric indigestion or flatulence or dyspepsia,
Peptic ulcer,
Ulcerative colitis,
Diverticulosis or diverticulitis,
Constipation,
Diarrhoea,
Dysentery,

Malabsorptive syndromes,
Tropical sprue, and
mellitus, phenylketonuria,
Metabolic disorders—diabetes
galactosemia, Wison's disease.

Dyspepsia

Dyspepsia or flatulence is a common abdominal disorder. It is defined as deranged digestion when the functions of stomach are affected. Symptoms of this disorder are bitter taste in the mouth, heartburn, nausea, loss of appetite, distention, betching, anorexia, acrid eructations, epigastric distress or pain, discomfort or pain in the stomach, vomiting and cardiospasm.

The causes of dyspepsia are many. The presence of air or gas in the stomach or intestine interferes with the motility of the intestine. It occurs either during or after the ingestion of food. This disease can occur due to organic diseases of gastro-intestinal tract, cardiovascular or kidney disease or malignant diseases. Functional reasons of stomach also produce flatulence. In the absence of organic reasons rapid eating, inadequate chewing, swallowing air through food, ingestion of undercooked foods or fried foods, gas forming vegetables like onion, cabbage, beans, radish, cauliflower, pulses, starchy foods, protein-rich animal foods, absence of bulk in the diet can produce the presence of air in the stomach or intestine. A considerable amount of air is taken if we suck or chew food, and while smoking and chewing betel leaves. If fermentation of the food in the intestine takes place it produces gas. Enzyme deficiency like disaccharidase deficiency results m poor absorption of sugar and thereby in gas formation. Too many spices and condiments, high residue and infestation with worms and parasite also produce gas. Finally, the emotional state influences the stomach activity. Aggressive emotions like anger, rebelliousness and excitement increase the motor activity of the stomach while depressive states like worry, fear and depression delay contraction and emptying of the stomach. There is a saying that the abdomen is the sounding board of emotions.

Dietary Modifications : Dietary regulations bring marked difference in the occurrence of flatulence. But individual variations are here for its occurrence and so the cause has to be located. Treatment must be directed to the patient as a whole and not to the disease. Dietetic treatment aims to supply all nutrients. The person must be instructed to avoid excessive amounts of food, saturated fats, highly spiced and seasoned foods. Good eating habits must be developed. The food must be consumed in a relaxed manner. The patient must be advised to chew the food properly. Air swallowing should be avoided. Foul smelling, undercooked or overcooked foods, putrefied foods and fibrous vegetables must be avoided. Though condiments and spices are restricted, garlic is good for flatulence and it inhibits the growth of bacteria in the colon. Fluid intake must be increased but sucking through a straw or bottle increases air sucking.

Pulses and beans, raw vegetable salads, roots, sweets, dried fruits, bakery items except biscuits, nuts, condiments and spices, papad, chutney or pickles are better avoided or restricted. Dinner must be taken at least an hour before sleep. Meals should be taken in a pleasant and relaxed atmosphere. All forms of excitement are harmful to normal digestion. Nervous dispepsia must be treated psychologically.

Diarrhoea and Dysentery

Diarrhoea is a condition where loose or watery stools are passed frequently. In dysentery unformed stools are accompanied by the passage of blood and mucus. Diarrhoea can be functional or organic. Neuromuscular overactivity creates diarrhoea. Consumption of irritating foods, fermented foods, unhygienically handled food, stale food, besides allergy, achlorohydria, nervousness, uraemia, and endocrine imbalances are the main causes of functional diarrhoea. Nutritional deficiency like kwashiorkor or pellagra or vitamin deficiency produce diarrhoea.

Diarrhoea can be acute or chronic in nature. Acute diarrhoea occurs mainly due to contaminated food consumption.

After an acute attack of dysentery or diarrhoea it may be

repeated often. This can lead to chronic diarrhoea. Infestation with giardial-amblia is a common cause of chronic diarrhoea.

Nervous diarrhoea occurs to some people when faced with fear of an examination or an interview.

Diseases of small intestine, lack of hydrochloric acid in the stomach, malabsorption syndromes, malnutrition, vitamin A deficiency, niacin deficiency and protein deficiency cause diarrhoea. Tuberculosis also produces chronic diarrhoea.

Dietetic Management : A very low residue diet is recommended. Residue is the bulk remaining in the intestine after food is assimilated. Milk is a high residue diet. In acute diarrhoea the alimentary canal must get complete rest. If vomiting is present no food is allowed. Saline with 5 per cent glucose can be given. Electrolytes like sodium and potassium with high fluid are recommended. Apple, tender coconut water and fruit juices, rice gruei and thin porridges without milk are prescribed. Arrowroot and sago are excellent for diarrhoea. Strained fruit juices or soups are allowed. Jaggery and honey are also good. Leafy vegetables and green vegetables may be avoided. Overripe or fibrous vegetables are excluded. Biscuits, soft desserts without milk or with, if tolerating, skimmed milk and soft cooked eggs are permitted. Fried items, fat, pulses, beans, vegetable salads, seedy fruits, sweets, dried fruits, nuts, condiments and spices are best avoided. Only double cooked mashed vegetables are allowed. Once normal food is tolerated poached egg, cereal, porridge, fruit juice, baked non-vegetarian items, mashed potatoes or soups, biscuits and arrowroot drinks can be given in the menu. Since the food intake is low at first minerals like iron, calcium and all vitamins have to be supplemented. In acute stage 1,500 kcals and in chronic diarrhoea or dysentery 2,500 kcals are added. Liberal intake of proteins from permissible foods is essential. A fluid diet is modified into a soft bland diet as the condition of the bowel improves.

Malabsorption Syndrome

In malabsorption syndrome, adequate digestion or intestinal absorption of a number of substances like fats, proteins, carbohydrates, vitamins, minerals and water are disordered. Nutritional deficiencies develop in such a condition and normal life processes are affected. Chronic under-nutrition brings ill-health, anaemia, steatorrhoea, tropical sprue and celiac diseases. Fibrosis of the pancreas, chronic pancreatitis, carcinoma in the pancreas and stones in the duct of wirsung are other diseases due to malabsorpuon.

In all these diseases normal digestion and absorption of carbohydrate, proteins and fats are reduced. Enzymatic actions are very poor because some of them are absent in certain diseases. Stools are dry, bulky, pale and greasy and often frothy.

Tropical Sprue : The exact cause of sprue is not known. Supplementation of nutrients like folacin or B12 shows improvement in this disease. In sprue, normal absorption of glucose, fats and fat soluble vitamins is impaired. Symptoms of sprue are anorexia or vomiting, sore tongue, diarrhoea, abdominal distention, macrocytic anaemia, low prothrombin production, rapid weight loss and muscle wasting, excessive calcium loss, weakness and hyperpigmentation. It is also assumed that an infection factor may be the reason.

Dietary Modifications : Non-tropical sprue patients showed improvement in a glutengliadin restricted diet. A high carbohydrate, high protein, low fat, low residue, low fibre, bland diet is recommended. In a high carbohydrate diet glucose and sucrose sources produce discomfort. Fructose sources are better tolerated. Honey and fruits are the best sources of fructose. Mineral and vitamin supplementation is essential.

Foods included in a sprue diet are weak tea or coffee, non-fat milk like skimmed milk, double cooked soft porridge, infant foods, milled cereals, and their products, tender vegetables, ripe fleshy fruits like banana, papaya, mango, apple, baked or canned fruits without seeds and skin, fruit juices, strained vegetable soups without seasoning, mashed pumpkin, carrots, peas, beetroot, strained beans, custards and puddings with non-fat milk, white bread, sponge cake, honey, jelly, eggs and biscuits.

Foods avoided are cereals, bread with bran, fruits with skin, seeds, fats, fried and crisp items, puddings with whole milk or other milk items, confectioneries with cream or ghee, sugar and sweet items, preparations where spices are used, stimulants like alcohol, flavoured drinks, vegetables with fibres, skins, seeds, sprouts, strong flavoured vegetables like cauliflower, cabbage, cucumber, onion, dried peas, lentils, beans, leafy vegetables and hard sweets and raw vegetables.

Miopathic Steatorrhoea : Steatorrhoea is characterised by loose motions containing large amounts of fat. The mucosa of the intestine is inflamed and the normal absorption of all nutrients is lowered. The cause of this condition is not identified clearly. Children with celiac diseases due to sensitivity of the intestine, especially gluten sensitivity, are prone to steatorrhoea in adult life. Family history also plays a role in its occurrence.

Treatment aims at removing irritation from dietary pattern. The faecal fatty acids are from fermented carbohydrates and unabsorbed dietary fat. Putrified foods, fried foods, and animal fats are restricted. Foods rich in fibres like whole cereals, millets and matured vegetables and spices are excluded in this diet. Diet prescribed for tropical sprue is given in this condition also.

Constipation

Constipation is characterised by infrequent and incomplete evacuation of the bowels. Hard, dried stools are difficult to pass. Autonomous nervous system normally controls the bowel movement. The type of food—high fibre or low fibre—also influences evacuation. For example, a vegetarian diet with increased roughage produces bulkier stools. Though most people have a bowel movement daily some people feel normal even with a bowel evacuation on every second or third day. Physical activity and ingestion of food provoke bowel evacuation. Fasting and inactivity produce constipation. Lack of exercise, poor personal hygiene in maintaining regular habits of evacuation, limited intake of fluids, consumption of concentrated foods, deficiency of fats and thiamine produce poor muscle tone and evacuation. Nervous disturbances like tension, anxiety, excitement of various forms and worry affect the normal muscular contraction and evacuation. Excessive use of laxatives and regular enemas deprive the muscles of the intestinal wall to have normal movements and develop constipation. Regular toilet habit must be inculcated from infancy.

Neglected constipation leads to piles and prolapse of the rectum. And it is dangerous for a heart patient to strain during defecation.

There are three types of constipation—atonic constipation, spastic constipation and obstructive constipation.

Atonic constipation is more common among people. The main reasons for atonic constipation are lack of fluids in the body, especially after perspiration for stool formation, lack of roughage which contributes to the lack of cellulose stool formation, deficiency of vitamin B1 which produces poor muscle tone, lack of potassium which reduces muscle tone, irregular evacuation habits and use of purgation agents. Due to any of the above causes muscular tone of the intestine is affected and peristaltic action is reduced. Bacterial action on stagnated food is more and symptoms of constipation develop.

Spastic constipation, on the contrary, occurs due to excessive muscle tone of the colonic muscles. The movement of the food is very irregular and often causes pain in the lower abdomen. Irritating foods, excessive use of purgatives or mental stress produce this type of constipation. Spastic constipation occurs as a complication of some other disease. Excessive use of alcohol, tea or coffee also produce this.

Obstructive constipation is due to malignancy or stricture of the colon.

Use of castor oil or other purgatives in infancy is a common practice in our country. It contributes to constipation in later life.

Modification of the Diet : The objective of dietary treatment is to encourage bowel movement and improve bowel evacuation. A well balanced diet with high B group vitamins and liberal fluid intake is recommended. Fibre or cellulose content of the diet must be high. Bland cooking is preferred. In spastic constipation high roughage is harmful. A normal diet with light mental altitude and proper exercise or physical activity is recommended for a constipation patient. Potassium-rich vegetables must be included in the diet.

A high fibre diet is characterised with coarse cereals, wholegrain with bran, pulses, fresh fruits, salad, vegetables, fibrous vegetables like ashgourd, snakegourd, pumpkin, leafy vegetables, roots and tubers, dried fruits and fluids. Highly refined and concentrated items like maida, fried foods, excessive sweetened pickles and papads and chutneys are not permitted. A regular time for meals is very important. Relaxed living enables proper bowel movement in the body. Exercises also enable proper bowel evacuation.

For spastic constipation, a soft bland diet is recommended. Small meals prevent stagnation of food mass in the intestine. Vitamin B supplements are essential. Daily 8 to 10 glasses of water must be ingested to help stool formation.

Constipation among Children : Continuous usage of castor oil or purgatives by infants and children to clean the bowels affects the muscle tone of the intestine. This leads to constipation. Instead of purgatives lots of water, fruit juices and fruits like banana, apple or guava or other fibrous fruits are better measures.

Sample Menu for a Constipated Patient

Time	*Meal*	*Menu*
6 a.m.		1 glass warm water. After some time coffee
8 a.m.		Breakfast Chapathi from whole wheat flour, Vegetable curry with peas, Banana
10 a.m.	Mid-time	Fruit juice

Contd...

Time	*Meal*	*Menu*
12.30 p.m.	Lunch	Whole wheat chapathi or millet roti, Dal Curry with spinach or fish curry, Vegetable salad, Beans pugath, Buttermilk, Fruit salad
2 p.m.	Mid-time	Vegetable soup
4 p.m.	Tea	Tea, Boiled groundnut
6 p.m.	Mid-time	Sweetened lime juice
8 p.m.	Dinner	Wheat dosa, Sprouted green gram curry, Vegetable salad
	Bed time	Milk beverage

At least 10 glasses of water must be taken.

Nutrition in Allergies

Allergy may be defined as the reaction of tissues to specific substances. The allergen is an external substance capable of producing specific antibodies in the body of the allergic person. Clinical manifestations of allergy are bronchial asthma, hay fever, hives, oedema, gastrointestinal symptoms, headaches, dermatitis and itching.

If ingestion of specific foods produce allergy it is termed as food allergy. Nausea, vomiting, urticaria, diarrhoea, colic or spastic constipation, headache, itching, oedema, dermatitis, circulatory collapse, asthma, shock or even death occur due to allergy. Food allergy is common among infants and young children. Most allergies are protein in nature. Protein foods like egg, milk, gluten of wheat, soyabeans and certain other protein foods commonly produce allergy. Denaturation of proteins often results in loss of their allergenic capacity. Raw or pasteurised milk may produce allergy but thoroughly boiled or evaporated milk may not produce allergy.

Diagnosis of the allergic food is difficult. Case history of all foods consumed must be tested using a food diary. Scratch or patch tests are also used to detect allergy.

Dietary treatment is mainly aimed to eliminate the foods which produce allergy. Trial diets including foods known to be allergenic are given to the patient. Exclusion of the allergic food from the dietary is the only effective means to prevent allergy. If infants are born with milk allergy, substitutes must be made through goat's milk or evaporated milk. Soyabean milk is used as a substitute since soyabean is very nutritious.

A normal well balanced diet excluding the allergic item can e given.

Problem of Obesity

Obesity or over-nutrition is a menace to health and it is a public health problem of the well-to-do people. Obesity is a condition in which there is excessive weight gain in the body. An increase of 10 per cent over the ideal weight or optimal weight is termed obesity. Excessive weight gain is mainly due to high intake of food. When more energy is taken through food and less is utilised through activities the excess energy is converted into fat which is deposited as adipose tissue.

Excessive weight is a predisposing factor for cardiovascular disease, osteoarthritis, diabetes, gout, liver and gall bladder disease and hernia. Surgery is always a risk with obese people. There is an old saying. "The longer the belt, the shorter the life". Modern medicine emphasises this statement. In obese persons physical activity is limited and fatigue, backache and foot aches are common after little exertion. Apart from physical handicaps it produces psychological setbacks. An obese person is very self-conscious and always lags behind in a group as the physical reflexes are slow. Their social involvements are poor because of overweight and its hazards.

The Causes

Obesity is mainly caused by excessive calorie consumption. If energy is not utilised for activities it accumulates as adipose tissues. If adipose tissues are formed even in early childhood they tend to produce obesity in later life. The number of fat cells will grow in size as the child grows and becomes obese. Thus overnutrition in childhood has an influence over obesity in later life. Now a chubby child is not considered as a healthy child for this reason.

More fatty cells in the body need not always be due to high calorie consumption. Endocrine imbalance, and genetic factors often cause this peculiar phenomena in the body.

Excessive intake of calories can often be due to physiological or psychological causes. Through physical examination, dietary history, living habits and family and social set-up have to be investigated before dietetic planning. In the hypothalamus in the brain there are two parts in nuclei, median and laternal, which regulate appetite in a person. Lesion in median nuclei increases the appetite while a lesion in the lateral nuclei reduces the appetite. Another cortical centre of the brain controls hypothalamus.

Endocrine glands like thyroid, pituitary and in females hormones influence the appetite and weight gain. Obesity is common among women after pregnancy and it can be due to causes other than those connected with nutrition. But obesity resulting from disturbances of glands are less than 5 per cent and the remaining are due to too much eating. Labour-saving devices at home and in industry and modern comfortable living contribute to the high occurrence of obesity. Those who engage in strenuous physical activity are less likely to become obese. Since obesity is common among people after the age of 35, it is related with food consumption and pattern of work. When physical activities are reduced food consumption must be reduced. But the consumption pattern remains unchanged while activities are reduced which results in obesity. The role of heredity in obesity is not well understood. Dietetic habits of the family rather than hereditary factors are always responsible for obesity. Food habits are more or less the same from one generation to another and children imitate their parents' dietary pattern. Eating too much or eating fattening foods are thus handed over as food habits from generation to generation.

In middle age especially, women feel lonely and unwanted and they find solace in eating. A person who is bored, unloved or discontented with worry or sorrow indulges in overeating to escape from his problems. Like any other addiction overeating is also an addiction and treatment for this requires psychological approach. Such people derive physical pleasure by eating and thus an outlet of their emotional disturbances. A poorly adjusted person feels rejected and thus derives oral gratification through eating and this type of obesity is called psychological obesity. Psychological obesity is of two types: developmental and reactive. Developmental obesity develops from childhood onwards and it depends on food intake, both qualitative and quantitative and the pattern of living. Reactive obesity initiates with some upsetting experiences like homesickness, illness, separation or death of a dear person, and other maladjustment problems in life.

The Treatment

Losing weight requires careful planning in diet. Reduced food intake and regular depletion of energy from the body for activities are the practical methods of reducing weight. Before reducing the weight one must know the ideal weight for various heights. For an adult, adjustment in the diet can be done based on body weight.

Standard Weight for Males and Females

Height in cms.	*Weight in kg. (males)*	*Over-weight limit*	*Under-weight limit*	*Weight in kg. (females)*	*Over-weight*	*Under-weight*
148	47.5	57.0	38.0	46.4	56.0	37.0
152	49.0	59.0	39.0	48.5	58.0	39.0
156	51.5	62.0	41.0	50.5	60.5	40.5

Contd...

Height in cms.	Weight in kg. (males)	Over-weight limit	Under-weight limit	Weight in kg. (females)	Over-weight	Under-weight
160	53.5	64.0	43.0	52.5	63.0	42.0
164	56.0	67.0	45.0	55.0	66.0	44.0
168	59.5	69.5	49.5	58.0	69.0	46.5
172	62.0	74.5	52.4	60.5	72.5	48.5
176	65.5	78.5	55.5	64.0	77.0	51.0
180	68.5	82.0	57.5	67.0	80.5	53.5

As the person grows old, a slight change in ideal weight is normal and that is why a limit is given for overweight. Gaining weight until late middle age is not physiologically necessary.

The treatment of obesity is a long range process and the patient's cooperation and efforts in dietetic discipline are the key factors in its success. It must be made clear to an obese person that obesity is less often due to what one inherits but due to what one ingests. Overeating becomes a habit and there is no mechanism other than strict control over diet which can reduce weight. All other efforts have little effect in reducing weight. Omission of one meal or the main meal has no advantage in weight reduction because it increases the appetite for the next meal. Usually obese people vehemently protest that they are not eating enough food, leave alone more food. The main meal may not be large in quantity but in between tit-bits or snacks or left-overs amount to a number of calories. To reduce weight one must be strict in- the matter of food intake and energy output through work. Increase the physical activity through brisk walking, gardening, household chores like mopping, washing and ironing and cycling or swimming. Self-control in dieting and patience to do work for a prolonged period only can show results. Bringing about changes in dietary habits aim at depleting body fat for energy purpose. One gram of body fat represents 9 calories. After comparing an obese person's weight with ideal weight a reducing diet has to be formulated. A determination to stick to a low calorie diet is an important factor in reducing weight. If 1,000 calories are reduced daily the weight reduction per week is about 770 gms, provided the person is active. Even this pattern will bring about reduction of only 3.1 kgs per month. One weeks's strict low-calorie diet pattern must be formulated in the presence of the patient and a strict follower of this regime can bring about weight reduction. Small helpings of calorific food in between definitely upsets the weight reduction pattern.

Keeping a weight chart and weekly recordings are very effective. Initial weight loss need not be from fat depletion. It can be from loss of salt and water. Motivation of the patient is essential to bear the initial problems.

Exercise in moderate form helps in losing weight. If cardiovascular diseases are affliciting an obese patient, exercises must be mild. As a rule obese persons cannot engage in hard exercise as they are less active. Massage or steam bath are not reliable or a permanent solution for obesity. Weight-reducing drugs or tablets can be harmful and only under medical supervision should a person consume them. Though formula diets with hydrophylic substances are effective a person cannot depend on them for ever. Fasting is not a healthy method for reducing weight because it affects the electrolyte balance, liver, hair and structure and functions of cardiac muscles. Nervous tissues are also affected which result in memory loss. Deviation of any form from a mixed diet is not advocated. Only restriction of certain nutrients is tolerated by the body. Even high reducing diets or rapid reduction in weight can produce hernia, gall-bladder diseases and peptic ulcer. Severe hunger or nervous exhaustion is not good for the body.

Dietetic Management : A reduction in diet aims at maintaining and restoring good nutrition along with gradual reduction in body weight. Low calorie foods must be included in the dietary pattern. An obese patient must be given information about low calorie items in the diet. A wide choice from daily food items provides confidence in following the dietetic instructions. About 20 kcals per kilogramme of ideal body weight is recommended for a sedentary worker and 25 kcals for a moderately active person. An obese person has to reduce the calories to an average of half of their requirements. Depending upon their body weight 800 kcals, 1,000 kcals, 1,100 kcals and 1,200 kcals diets are prescribed. Cereals and cereal products which make the main items of our meals have to be reduced considerably. Sweets, súgar, chocolates, jaggery, jam, honey, syrup, fruit preserves, cakes, pastries, puddings, fried items, roots like potato, tapioca, yam, banana, apple, whole milk, dried fruits, papad, chutney, pickles, nuts, alcoholic drinks and soft drinks, creams, coconuts and fatty foods and oils are avoided in the regime of low-calorie diet. Foods to be included are unsweetened lime juice, clear soups without seasoning, strained vegetable soups, all green leafy vegetables, carrots, onions, brinjals, drumsticks, tomatoes, bittergourd, pumpkins, cauliflower, ladiesfinger, ashgourd, cucumber, french beans, green mango, plantain flowers, snakegourd and prescribed amounts of cereals and pulses. An accustomed dietary pattern with less carbohydrate and fat but balanced in all other nutrients only makes it workable because reducing diet is used for a prolonged period. Judicious selection is essential. The patient must be educated on the calorific value of foods. For example, the breakfast items used in an Indian diet and their calorific value can be compared.

Food items	*Calorie supplied*
One thin chapathi	80 kcals
One slice of bread	60 kcals
One thin dosa	130 kcals
One idli	100 kcals
One bun	280 kcals
Two parathas (thin)	275 kcals
Two puris	245 kcals

Contd...

Food items	Calorie supplied
Three tablespoon rice, cooked (60 gm)	70 kcals
Three tbs-uppuma (100 gm)	230 kcals
Rava puttu (100gm)	230 kcals
One cup coffee with sugar	65 kcals
One cup coffee without sugar	25 kcals
One cup milk	100 kcals
1/2 cup sambar	105 kcals
1/3 cup dal (for chapathi)	92 kcals
One banana	153 kcals

From this any breakfast item can be selected but the calorific value must be adjusted. For lunch, tea and dinner, various familiar items in small quantities are practicable. Salads or steamed leafy vegetables can be liberally included so as to give bulk and fullness to the meal. Non-vegetarian items are rich in fat and so they must be included in small quantities in a reducing diet. Preparation of non-vegetarian dishes again contributes more calories compared to other food groups. Defatted skimmed milk can be included to provide protein and other nutrients.

One gram of protein per ideal weight is essential to meet the protein requirements. Fat is restricted but vegetable oils other than coconut and palm supply essential fatty acids and little cooking fat is permissible.

One important aspect in prescribing low-calorie diet for an obese person is that the diet must provide satiety value or a sense of satisfaction and well-being to the patient. Reducing diet pattern should not be thrust upon him. He must wholeheartedly follow the regime. In a 1,000 kcals diet mineral and vitamin supplementation is necessary.

Sample Menu for an Obese Person (1,200 kcals-vegetarian)

Time	*Meal*	*Menu*		
6 a.m.	Bed coffee	Coffee (without sugar)		
8 a.m.	Breakfast	Dry Chapathi, Spinach Curry (50 gm), Coffee (without sugar)		
10 a.m.	Mid-time	Buttermilk		
12.30 p.m.	Lunch	Rice or chapathi (50 gms rice or flour), Beans pugath, Dal curry, Tomato-beetroot salad, Butter-milk		
4 p.m.	Tea	Coffee (without sugar), Baked vegetable cutlet, Papaya		
8 p.m.	Dinner	String hoppers or phulkas (50 gm), Cucumber salad, Fruit cup		
The above diet supplies		kcals	-	1,186 kcals
		proteins	-	48 gms
		fat	-	27 gms

12

Diet Therapy

Therapeutic Modifications

"The best doctors in the world are Doctor Diet, Doctor Quiet and Doctor Merryman," said Jonathan Swift. Though it is an old saying it is very apt in the case of certain diseases. For, in certain diseases, dietary modification is more important than medical treatment. In some other diseases, diet therapy goes hand-in-hand with medical care. In deficiency diseases dietary modification alone is enough. Quantitative and qualitative modifications are done for various diseases. Elimination or addition of certain nutrients, or alteration in the normal pattern of diet and cooking methods are also employed in some conditions.

The main objectives of diet therapy are to maintain good nutritional status of a sick person, to correct deficiencies, if any, to restrict some nutrients, to change the cooking methods so as to give rest to digestive organs or to give rest to certain organs in the body, to reduce or increase the body weight whenever necessary.

There are certain principles in diet therapy. One important aspect is that all therapeutic diets are adaptations of the normal diet and skeletal structure of the therapeutic diets must be based on the requirements of a healthy person. The person in charge of dietetic planning also must consider the patient as a person and consideration must be given to the economic status, dietary pattern, likes and dislikes, family environment, preferences, religious status and availability of items. Dietetics must always give room for flexibility. Rapport with the patient is essential to make dietetic regimen a success. As a rule therapeutic diet must be easily digestible, soft, liquid, clear fluid or bland based on the conditions. Best sources must be selected to ensure maximum utilisation from the food consumed because as a whole a patient has poor appetite. Along with the discomfort of disease it is always difficult to implement a strict dietetic regimen. Confidence and cooperation from the patient are essential for the success of diet therapy. The patients must be educated on the importance of modification in the diet for quick recovery and the consequences of uncontrolled diet in special conditions. The dietetic history of the patient must be collected to know of any intolerance of food or allergic manifestation in the patient. Working conditions and dietary habits at work place also must be considered before dietetic instructions are given.

Common modifications in diet therapy are changes in consistency by adopting a full liquid diet, clear liquid diet, nasal feeding or tube feeding or soft diet. Changes in the preparation are made by avoiding all condiments and spices and suggesting bland diet which is chemically, mechanically and thermally non-irritant in nature. High calorie diets are also prescribed for underweight persons or in fevers or in hyperthyrodism. High protein diets are recommended for protein calorie malnutrition, cirrhosis of liver, peptic ulcer, tuberculosis, typhoid, nephrotic syndrome, celiac diseases and during pregnancy and lactation. Low-protein diets are suggested for hepatic coma or failure, kidney diseases like uraemia or nephritis.

Fats are restricted in a low-caloric diet, in liver diseases and in hypertension. Modifications are also necessary in fat in steatorrhoea, malabsorption syndrome and in undernutrition.

A mineral like calcium is essential in the treatment of rickets and osteomalacia and is restricted in renal calculi. Sodium is restricted in hypertension and in cardiac diseases. In kidney diseases also sodium chloride is restricted.

In all therapeutic diets high vitamin content is recommended. Restriction of various items in diet will result in deficiency or one or two vitamins and so their supplementation is essential.

Fibre content in the diet should be increased to remove constipation while it should be reduced in peptic ulcer, ulcerative colitis, celiac diseases, diarrhoea and dysentery.

Chemical constituents like purine are restricted in the treatment of gout and a low oxalic diet is prescribed for renal calculi.

Diet consistency is often modified depending upon the nature and condition of various diseases. Liquids are used for oral or nasogastric feeding. After surgery or in conditions where the patient has difficulty in swallowing foods or in inflammatory conditions of gastro-intestinal tract liquid diets are advocated. Soft and bland diets are given later on.

Liquid Diets

Liquid diets are suitable for post-operative diabetes mellitus, intragastric and jejunostomy feeding, constriction of oesophagus due to carcinoma or bums, fevers, acute diarrhoea.

If food is taken by mouth, wheat flour or the equivalent dry weight of other cereal may be given as thin conjee or gruel. This should be carefully strained in cases of constriction of the oesophagus and diarrhoea. If butter is prescribed, this may be added during cooking. Skimmed milk powder may be reconstituted with water or beaten into fresh milk. Tea, coffee or cocoa may be added as flavouring unless contraindicated.

Eggs may be given an egg flip. Fruit juice should be prepared fresh as required and carefully strained in cases of constriction of oesophagus and diarrhoea.

If food is required for tube-feeding, milk feeds may be prepared using proportionate quantities of foods prescribed.

Preparation of Milk Feeds : Mix wheat flour with cold water to a thin paste. Boil the milk and add it to the wheat paste, stirring continually, then return to the fire and cook for two minutes, stirring all the time. Add butter, if prescribed, and stir until melted and well mixed. Cool to near body temperature and beat in egg, skimmed milk powder, sugar and salt Dilute if necessary to a consistency which will pass through the tube. Strain and administer at body temperature.

If using wheat flour, and the mixture is found to be too thick to pass through the tube, skimmed milk powder may be substituted, using the same dry weight. This will mean a decrease in the carbohydrate value of the total diet, but an increase in the protein value.

Liquid Diet 1000 kcals

Summary of Diet	*gm* C	*gm* P	*gm* F	*kcals*
Oranges 6 (juice only)	60	...	...	240
Sugar 4 ozs	120	...	...	480
Milk 16 ozs	22	14	16	288
	202	14	16	1008

Additional fluid as water or barley water may be used as desired unless fluid restriction is recommended.

Liquid Diet 1200 kcals : Quantities are the same as for the Liquid Diet of 1000 kcals, with the addition of one of the following:

Milk 10 ozs	giving additional 9 gms protein
Milk 6 ozs and eggs 2	giving additional 12 gms protein
Skimmed milk powder 2 ozs	giving additional 20 gms protein

Liquid Diet 1500 kcals

Summary of Diet	*gm* C	*gm* P	*gm* F	*kcals*
Oranges 6 (juice only)	60	...	...	240
Sugar 2 ozs	60	...	...	240
Milk 30 ozs	42	27	30	540
Wheat flour 1 ozs	33	4	...	200
Eggs 3	...	10.5	10.5	135
Skimmed milk powder 2 gms	30	20		200
	225	61.5	40.5	1505

For tube-feeing, administer as follows:

Four feeds, each consisting of: Milk 7 ozs

Skimmed milk powder 1 oz Wheat flour 1 oz (in each of three feeds) Egg 1 (in each of three feeds) Sugar 1 oz Salt (one) level teaspoon (unless restricted).

Orange juice and remainder of sugar should be given between the milk feeds during the day, with additional fluid (water or barley water) as desired.

Liquid Diet 2000 kcals

Summary of Diet	*gm* C	*gm* P	*gm* F	*kcals*
Oranges 6 (Juice only)	60	...	...	240
Milk 40 ozs	56	36	40	720
Wheat flour 2 *ozs*	55	7	...	250
Eggs 3	...	10.5	10.5	135
Skimmed milk powder 2 ozs	37	25	...	250
Sugar 3 ozs	105	...	...	420
	313	78.5	50.5	2015

Five feeds each consisting of: Milk 8 ozs Wheat flour 1 oz Skimmed milk powder 1 oz Egg 1 (in each of three feeds) Sugar 1 oz Salt, 1 level teaspoon (unless restricted)

Orange juice and remainder of sugar should be given between the milk feeds during the day, with additional fluid (water or barley water) as desired.

Liquid Diet 2500 kcals

Summary of diet	*gms* C	*gms* P	*gms* F	*kcals*
Milk 40 ozs	56	36	40	720
Wheat flour 2 ozs	57	7	...	250
Eggs 3	...	10.5	10.5	135
Skimmed milk powder 3.75 ozs	56	37	...	375
Sugar 4 ozs	120	...	...	480
Orange 3 (juice only)	30	...	...	120
Butter 2 ozs	...	...	48	432
	319	90.5	98.5	2512

For tube-feeding, administer as follows:

Milk 8 ozs

Wheat flour 1 oz

Egg 1 (in each of three feeds)

Skimmed milk powder 3/4 oz

Sugar 1 oz

Butter 1 oz (in each of four feeds)

Salt, 1 level teaspoon (unless restricted)

Orange juice and sugar should be given between milk feeds.

Liquid Diet 3000 kcals

Summary of Diet	*gms* C	*gms* P	*gms* F	*kcals*
Milk 40 ozs	56	36	40	720
Wheat flour 3 ozs	66	9	...	300
Eggs 3	...	10.5	10.5	135
Skimmed milk powder 6 ozs	90	60	...	600
Sugar 4 ozs	120	...	...	480
Oranges 3 (juice only)	30	...	...	120
Butter 3 ozs	...	...	72	648
	362	115.5	122.5	3003

For tube-feeding, administer as follows:

Six feeds each consisting of: Milk 6 ozs Wheat flour 1 oz Egg 1 (in each of three feeds) Skimmed milk powder 1 oz Sugar 1 oz Butter 1 oz Salt, 1 level teaspoon (unless restricted).

Orange juice and remainder of sugar should be given between the milk feeds during the day, with additional fluid (water or barley water) as desired.

Liquid diets are usually used for relatively short periods. If liquid diet is to be used for prolonged periods supplementation of some vitamins and minerals is essential. The main purpose of liquid diets is to reduce effort for digestion and absorption and not to satisfy the requirements. All nutrient sources cannot be planned in a liquid diet satisfactorily. Enriched or pre-cooked infant cereal foods can be incorporated to contribute iron, thiamine and niacin.

Soft Diet

Soft diets are recommended for patients with gastro-intestinal disorders or in post-operative cases. In acute infection, where loss of appetite and vomiting persist, soft diets are recommended. The nature of the diet is soft but it is neither fluid nor a normal diet but in between these two. For patients who cannot masticate or chew, a soft diet is suggested. Soft diet contains no fried foods, strongly flavoured vegetables, raw foods, fibre, spices or condiments. Depending upon the disease condition, sources of nutrients can be selected. Milk and milk products, fruits, eggs and cereals can be incorporated with one another to give variety and good taste, since condiments and spices are used less in soft diet. Restrictions of various nutrients differ according to the symptoms of disease.

Characteristics of a Soft Diet : As a whole the soft food needs no mechanical action to digest it. Cereals as porridge, pre-cooked infant cereals available in the market or soft chapatis of wheat, rice, jowar or bajra, double-cooked rice and sweet cereal preparations are included in the soft diet. Rice flakes, puffed rice, noodles, strained oatmeal and macaroni are the other cereal items that can be included in a soft diet. Pulses can be included as dal soup or mashed dal. Vegetables are used as vegetable purees (cooked and mashed) or soups or boiled in various preparations. Meat or fish can be included in a soft diet as baked or minced items, strained unseasoned soup, boiled or roasted forms. Milk in any form is allowed. Egg as soft-boiled, scrambled, poached or in baked form is permissible. Fruits in the form of fruit juices and cooked or baked form are included in the soft diet. Steamed items are better digested.

Bland Diet

Bland diet is used for diseases of gastro-intestinal tract. In peptic ulcer and in gastric ulcer a bland diet is used. In this diet, mechanical, chemical and thermal irritations are avoided. Seeds, skin, peel, fibre and hard solid foods produce mechanical irritation. Chemical stimulation occurs on consuming meat extracts, condiments and spices, alcohol, acid-producing foods, strongly flavoured vegetables and fruits.

Muscular tone and mobility of intestine are increased by hot and warm foods, liquid, fibrous or concentrated sweets. Cold foods, dry foods and low fibre foods reduce the motility of the intestine. Therefore, thermal irritation by cold or heat has to be avoided for gastro-intestinal disorders. Emotional attitude of the patient influences the enzyme production, muscle tone and motility and also affects digestion of food. Fear, anger, worry, pain and discontent have negative attitude in the patient towards food. Neurosis is to be handled first in the gastric diseases for effective dietary treatment.

Common diseases where dietetics plays an important role in the treatment can be grouped as (1) Deficiency diseases like kwashiorkar, marasmus, anaemia, (2) Gastro-intestinal disorders like peptic ulcer, ulcerative colitis, constipation, diarrhoea, (3) diseases of liver, biliary tract and pancreas like cirrhosis, infantile biliary cirrhosis, jaundice, and viral hepatitis, hepatic coma and coma, pancreatitis, (4) kidney diseases like nephritis, chronic renal failure or uraemia, calculi, (5) metabolic disorder like diabetes mellitus and obesity, gout and (6) heart diseases like high blood pressure and congestive cardiac failure.

Acidic and Alkaline Foods

The mineral element left after the combustion of food is known as ash. Ash, sodium, potassium, calcium and magnesium are alkaline radicals. Chloride, phosphate and sulphate are acid radicals. The reaction of blood is maintained slightly alkaline by kidneys. Kidneys excrete acid or alkaline urine to make the blood pH. In kidney diseases the alkali reserve of the blood may be affected. In urinary calculi especially, in calcium phosphate, for crystal formation diet has an influence.

Alkaline Foods	*Acid-producing Foods*
Whole wheat	Fruits like apple, apricots
Bread	banana, berries, dates
Cornmeal	Grape juice
Oatmeal	Lemon juice
Puffed rice	Olive

Contd...

Alkaline Foods	*Acid-producing Foods*
Puffed wheat	Pumpkin
Egg	Spinach
Egg yolk	Tomato
Groundnut	Oranges
Chocolate	Peach
Fish	Pineapple
Mackerel	Raisins
Oysters	Milk
Salmon	Asparagus
Pomfret	Beetroot
Meat	Carrots
Poultry	Cabbage
Beef	Cauliflower
Kidney	Cucumber
Liver	Beans
Chicken	Lettuce
Mutton	Onion
Pork	Green peas
Rabbit	Potato

Potassium-rich Foods		
Bread	Kidney	Whole
wheat	Liver	Bran
Pig	Wheat germ	Pork
Eggs	Salmon	Milk
Sardine	Apricots	Tuna
Banana	Coconut	Groundnut
Duck	Cherries	Peanut butter

Berries	Chocolate	Raisins
Soyabeans	Dates	Sweet potato
Oranges	Tomatoes	Pineapple
Plums	Strawberries	Beef
Brain	Chicken	

Sodium-rich Foods

Commercial foods made with milk, salt

Chocloate milk	Frozen limabeans
Condensed milk	Potato chips
Ice-cream	Glazed fruits
Malted milk	Dried fruits with sodium
Greens, spinach	sulfite added
Beets, carrots	Yeast bread, canned
Frozen peas with salt	foods, enriched cereals
Milk mixes	

Bakery items with baking soda, salted popcorn, salted readymade items, shell fish, crab, oysters, peanut butter, salted butter, beverages with flavoured powders, animal foods and commercial sweetened desserts.

Items at Work

The studies leading to the discovery of biotin began when it was observed that rats fed a ration rich in raw or slightly cooked egg white developed a peculiar skin disorder, showed extreme loss of body hair, and finally died. This condition was referred to as "egg-white injury," and the toxic factor in the egg-white protein which was responsible for the disorder was identified and called *avidin.* Avidin is destroyed when eggs are cooked. Then, a protective factor that counteracted the toxic effect of the avidin was found in such foods as liver and yeast, but it was called by many names such as vitamin H, Factor X, and others before its identification as biotin was established. Now, it is known that the "egg-white injury" occurred when the biotin from a food combined with the avidin of the egg white to form an insoluble substance that could not be absorbed from the intestinal tract.

This was originally included in bios and was later known as vitamin H (from Haut = skin) because deficiency caused changes in the skin of rats. It was isolated in 1936 and synthesized inl943 (Harris and others, 1943).

Biotin is present in every type of living cell but in very low concentration. It is, however, one of the most highly biologically active substances known. The richest natural sources are liver and kidney, yeast and cereals.

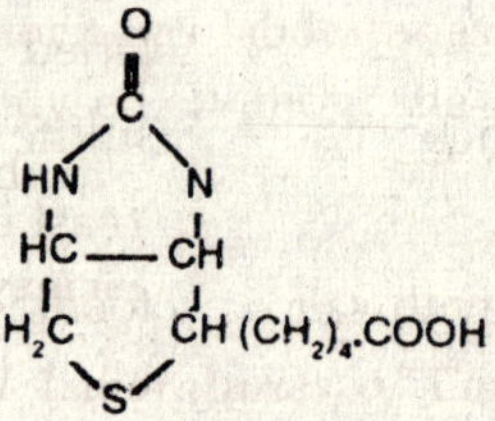

```
        O
        ‖
        C
      /   \
    HN     N
    |      |
    HC ——— CH
    |      |
    H2C    CH (CH2)4.COOH
      \   /
        S
```

BIOTIN

Biotin

Since 1941 a sulfur-containing substance called biotin has been considered as another of the B-group of vitamins. It first attracted attention as preventing the so-called "egg white injury" and has since been found to be necessary in the nutrition of several species of animals. Apparently the substance that causes the injury because of excessive egg white is a protein called *avidin* or *avidalbumin;* which combines with biotin, making it unavailable to the body.

Biotin apparently has important functions in intermediary metabolism. It has been considered as a coenzyme in the synthesis of aspartic acid, which plays a part in a deaminase system; and in several other processes involving the fixation of carbon dioxide.

It is still (1951-52) uncertain whether biotin is apt to be of practical importance in human nutrition.

Function of Biotin : To date, the exact function of biotin in man is not known, but it appears that this nutrient is an essential part of certain coenzymes. There is evidence that biotin is involved in carbon dioxide fixation reactions and in the reverse of this reaction, decarboxylation. An example of carbon dioxide fixation takes place in the conversion of pyruvic acid to oxaloacetic acid, an important step in carbohydrate metabolism. Carboxylation reacticns are involved in the synthesis of fatty acid and formation of urea. Biotin appears to be necessary for biosynthesis of folic acid and is closely related metabolically to folic acid and pantothenic acid.

Biotin Deficiency

In Animals : The symptoms of biotin deficiency in animals are quite similar from species to species. In the early stages of biotin deficiency in rats, the animal loses hair around the eyes, which produces a characteristic "spectacle eye conditions," and as the disorder progresses there is a general loss of hair over the entire body (Fig.). Loss of weight, abnormal posture, and a spastic gait are observed in the advanced stages of the deficiency, and death will occur if biotin is not restored to the rat's ration.

In Man : *A* biotin deficiency in man has been induced experimentally by feeding male subjects a low biotin diet that contained 30 per cent of the total Calories in the form of egg white. By the end of the first month on the experimental diet, all the subjects had developed a fine scaliness on their skin. During the ninth and tenth week of the deprivation, the men experienced mild depression, extreme weariness, sleepiness, pains in the muscles, and highly sensitive skin. Later, however, they developed anorexia and nausea. Because the symptoms of the deficiency state disappeared so quickly after the restoration of biotin to the diets of the subjects, it was concluded that this vitamin is in essential nutrient for man.

Recommended Allowances : As yet recommended allowances for biotin have not been established, but it has been suggested that probably between 0.150 and 0.300 mg of the vitamin provide the daily needs. Because biotin is widely distributed in foods, with the average diet supplying the suggested daily need besides being synthesized in the intestinal tract, it is very unlikely that a deficiency of the nutrient occurs in man.

Food Sources : Biotin is found in many foods of both plant and animal origin. The richest food sources of the vitamin are found in kidney and liver, and good sources of biotin include eggs, most fresh vegetables, and some fruits. Meat, wheat products, and corn products, however, are considered to be poor in biotin.

Pantothenic Acid

About 1940, pantothenic acid received a great deal of publicity because of its possible use as a remedy to overcome the graying of hair in human beings. Based on the observation that the fur of a black-haired rat would gray when it was deprived of the vitamin, studies were undertaken to observe the effects of adequate intakes of pantothenic acid on individuals with prematurely graying hair and on elderly people with gray hair. The findings from these studies indicated, however, that the vitamin had no consistent effect on relieving the process of graying hair in man.

This too, is one of the factors necessary for the growth of yeast cells and known now to be needed also by certain bacteria.

It was synthesized in 1939 (Woolley and others, 1939), and calcium pantothenate is now available as a pharmaceutical preparation.

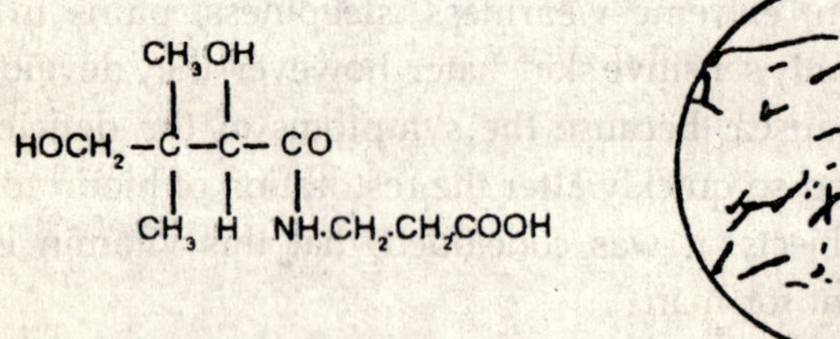

PANTOTHENIC ACID

In 1933 R.J. Williams coined the name *pantothenic acid* to indicate universal occurrence of this substance in all organisms which have been adequately examined. It is probably due to the wide natural distribution of this substance that there is as yet no consensus as to whether it need be supplied to human beings through their food, or is formed adequately in our bodies or the micro-organisms to which our bodies serve as hosts.

Like several other vitamins, pantothenic acid is an essential component of an enzyme system, in this case, of a system controlling acetylation processes (such as the formation of acetyl choline) in the body.

Vernon (1950) described and discussed a syndrome of painful "burning" sensation in the feet, observed in prisoners of war, which he thought had been frequently observed but "inadequately reported and referred to as dry beriberi." Vernon follows Glusman in calling the disease *nutritional melalgia* and further characterizes it as *a deficiency vascular disease.* Vernon writes, "It may represent a pantothenic acid deficiency," and according to him, the work of Gopalan indicates that calcium antothenate yields significant therapeutic results and "seems to establish a relationship of pantothenic acid" to the symptom of "burning feet."

Gopalan (1946) describes the deficiency disease in his "burning feet." It has certain well-marked and constant clinical features and is a definite clinical entity. It seems to be common among the poor of South India-decidedly more common than "peripheral neuritis" associated with thiamine deficiency.

"Outbreaks of 'burning feet' have previously been reported among malnourished populations and have often occurred in jails. The disease has not, however, hitherto been adequately observed and described and has often been confused with peripheral neuritis."

Signs suggestive of riboflavin deficiency were almost always present in the "burning feet" patients, but Gopalan considers the two diseases distinct.

Definite improvement resulted in all of 10 patients who were given calcium-pantothenate only. This improvement was more striking and rapid than that resulting from the yeast concentrate treatment which, however, was also effective.

The explanation for the close association signs of riboflavin deficiency with signs of pantothenic acid deficiency may lie in the fact that functions of these two vitamins in human nutrition are closely interrelated, and possibly in a similarity of their distribution in food. The observation of Spies and his associates (1940) that the injection of pantothenic acid causes a rise in the blood level not only of pantothenic acid but also of riboflavin, and similarly that the injection of riboflavin causes a rise in the blood level not only of riboflavin but also of pantothenic acid, is suggestive of a close interrelationship of the two vitamins.

Functions of Pantothenic Acid : Pantothenic acid functions in the body as a part of the coenzyme called coenzyme A. This coenzyme mediates acetylation, the transfer or acceptance of the acetyl group (CH_3CO). Certain fats and amino acids can be formed from the intermediate products of carbohydrate metabolism by splitting off or adding an acetyl group (s). Coenzyme A is one of the enzymes involved in the series of chemical reactions that are necessary to break down carbohydrates and fats for the production of energy. The formation of the porphyrin part of the hemoglobin molecule requires coenzyme A. Pantothenic acid, a part of coezyme A, is thus of importance in many phrases of cellular metabolism.

Effects of a Pantothenic Acid Deficiency

In Animals and Birds : The symptoms of a pantothenic acid deficiency in birds and animals vary from species to species. The chick shows growth failure and then develops a characteristic type of skin lesion which involves the eyelids and the mouth, whereas the fur of a black-haired rat will turn gray when the animal's ration is low or deficient in this nutrient (Fig.). Other characteristic symptoms that have been observed when rats are deprived of the vitamin, are the failure to grow and the degeneration of the cells of the outer layer, the cortex, of the adrenal gland.

In Man : The absence of pantothenic acid in the diet, done, has not been effective in producing an experimental deficiency in man. Only when human subjects were fed an antagonist of the vitamin (omega-methyl pantothenate) in a diet deficient in other nutrients as well, were symptoms produced. Symptoms developed early in the experiment with the men showing signs of rapid heart beat on exertion, dizziness, and a lowered blood pressure. Because they became fatigued easily, the men slept more during the day than was normal. During the third week of vitamin deprivation, both anorexia and constipation developed, while in the following week the men became quarrelsome and discontented. As the deficiency progressed, the subjects complained of numbness and tingling in the hands and feet and showed definite signs of muscular weakness. When pantothenic acid was restored to their diets, however, it alone did not immediately improve all the symptoms of the deficiency state. Consequently, it is believed that the deficiency effects observed might have been due to the toxicity of the antagonist rather than to a complete lack of pantothenic acid; only the use of a diet supplemented with all the vitamins brought about complete recovery in all the subjects.

Recommended Allowances for Pantothenic Acid : Although the daily allowance for pantothenic acid is not yet known, it has been suggested to be about 10 mg per day. The average amount in the adequate American diet has been reported to be between 16.3 mg (high-cost diet) and 14.2 mg (low-cost diet) per day and about 6 mg per day in inadequate diets.

Food Sources of Pantothenic Acid : Inasmuch as this vitamin is found in all plant and animal tissues its name, which was coined from the Greek and means "from everywhere," is appropriately chosen. The richest amounts of the nutrient have been found in liver, kidney, yeast, egg yolk, and fresh vegetables. Like other B-vitamins, whole-grain cereals contain appreciably more pantothenic acid than do refined cereal products. Milk, also, is an important carrier of the nutrient in the diet (1.5 mg pantothenic acid per pint).

Folacin

It is also known as *vitamin M (Pteroylglutamic acid).*

Folic acid, first designated as vitamin M, is now chemically identified as pteroylglutamic acid (or glutamates); vitamin B_{12} is now held to be the specifically antipernicious anemia substance; and the citrovourm factor, into which folic acid is converted *in vivo* in the animal organism, is a substance required for growth by the bacterium *Leuconostoc citrovorum.*

Long before folacin was either isolated or synthesized, its deficiency symptoms had been described in man, animals, and microorganisms. Many laboratories had independently studied the effect of a folacin deficiency in a variety of species, and different names for this nutrient such as vitamin M, vitamin B and L. *casei* factor had been reported. Now it is known that there is a series of biologically active derivatives of folacin (pteroylglutamic acid) that make up the folic acid group of vitamins. Members of this group include folacin, pteroyltriglutamic acid, pteroylhepta-glutamic acid, and folinic acid or citrovorum factor, a derivative of folic acid (9). It appears that folinic acid is the biologically active form of the vitamin.

This was first discovered in 1941 (Mitchell and others, 1941) as a factor in green leaves (folium = leaf) needed to protect chicks from a variety of anaemia. Later similar factors were described which were needed for the growth" of micro-organisms. These were grouped together as folic acid when an active compound was synthesized in 1945.

```
                                                        N       N
COOH            HC—CH                     HC     C     C—NH2
CH—NH—CO—C           C—NH—CH2—C       C     N
CH2             NC═CH                      N     C
CH2                                                     OH
COOH
```

Day, Langston, Darby and coworkers found previously unknown substance to be needed in the nutrition of the monkey. This they designated *vitamin* M. Other groups of workers used folic acid, vitamin B_c, and still other designations for what finally proved to be essentially the same substance in antianemic activity.

Chemically it was found to be pteroylglutamic acid and its formula was established as;

The B vitamins are of interest in having another feature in common. Many of them can be synthesized by bacteria and other micro-organisms such as moulds. It is normal for certain bacteria to inhabit the intestinal tract of man and other animals. These cause no harm and must not be confused with disease producing bacteria or germs. Some of these obtain their own nourishment from the intestinal contents of their host and in turn they synthesize B vitamins, which thus become available for the host. this process reaches its highest development in ruminants such as the cow. The rumen contains a large volume of semi-fluid material at a temperature ideally suitable for the bacteria to function and considerable quantities of some of the B vitamins are manufactured there.

Vitamin B_1, riboflavin, nicotinic acid and pyridoxin are all synthesized in this way and also in other sites in the intestinal tract. Vitamin B_{12} seems to be the only vitamin known to be synthesized only by micro-organisms. It is not found, even in small quantities, in plants.

Folic Acid in Nutrition : In 1948 King reviewed in Reprint 129 of the National Research Council Reprint and Circular Series three lines of evidence that this substance (folic acid, pteroylglutamic acid, vitamin B_c, L. *casei* factor, or vitamin M) is essential to normal human nutrition:

> "(1) Numerous widely distributed instances have been found in which individuals who revealed no other basis for functional impairment characterized by macrocytic anemia and associated tissue changes,

responded promptly to folic acid therapy, using either the synthetic or the highly purified natural product (pteroylglutamic acid). The dietary histories of these patients have been characterized, in most cases, by an intake of foods that would provide only very small quantities of folic acid.

"(2) The characteristic macrocytic anemias identified in infants, children, adult women, and adult men, most logically interpreted in terms of an etiology of folic acid deficiency, have been strikingly similar to conditions established by folic acid deficiencies in controlled animal experiments.

"(3) Attempts to deplete volunteer subjects of their tissue reserves of folic acid by supplying diets adequate in other essential nutrients but low in folic acid have met with varying success. Some investigators have not found a characteristic depletion in blood, urinary, or fecal concentrations of folic acid, but in other instances there has been evidence of a slow depletion, such as would be anticipated on the basis of animal experiments and clinical observations of individuals in an uncontrolled environment. Synthesis of folic acid by micro-organisms in the intestinal tract apparently accounts for a major part of the irregularity in depletion experiments. The incidence of clinical deficiencies, however, affords evidence that intestinal synthesis should not be relied upon as a source of this nutrient.

"The quantitative requirement cannot be estimated closely from published evidence. Doan, et al observed a hematologic response from a dosage of 2 mg. of synthetic folic acid per day; Kurnick observed improvement after a dosage of 2.5 mg. per day of folic acid; and Moore, et. al. observed a response from 2 mg. per day.... Comparative studies with monkeys, chickens, and turkeys, on a caloric basis, provided an indirect basis for estimating a human requirement in the range of 0.1 to 0.2 mg. per day. Many investigators suggest that estimates of requirement should be based upon studies of nutritional macrocytic anemias and directly related cases rather than upon protection from pernicious anemia."

Folic acid is active hematologically in macrocytic anemias, but it pernicious anemia neither prevents nor alleviates neurological symptoms. However, in macrocytic anemias of infancy and prequancy nutritional macrocytic anemia, and in sprue it is a highly effective therapeutic agent.

Distribution of Folic Acid : According to R.J. Williams and coworkers the available data on quantitative distribution of folic acid " are too low by a variable and unknown amount" because when these data were determined enzymes capable of freeing folic acid completely from tissues were not known.

More recently, however, Toepfer (U.S. Department of Agriculture), in work more especially directed to the quantitative aspect, has determined the folic acid content of many foods, representative cases of which are included in Table.

Total Folic Acid Content of Foods

Approximate averages or representative values: milligrams per kilogram (parts per million)	
Almonds	0.45
Apples	0.01
Asparagus (Fresh)	0.86
Bananas	0.10
Beans, green	0.23
Lima (fresh)	0.34
Wax	0.36
Beef, round, I	0.07
Beef, round, II	0.09
Beef, round, III	0.10
Beets	0.16
Bran	1.0

Approximate averages or representative values: milligrams per kilogram (parts per million)	
Brazil nuts	0.05
Broccoli	0.33
Cantaloupe	0.04
Carrots	0.06
Cauliflower	0.13
Celery	0.08
Cheese (Cheddar type)	0.12
Chicken, light meat	0.03
Chicken, dark meat	0.03
Chuck(Texas study)	0.15
Corn, sweet	0.14
Eggs	0.03
Filberts	0.71
Heart	0.03
Kale	0.42
Kidney	0.58
Lamb	0.03
Liver	2.94
Milk (butter milk)	0.11
Mustard greens	0.38
Oatmeal	0.31
Oranges	0.05
Peanuts	0.61
Peas, green, fresh	0.25
Peas, dry blackeye	4.9
Pecans	0.34
Potatoes	0.06
Pumpkin	0.04
Tomatoes	0.04
Walnuts	0.78
Wheat, entire, I	0.45
Wheat, entire, II	0.41
Yams	0.19

Vitamin B_6, Pantothenic acid, Biotin, Folic Acid, and Choline Content of Selected Foods[1]

Food	Protion Amt	Wt, gm	Vit B_6 µg.	Pantothenic Acid, µg.	Biotin, mg	Folic Acid, µg.	Choline, mg
Bread, white	1 sl	23	23.0	0.101	0.3	3.4	—
Bread, whole wheat	1 sl	23	96.0	0.182	0.4	6.9	—
Cheese, Cheddar	1 oz	30	18.7	0.114	1.0	4.5	13.6
Egg	1	50	126.0	0.795	11.2	2.5	252.0
Milk, whole	1 c	244	87.8	0.756	11.5	1.5	36.6
Apple	1	130	39.0	0.130	1.2	2.6	—
Banana	1	100	320.0	0.310	4.4	9.7	—
Orange	1	100	31.0	0.220	1.9	5.1	—
Apricots, canned	½ c	125	67.5	0.125	—	0.6	—
Pineapple, canned	Ke	125	88.7	—	—	1.0	—
Beef, liver	2 oz	57	378.5	5.324	54.7	167.6	290.7
Beef, round	3 oz	100	495.0	0.520	2.6	10.5	68.0
Ham	3½ oz	100	440.0	0.640	5.0	10.6	122.0
Chicken, dark		100	25.0	0.692	10.0	2.8	—
Chicken; white	3½ oz	100	130.0	0.804	11.3	3.0	—
Tuna, canned	3½ oz	100	670.0	0.420	3.0	1.8	—
Beans, Lima	3½ oz	100	170.0	0.450	—	34.0	—
Beans, snap, green	3½ oz	100	63.0	0.200	—	27.5	42.0
Broccoli	2/3 c	100	171.0	1.290	—	53.5	—
Carrots	½ c	55	66.0	0.150	1.4	4.4	7.0
Peas, green	3½ oz	100	150.0	0.820	9.4	25.0	75.0
Spinach	3½ oz	100	198.0	0.310	6.9	75.0	22.0

Function of Folacin : The folic acid group functions as coenzymes in the transfer of one carbon unit which is important in the metabolism of many body compounds. Purines and pyrimidines, examples of these types of compounds, are utilized in the building of nucleoproteins and are found in the nucleus of every cell. Folacin is necessary for normal blood formation (hematopoiesis) because of its presumed function in the formation of purines and pyrimidines. In a study of megaloblastic anemias Vilter reported that "all evidence points toward a dominant chemical role for the folic acid coenzymes in hematopoiesis, with vitamin B_{12} and ascorbic acid playing dependent parts."

Average Content of Selected Nutrients in High-Cost, Low-Cost Adequate, and Poor Diets as Calculated from Food Composition Tables and Determined by Microbiologic Assays

Nutrients per Day lated	*High Cost*		*Low Cost*		*Poor*	
	Calcu- zed	*Analy- lated*	*Calcu- zed*	*Analy- lated*	*Calcu- zed*	*Analy-*
Calories	3013		2439		1117	
Protein, gm	126	130	112	116	32	31
Folic acid, ug	120.4	193.4	117.0	157.4	30.8	47.3
B_6, mg	—	2.0	—	2.7	—	1.0
Pantothenic acid, mg	11.0	16.3	8.9	14.2	4.1	6.0
B_{12}, ug	—	31.6	—	16.0	—	2.7

Adapted from Mangay Chung et al. Am. J. Clin. Nutr. 9:578, 1961.

Folacin Deficiency

In Birds and Animals : Although all animals have a need for folacin, the amount required in the daily ration varies from species to species, because some of them can produce the vitamin by intestinal synthesis. The dog, rabbit, and rat meet their need for the vitamin by intestinal synthesis, but chicks and monkeys must have folacin in their feed, otherwise a deficiency will occur(Fig.).

In Man : Folacin is effective in the relief of certain types of human macrocytic anemias. In order to show better the cause and effects of this type of anemia, a brief description is given of the development and growth of the red blood cells. After the red blood cells are produced in the marrow of the bone, they must undergo a process of growth and development called *maturation* before the cells are discharged into the blood stream ready to carry on their function in the body. In the first stages of their development, the immature red blood cells are large, nucleated, and contain little or no hemoglobin. A *megaloblast* is an example of this type of immature cell. As maturation proceeds, the nucleus becomes smaller, more and more hemoglobin is formed, and the size of the cell is reduced. The mature red blood cell is called an *erythrocyte.* The process of maturation is dependent on the action of certain enzyme systems, and it is believed that it is in this role, as part of a coenzyme, that folacin functions in hematopoiesis.

A person suffering from a macrocytic anemia caused by a folacin deficiency shows a characteristic blood pattern as well as other typical symptoms of the disorder. In the blood stream there are many large, immature megaloblasts and relatively few mature erythrocytes. Because of this condition, the oxygen-carrying capacity of the cells, which have not formed adequate amounts of hemoglobin, is greatly reduced and results in symptoms of weakness, rapid breathing, and a slowing down of the body processes. The normal growth and development of other blood factors, the white blood cells *(leucocytes)* and blood platelets *(thrombocytes)* are also altered during a folacin deficiency. A decrease in the leucocytes, which are the body's chief defense against micro-organisms, will result in less resistance to disease on the part of the aneima patient, and his normal process of blood coagulation may be affected by the lowered number of thrombocytes. Besides the effects caused by an alteration of certain blood constituents, the macrocytic anemia patient may show weight loss, inflammation of the tongue, and disturbances of the intestinal tract.

Folacin has been shown to be effective in relieving the symptoms in patients with tropical and nontropical sprue, nutritional macrocytic anemia, macrocytic anemia of pellagra, megaloblastic anemia of pregnancy, and megaloblastic anemia of infancy. Also this nutrient has been shown to improve hematopoiesis in pernicious anemia but "it is an incomplete treatment for this disease." Folacin has no effect whatsoever in relieving the neurological manifestations characteristic of pernicious anemia; actually it seems to aggravate the neurological lesions that involve the degeneration of the nerve cord. The macrocytic type of anemia does not respond to folacin therapy.

That combined deficiencies of folacin, vitamin B_{12}, and ascorbic acid are much more common than a single deficiency of any one of these nutrients has been proposed. Vilter et al. believe that "the usual defect responsible for a megaloblast is an abnormality in folic acid metabolism which reduces the amount or the activity of the folic acid coenzymes. Deficiencies of vitamin B_{12} and ascorbic acid adversely influence formation of these coenzymes..."

A variety of antagonists of folacin has been identified. When these antivitamins, such as aminopterin, are fed to animals, one of the early alterations in the process of hematopoiesis is a reduction in the number of leucocytes or white blood cells produced. Because of this finding, the administration of folacin antagonists has brought temporary relief, but not a cure, in cases of human leukemia, a disease in which there is a marked increase in the production of leucocytes.

Recommended Allowances for Folacin : So far the National Research Council has not suggested a folacin allowance for man. However, based on the folacin analysis of adequate diets (0.193 and 0.157 mg per day) and inadequate diets (0.047 mg per day) in the United States, it has been stated that a ".... diet containing 0.15 mg total folic acid activity should supply at least 0.05 mg folic acid which is active for human beings."

Because folic acid in amounts greater than 0.1 mg per day mask the neurological symptoms of pernicious anemia, the sale of the vitamin without prescription in amounts recommending doses greater than 0.1 mg per day is prohibited in the United States.

Food Sources : Folacin is widely distributed in nature, especially in the green foliage of plants; hence the name folacin. The richest food sources are found in chicken livers and vegetables such as asparagus, broccoli, endive, leaf lettuce, and spinach. Liver, legumes, and other leafy-green vegetables are good contributors of the vitamin.

Fat-soluble Vitamins

Vitamin E (Tocopherols)

Almost simultaneously with the full establishment of vitamin D as a fat-soluble essential distinct from vitamin A, different investigators, prominent among them being Evans and his coworkers at the University of California and Mattill, working first at the University of Rochester and later at Iowa University, found evidence that for normal reproduction a further fat-soluble factor was nutritionally essential. This came to be known as vitamin E, then *tocopherol,* and more recently *alpha-, beta-, gamma-,* and *delta-tocopherols.*

The four known natural tocopherols are so closely related that custom continues to use the collective-singular term, vitamin E.

Research that eventually led to the discovery of vitamin E was conducted in the early 1920's by Mattill, Evans, and Sure. During an investigation of the influence of diet on the reproductive cycle of the rat, it was found that rats became sterile when reared on a purified diet which contained all the then-known nutrients. Even though the experimental animals fed with this ration seemed to be quite healthy, they were not able to produce young. When fresh green leaves or dried alfalfa were fed to these sterile animals, reproductivity was restored in the female but not in the male of the species. The unknown factor, which prevented sterility, was first called substance X and later was named vitamin E.

Synthetic alpha-tocopherol acetate has been adopted as the International standard for vitamin E; and the International Unit has been defined as the specific activity of 1 milligram of the standard preparation. Vitamin E is rather widely distributed in nature where it is largely associated with anti-oxidants.

Properties of Vitamin E : The chemical name for vitamin E is tocopherol (from Greek *tokos,* childbirth; *perhos,* to bear; and the chemical suffix -ol, signifying an alcohol). Actually there are six different tocopherols, which collectively are called vitamin E. The biological activity of the tocopherols varies, with alpha being the most potent. The number and position of the methyl (CH_3) groups within the molecule seem to influence biological activity. This conclusion is reached because the only difference among the tocopherols is in the structure of the molecule.

Vitamin E occurs as a yellow viscous oil that is insoluble in water but soluble in all the fat solvents. Although it is quite stable to acids and heat (in the absence of oxygen), it is readily destroyed by ultraviolet light, alkalies, and oxygen.

Though Vitamin E is stable to heat but is destroyed when fats or oils containing it become rancid. It is thus safe from destruction as long as it remains in the intact cells but when the seeds are crushed or the oil is expressed, rancidity may develop with loss of vitamin activity. Vitamin E is also readily oxidized by ferric salts.

Sources of Vitamin E : The chief vegetable oils which contain vitamin E are wheat germ oil, cotton seed oil and rice germ oil. A little also occurs in the small quantities of oil present in certain green leaves, e.g. lecttuce and alfalfa.

It was isolated in crystalline form in 1936 by Evans and since then several varieties have been identified, i.e. a-, B-, y -and 8-tocopherol. Mixtures of these seem to exist in natural sources in a state of equilibrium, but some plant products are richer in one and some in another a~tocopherol, which is most active biologically has also been synthesized.

VITAMIN E

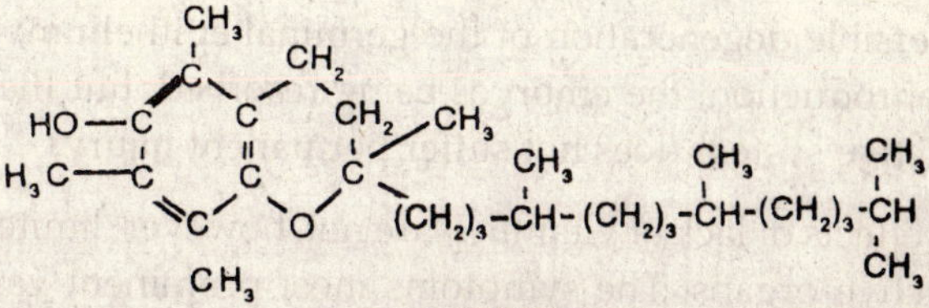

TOCOPHEROL

Vitamin E is widely distributed in foods but not in high concentration. Bread contains it if made from the whole grains but not if the germ has been removed. The animal foods containing the largest quantities are eggs and lean meat—the latter because vitamin E is found in the animal body in association with muscle.

Food Sources of Vitamin E : Inasmuch as vitamin E occurs mainly in plant materials, the richest sources of the vitamin are found in vegetable oils (such as wheat germ oil and cotton seed oil), leafy-green plants and vegetables, as well as whole-grain cereals. Although animal products contain little of the vitamin, liver, heart, kidney, milk, and eggs are the best animal sources of vitamin E.

Function of Vitamin E : It has long been believed that the function of vitamin E in the animal organism is directly related to its antioxidant property. Besides its possible function as an activator in certain enzymatic reactions, vitamin E plays an important role in the protection of vitamin A, carotene, and ascorbic acid from oxidation both in the digestive tract and in the body cells. Because of the protective property of vitamin E more efficient use can be made by the body of vitamin A and ascorbic acid.

Chemically, this association with anti-oxidants in natural occurrence correlates with the fact that vitamin E, while relatively stable in several respects, is rather easily destroyed by oxidation.

The oxidative destruction of vitamin E is catalyzed by iron salts. Hence a food mixture for experimental purposes can be made deficient in vitamin E by moistening with a solution of iron salt and then heating to dryness.

When rats are fed diets otherwise adequate to their needs but lacking vitamin E, the males become permanently infertile through an irreversible degeneration of the germinal epithelium; females fail in reproduction, the embryos being resorbed, but the female reproductive system does not suffer permanent injury.

The effects of lack of vitamin E are not, however, limited to the reproductive organs. The symptoms most prominent vary from species to species, and with the age of the individual, but in one or another species may include failure of growth, muscular dystrophy, injury to the central nervous system, interference with normal heart action, and possible endoctrine disturbances.

Whether the counterpart of any of these conditions occurs in human beings is still controversial.

Evans (1939) pointed out the occurrence of degeneration of the cross-striated musculature in vitamin E deficiency. It has also been suggested that this may be the cause of the failure of development of the fetus. Compare Mason (1944).

Puppies, rabbits, guineapigs, and rats have developed muscular dystrophy when kept for long periods on vitamin-E deficient diets, and in some cases this has been cured by giving synthetic alphatocopherol.

Vitamin E has also been found to have in some sense a sparing effect upon vitamin A. The converse may 'also be true.

Vitamin E occurs abundantly in wheat germ oil, but may not be its only influential constituent as has been assumed by some experimenters. Other vegetable oils also are rich sources of vitamin E.

Because of its wide distribution in foods and the improbability of its being a limiting factor in human nutrition, it seems probably unnecessary and possibly misleading to lay emphasis upon vitamin E in practical considerations of food values. Though, there are numerous reported cases in which vitamin E seemed to be helpful in the treatment of cert ·in muscular and nervous diseases but it should be noted carefully that the Council on Pharmacy and

Chemistry of the American Medical Association has warned against regarding the value of vitamin E for man as established, and has emphasized the need of more fully controlled investigation.

Effects of a Vitamin E Deficiency

In Animals and Birds : Vitamin E has been shown to be essential for animals and birds, including the rat, rabbit, dog, guinea pig, chick, and duck. The most characteristic deficiency symptoms, however, occur in the rat and in the rabbit.

When rats are fed rations deficient in vitamin E, permanent sterility in the male and temporary sterility in the female result. The permanent sterility of the male rat, that is caused by a degeneration of the cellular material of the testes, cannot be relieved by vitamin E therapy. In contrast to this, conception does occur in the deficient female rat, but about the eighth day of pregnancy the fetuses, or unborn animals, die and are resorbed. However, if vitamin E is added to the rations of these sterile females, their next pregnancy will be normal and they will produce living, healthy young. One of the reasons postulated for the death of the unborn young is the lack of an adequate blood supply to the fetus because of a change in the permeability of the reproductive tissues.

Young rabbits develop a condition known as muscular dystrophy when they are fed a ration deficient in vitamin E. This disorder, that is characterized by a loss of muscle tone and a general weakening of the muscles, is quickly relieved when vitamin E is added back to the ration.

In Man : As yet there is no conclusive evidence to indicate that vitamin E is essential to man. It should be noted, however, that the plasma level of alpha tocopherol is lowered in normal adults after maintenance on a limited intake (2 mg daily in contrast to an estimated average of 15 mg daily for the supplemental group) for a period from 10 to 22 months. No clinical or physiological effects accompanied the lowered plasma level during the period of observation. Vitamin E seems to have no effect on the relief of sterility in human beings or on the cure of human muscular dystrophy. Horwitt reported a relationship between serum levels of vitamin E and hemolysis of the red cells (erythrocytes) in the presence of hydrogen peroxide. Subjects who received the smallest amounts of vitamin E showed the greatest degree of red cell hemolysis.

Recommended Allowances

The Food and Nutrition Board states that until more is known about the antioxidant needs of the body and the role that selenium and other nutrients play in decreasing vitamin E needs, it is difficult to make any recommendation other than the vitamin E requirement will vary between 10 and 30 mg daily for adults. Because vitamin E is so widely distributed in the foods of the diet, it is doubtful that a vitamin E deficiency would ever develop in the human being. It is estimated that the average daily adult diet contains about 14 mg of vitamin E.

Horwitt and associates are conducting a long-term study of the human requirement for tocopherol. Some of the conclusions from their work are :

(1) The tocopherol requirement is a function of the amounts of polyunsaturated lipids in the diet and in the tissues.

(2) When polyunsaturated fatty acids in the diet are low, the need for tocopherol decreases to very low levels, but past dietary habits which have affected tissue composition must be taken into consideration in evaluating tocopherol needs.

(3) The time of erythrocyte survival is shortened in man when a diet with a relatively low tocopherol to linoleic acid ratio is fed for prolonged periods.

Vitamin K

In 1929 Dam, a Dinish scientist, reported that chicks raised on a synthetic diet developed hemorrhages under the skin that could not be relieved with the addition of ascorbic acid to the ration. This disorder, which was characterized by a prolonged blood clotting time, disappeared when a mixture of cereals or natural foods was given to the birds. Later Dam found that this antihemorrhagic factor was present in the fat-soluble fraction of certain foods. He suggested it be called vitamin K, derived from the Danish term "Koagulation Faktor."

Sources of Vitamin K : This occurs naturally in green leaves, especially those of leguminous plants such as lucerne and alfalfa — also in such an unrelated substance as fish meal. It was first described in 1935 and was synthesized in 1939-40. Certain chemically related compounds (analogues), which can be produced in the laboratory have the same biological activity and these are the compounds chiefly used in medicine. The fat-soluble analogue is menaphthone, and there is also a water-soluble compound menaphthone bisulphite.

SYNTHETIC VITAMIN K

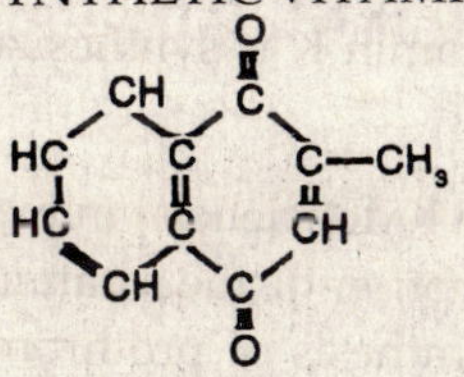

MENAPHTHONE

Food Sources of Vitamin K : Vitamin K occurs in plants; good sources are alfalfa, cauliflower, cabbage, spinach, kale, and soyabean. In contrast, fruits, cereals, and animal products contain little vitamin K. The occurrence of vitamin K in a wide variety of commonly eaten plant foods, its synthesis by bacteria in the intestinal tract, its stability, and its insolubility in water make a deficiency of this vitamin in the normal person quite improbable.

Properties of Vitamin K : Two forms of vitamin K are found in nature: K_1 occurs in green leaves, and K_2 is produced by bacterial synthesis. These yellow-coloured vitamins are stable to heat, unstable to alkalies, strong acids, oxidation, and light. Many structural modifications of vitamin K have been synthesized; one water-soluble form, menadione, is more potent and more widely used than the natural vitamin K.

Function of Vitamin K : Vitamin K is essential for the synthesis of prothrombin which is a precursor of thrombin, one of the factors needed for normal blood coagulation. Even though the production of prothrombin apparently occurs in the liver, the exact function of the vitamin in this synthesis is not known. It has been suggested, however, that vitamin K may be an essential part of the enzyme system involved in the production of this blood clotting factor.

Effects of a Vitamin K Deficiency

In Birds and Animals : Chicks fed a ration deficient in vitamin K develop a fatal bleeding disorder which is characterized by a prolonged clotting time of the blood. This disorder, however, may be relieved by the administration of vitamin K. It is commonly believed that vitamin K deficiency is an avian characteristic. In some studies with rats maintained on a vitamin-K-free diet, when access to their faces was completely prevented, a bleeding tendency developed. Some vitamin K is synthesized in the small intestine by bacteria.

In Man : Vitamin K deficiencies in man result most often from either a faulty absorption of the vitamin or liver disorders that interfere with the synthesis of prothrombin, rather than from a dietary lack of the nutrient. Inasmuch as vitamin K is supplied to the body by the food intake plus the synthesis by microorganisms in the intestinal tract, there usually is an adequate supply of the vitamin available to the body. Sometimes however, the intake of large amounts of sulfa drugs or other antibiotics may destroy the micro-organisms which synthesize the vitamin and the supply then may become low.

Because vitamin K is fat soluble, the presence of bile is necessary for its absorption as is true with the absorption of fats and other fat-soluble vitamins. Therefore, when disorders of the liver or gall bladder interfere with the secretion of the bile fluid, a vitamin K deficiency may occur. For example, in cases of obstructive jaundice, where a blockage of the bile duct prevents bile from flowing normally into the intestine, vitamin K is not adequately absorbed. On the other hand, in certain liver disorders, such as cirrhosis, adequate vitamin K may be absorbed, but the synthesis of prothrombin does not occur because of the damage to the liver cells themselves.

Newborn infants may have inadequate vitamin K supplies because micro-organisms of the right type may not have had time to become established in the intestinal tract.

Recommended Allowances for Vitamin K : The Food and Nutrition Board states that "with the exception of newborn infants, the average diet plus synthesis by intestinal bacteria provide adequate amounts of vitamin K."

The newborn infant has low blood serum levels of prothrombin, which decrease further during the first week of life, but spontaneously return toward the adult level in subsequent weeks. As a consequence, it has been a fairly common practice to routinely administer vitamin K to the mother prior to delivery or to the new born shortly after delivery. The practice has been questioned — it has been difficult to demonstrate that decreased levels of coagulation factors are a direct cause of hemorrhage of the newborn (neonatal), and there is not complete agreement that routine administration of vitamin K in pregnancy affects the incidence. So the Board has recommended that:

Vitamins K_1 and K_2 : As early as 1929 it had been observed by the Danish investigation Dam that chickens raised on certain artificial diets were subject to sub-cutaneous and intramuscular hemorrhages; and further study of such a hemorrhagic chick showed an abnormally long time required for the clotting of the blood. Others confirmed these observations; and Dam (1935) extended his work to the finding of experimental evidence that the hemorrhagic tendency and abnormally prolonged clotting time were attributable to shortage of a fat-soluble "vitamin K."

The work of several investigators showed that such a factor is widely distributed in green leaves.

One form of anti-hemorrhagic vitamin, obtained from alfalfa leaf meal and designated as vitamin K_1 or phyllochinon (phylloquinone), has been identified chemically as 2-methyl-3-phytyl-l, 4-naphthoquinone.

A second form of anti-hemorrhagic vitamin (vitamin K_2) was isolated by Doisy and coworkers from putrefied sardine meal.

In addition to these forms of vitamin K known to occur naturally, many synthetic products show anti-hemorrhagic properties in greater or lesser degree.

Bile salts appear to be highly important if not absolutely necessary to the absorption of (natural) vitamin K. For this reason, patients with diseases of the biliary tract in which bile flow to the intestine is impaired are apt to develop a condition of low blood-clotting ability which is really a K-avitaminosis, notwithstanding the fact that their diet may have contained normally adequate amounts of anti-hemorrhagic factor. Numerous clinical tests show that the hemorrhagic tendency in such conditions may be controlled either by the oral administration of bile salts with vitamin K concentrates or by the injection of anti-hemorrhagic vitamin.

The low clotting-power of the blood in vitamin K deficiency has been traced to an abnormally low content of *prothrombin* (a normal protein constituent of the blood which, with calcium ion and the cephalin-containing thromboplastic factor, gives rise to blood clot). Hypoprothrombinemia has been found clinically in various conditions of impaired digestive function and treated effectively in most instances as a K-avitaminosis. Since diminished clotting power due to low prothrombin content appears to be usual in the blood of newborn infants, clinicians generally recommend administration of vitamin K either to the mother before delivery or to the infant at birth.

The National Research Council's circular on *Recommended Dietary Allowances*, Revised 1948, comments upon vitamin K in part as follows:

> "The requirement for vitamin K usually is satisfied by any good diet except for the infant in utero and for the first few days after birth. Supplemental vitamin K is recommended during the last month of pregnancy. When it has not been given in this manner, it is recommended for the mother preceding delivery or for the baby immediately after birth.... Pregnant women usually are found to have normal amounts of prothrombin in the blood, but many newborn infants

have abnormally small amounts. Although little relation seems to exist between the amount of prothrombin in the blood of the mother and that of the infant at birth, the amount of prothrombin in the blood of her infant in utero. Seldom does the mother receive enough dietary vitamin K to prevent an important decrease in the prothrombin level of the blood of her infant during the first few days after birth. The available evidence warrants increased attention to the vitamin K intake of the mother during the latter part of pregnancy ... (and) it is suggested that vitamin K be given to pregnant women during the last month of pregnancy."

Vitamin P

Since 1936 various experiments have suggested the existence of another factor besides vitamin C in the juice and rind of the lemon. This was at first called citrin and was later found to consist of several related compounds, chemically known as glucosides, among which the best known is *hesperidin*. Another glucoside with similar activity is *rutin* found in buckwheat and in the flowers of elder, violet, tobacco and forsythia.

Vitamin P activity is concerned with the control of bleeding from capillaries but is not identical with the action of ascorbic acid. There is still some doubt about its true nature and it was recommended in 1950 (Committee on Biochemical Nomenclature) that the term vitamin P, should no longer be employed. However, pharmaceutical preparations are available and are being tested for their value in treatment and on the results of these will ultimately depend the status of 'vitamin P.'

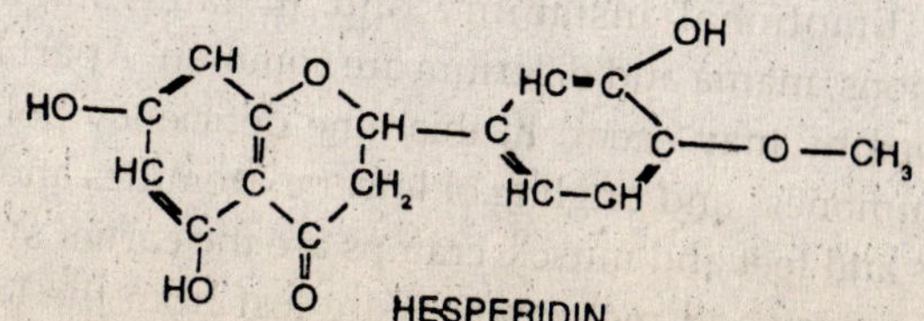

HESPERIDIN

13

Special Diet

During Nervous Disturbances

Research work in the science of nutrition has brought to light a greater relationship between nutrition and the functions of the nervous system. Glucose, B complex vitamins like thiamine, riboflavin, niacin, choline and B6 are essential for normal health of the nervous system. Choline and B6 deficiency affect the impulse-transmitting capacity and produces epilepsy and convulsions if the deficiency is prolonged. Thiamine depleted diets in experimental cases produced irritability, depression and quarrelsome nature. They were suspicious, non-cooperative and fearful in their nature. Administration of thiamine cured all these symptoms. Niacin deficiency produces pellagra. In pellagra nervous disturbances occur. Anxiety, loss of appetite, insomnia, depressions and tension status are the first symptoms of nervous disorder. Emotional instability and in later stage fearful hallucinations, mania and delerium are common. Apart from this encephalopathy may occur. In thiamine deficiency polyneuritis results. Numbness and tingling of lower extremities and burning of the toes and feet and muscle cramps are the earlier symptoms. Later on sensory and motor senses are lost from the legs.

Apart from all these deficiency symptoms dietary treatment is used for mental disorders like convulsion, anorexia nervosa, epilepsy and hysteria and in severe alcoholism.

Epilepsy

In idiopathic epilepsy the central nervous system is affected. This condition is characterised by loss of consciousness for short intervals which is accompanied by severe convulsions and spasms.

A ketogenic diet is very useful in its treatment. In such a diet complication may arise if kidney troubles are present in the patient. A very high fat diet is recommended in a ketogenic diet. The aim of including a ketogenic diet is to produce acidosis by reducing glucose content in the diet. When high fat intake is included it prevents complete combustion of fat and results in the formation of the ketone bodies, acetone, acetoacetic acid and hydroxybutyric acid. Fluid content is reduced leading to progressive dehydration and accumulation of ketone bodies. Since this disease is common among children, it is difficult to implement ketogenic diet because it is unpalatable and deficient in many nutrients. Severe pyridoxine deficiency also produces epileptic form of convulsions and abnormal electroencephalograph especially among children. Administration of high doses of pyridoxine and foods rich in pyridoxine are useful in its treatment. Ketogenic diet is recommended only when drug therapy is not effective in the treatment of epilepsy. About 1 gm of protein/kg of body weight and only 10 gms carbohydrate is allowed in a ketogenic diet. A ketogenic diet is deficient in calcium, iron and in water soluble vitamins, therefore supplements of those nutrients are essential.

Often a patient may feel nausea and vomiting on a ketogenic diet. Sudden transfer from a normal diet produces these symptoms. Gradual change from normal diet to ketogenic diet reduces these symptoms.

Egg, meat, butler, cream, fruits, vegetables, poultry, fish and all other fats are allowed. Preparations with cereals, starchy roots and tubers, sugar, fruits and vegetables rich in carbohydrates are restricted. Milk is not allowed because of its lactose and sugar content. So are desserts and puddings.

Anorexia Nervosa : Prolonged malnutrition and anxiety can produce some other psychiatric disorders and so çareful planning is essential in psychoneuroses, psychosis and addiction. Anorexia nervosa is common among nervous people. Hysterical manifestation and self-imposed starvation to combat emotional conflicts are common among young people, especially in women between 15 and 40 years. Fear, anxiety, conflicting emotion in the patient and immaturity in adolescence are the causes. Rapport with the patient helps to reach the root cause of the symptoms.

Dietary treatment along with psychiatric treatment is essential. Small, hourly feeds of a high protein, high vitaminised fluid diet is recommended. If self-feeding is not possible nasal feeding is essential.

In Alcoholism

Chronic alcoholism may be considered as a psychosomatic disease. Ethanol which is present in ethyl alcohol contains 7 calories per gram and it acts as a drug. Ingestion of ethanol distributes in total body water and blood, body tissues and body secretions are affected. Ingested alcohol is eliminated from the body mainly by oxidation with small quantities appearing in breath and urine.

Alcoholic's metabolic pathways, especially carbohydrates and fat metabolism, are affected adversely if supplementation of other nutrients are not done. Alcoholics have an unduly high requirement of B complex vitamins. Therapeutic doses of B complex vitamins are essential. Alcoholics as a group are peptic ulcer prone and chronic alcoholism results in gastrointestinal disturbances. Alcohol intake is associated with liver changes, especially in the form of fatty liver. Ethanol has an ill-effect upon mobilisation of fatty acids from adipose tissues and often increases the level of plasma non-esterified fatty acids. Hepato toxins produced by alcohol and mainly chloroform and carbon tetrachloride reduce the ability of the liver to secrete lipo proteins. Chronic alcoholism has been associated with deficiency diseases. Prevalence of cirrhosis of liver is often due to deficiency of certain essential nutrients. Protein deficiency produces fatty liver, hypo albuminemia, hypocholesterolemia, oedema, and normocytic anaemia. Vitamin A deficiency occurs most rapidly. Thiamin deficiency is the most common vitamin deficiency which results in ophthalmoplegia, palsy, ataxia, confusion, coma and peripheral neuropathy and often cardiac failure. Cardiac muscle metabolism is affected and lower extremities are badly affected. Depressed tendon reflexes, muscle cramps and weakness, pain and discomfort in the feet also occur.

Riboflavin deficiency is seen in an alcoholic. Dermatitis, angular stomatitis, and cheilosis are common. Pyridoxine deficiency produces convulsions, irritability, insomnia, mild ataxia and skin lesions. Folic acid deficiency produces macrocytive anaemia. Magnesium deficiency is common and potassium deficiency upsets the electrolyte balance.

Dietary Modification in Alcoholism : Deficiency of protein, B complex and minerals are common among alcoholics. Therefore, a well balanced diet high in protein and water soluble vitamins improves the health of an alcoholic. Without an adequate diet the liver of the alcoholics is likely to be damaged. Alcohol stimulates secretion of gastric juice and if enough food is not taken it leads to gastritis. In an empty stomach, if alcohol is consumed, peripheral blood vessels are dilated giving a visible flushing in the skin. Iron is usually accumulated in the body as alcoholic beverages are rich in iron and the drink stimulates iron absorption. Generally the intake of food is decreased and anorexia takes place. Coupled with B vitamin deficiency toxic substances are left out on the nerves which results in alcoholic polyneuropathy. Amnesic syndromes develop gradually. Fatty liver, alcoholic hepatitis, cirrhosis and haemochromatosis, gout and pancreatitis are the diseases common to alcoholics. Dietetic treatment depends on the complication in the person.

In Gout and Osteoarthritis

Gout : Gout is a hereditary disease which occurs mainly among males. This condition is characterised by disturbed purine metabolism and abnormal uric acid deposition in the joints. In the cartilages and articular cartilages of joints sodium-urate is deposited. Recurrent attacks of pain and swelling occur. Over-production or inadequate excretion of uric acid produce this condition. Certain vegetable and animal foods contain nucleo proteins which are broken down to proteins and nucleic acid. One byproduct of such a breadown is purine. Purines are oxidised to uric acid probably in the liver. Apart from this endogenous uric acid or the exogenous uric acid from food sources, the human body can synthesis uric acid from carbon and nitrogen compounds from the metabolic pool. Animal foods and organ meats are rich in uric acid. About 200 to 500 mgs from animal foods and 300 to 600 mgs even from a purine-free diet is derived by the body. Normal serum uric acid level is 3 to 5 mgs per 1 pp ml. But in a gout patient the serum uric acid level is 6 mgs or more per 100 ml of blood from men and 5 mgs per 100 ml for women. Administration of lactose results in decreased urinary urate excretion and serum uric acid level. Fasting increases the uric acid level in normal and gout persons. Little alcohol with low purine diet decreases the urate level in serum but large quantities produce high serum uric acid level. Among vegetarians the occurrence of gout is less.

The uric acid is deposited in and around the joints, the metatarsals, knee and toe joints. In acute and chronic forms gout attacks. Acute attacks are often mentioned as gout arthritis. Monosodium urate monohydrate crystals are formed from the phagocytes during gout attacks. Thus precipitation of urate crystals and leucocytic activity are presumed responsible for gout arthritis. Since the concept of gout is changing, dietary modifications are also changing. In a gout patient's diet purine rich foods are avoided. Fish roe, sweet breads, sardines, meat extracts, soup, herring, salmon, liver, kidney, pomfret, prawns, chicken, meat, green peas, lentils, spinach, mushrooms, cauliflower, brinjals, pulses, oatmeal, custard apple are rich to moderate sources of purine which must be avoided. Coffee and tea contain methylated purines which are oxidised to methyl uric acid, but usually this is excreted through urine. Still coffee and tea are to be minimised. All vegetables and fruits except those mentioned above are allowed. An overweight person must reduce weight; therefore a low calorie diet is recommended; 1,200 to 1,500 kcals are enough.

The protein content must be moderate to low, preferably milk protein, or vegetable proteins are recommended; 40 to 60 gms are harmless. Fats enable the deposition of urates and a low fat diet is recommended. Liberal fluid intake so as to excrete 1,200 ml of urine is recommended. About 3 litres of fluid can be given. Tea or coffee has to be limited to 2 to 3 cups daily. Alcoholic beverages are to be limited because after the ingestion of alcohol gout attacks are common. Beer is very harmful.

A low purine, low fat, low protein diet with moderate calorie content is recommended for a gout or gout arthritis patient. High fluid and vitamin content are essential.

Foods allowed are bread or chapathi or wheat, rice, maize, bajra or ragi, breakfast cereals, rice, egg, milk or milk products, vegetable soups, low purine vegetables, little fat, desserts without cream or much fat, fresh fruits, and pulses (limited amount), meat or fish (permitted items only when there is no gout attack).

Condiments and spices, papad, chutney, pickles and nuts are not allowed. Milk and milk products are restricted.

Osteoarthritis : Osteoarthritis is also known as degenerative arthritis. It is a chronic progressive disorder where the weight-bearing joints are degenerated. It is common among obese people, especially the middle aged. Knees, hips, lumbar and cervical spine are the common places where degenerative changes occur. Weight reduction takes off the strain from joints. Low calorie, low purine, low fat, low protein diet with high fluid and vitamin supplements are recommended.

A Sample Diet for a Gout Patient

Time	Meal
6 a.m.	Milk (skimmed milk)
8 a.m.	Chapathi, Vegetable stew, Coffee (skimmed milk)
10 a.m.	Pineapple juice
12.30 p.m.	Rice or soft chapathi, Dal curry, Amaranth pugath, Buttermilk.
2 p.m.	Barley water
4 p.m.	Vegetable cutlet, Coffee
8 p.m.	Broken wheat gruel, Plantain, Bread pudding (skimmed milk).

In Fevers

Fever may be defined as an elevation of body temperature above normal, i.e., 98.4°F and is the most important sign of an infection. Infection, inflammation or unknown causes manifest themselves as fever. Bacterial or fungi infections, antigen antibody reaction, malignancy or graft rejection are the main causes of it. When an exogenous factor causes fever it activates phagocytes in the bone marrow to release a fever hormone pyrogen. This endogenous hormone induces synthesis of prostaglandins which affect the thermo-regulatory centre in the anterior hypothalamus to increase body temperature. Drugs inhibit prostaglandis synthesis.

Fevers may be classified as (i) Acute, (2) Chronic, and (3) Recurrent.

The acute infections are of strong but short duration and they occur along with colds, pneumonia, influenza, measles, chickenpox, scarlet and typhoid fevers. All these diseases manifest fever as the first symptom. The duration of most acute infectious diseases is reduced by the use of antibodies.

Chronic infections may continue for months and stretch into years. Tuberculosis is an outstanding example. Fever accompanies it.

Recurrent fever is observed in malaria.

Metabolic Changes in Fevers : In most febrile conditions the metabolic rate is increased. The increase in metabolic rate is proportionate to body temperature and the duration of fever. An increase of 7-7.2 per cent in the metabolic rate per degree rise in Farenheit is observed. If the temperature is high about 40 per cent increase in metabolic rate occurs.

Glycogen stores are decreased. And catabolism of proteins is increased. This is very evident in the case of typhoid fever, malaria, typhus fever, polio-myelitis. Nitrogen waste is increased and it exerts a burden on the kidneys.

Water metabolism is also affected. Excessive perspiration and excretion of body waste increases the loss of body water. Electrolytes like sodium and potassium are also lost.

Accumulation of basic products in the body is another characteristic of fever due to infection.

Loss of appetite and nausea and vomiting are the other symptoms of fevers.

General Modification in Diet during Fevers Dietary modifications vary according to the nature and severity of the fever and length of convalescence.

Energy utilisation is high in fevers due to the high metabolic activities. The calorie requirement is increased about 50 per cent. If loss of appetite, nausea and vomiting persist it will be difficult to administer a high calorie diet. High carbohydrate drinks and cereal gruels can be included in frequent small feedings to meet this demand.

In prolonged fever 100 gms of good quality proteins have to be included. Protein supplements can be incorporated in fruit juices. High protein beverages and soups are the other means of high protein liquid sources.

Glycogen stores are depleted and so a liberal intake of carbohydrate is recommended. Glucose can be used for sweetening beverages, starchy gruels also supply carbohydrates.

Even though fats are rich sources of energy, a judicious use of fat is essential as it may interfere with digestion.

Electrolytes, especially sodium choloride, have to be supplemented. Salty juices and soups can meet this demand. Even though potassium is abundantly present in most of the food items, limited food intake restricts its availability and so in prolonged fever it has to be supplemented. Fruits juices and milk beverages can contribute considerable quantities.

Vitamin requirement increases during fever. Vitamin A and ascorbic acid have to be supplemented; B complex vitamins intake have to be adjusted with calorie intake: 0.5 mgs. per 1,000 kcals is the correct requirement.

Fluid intake must be liberal so as to meet the additional loss during fever. At least 3-5 litres of fluid intake is essential.

Modification in food preparation is also necessary. Bland, easily digestible foods must be used for febrile conditions. If it is necessary, a full liquid diet is prescribed. Since it produces abdominal distension a soft diet is more appreciated.

Instead of a four-meal pattern frequent small feedings are recommended.

Typhoid Fever : Typhoid fever is an infectious disease caused by salmonella typhosa and is usually transmitted by drinking water or milk contaminated with intestinal contents or carriers. Improved hygiene and prophylatic public health measures have greatly reduced the incidence. The length of convalescence depends to a great extent on nutritional therapy.

The symptoms include severe headache, high temperature, acute stomach pain, diarrhoea, and peyers patches are found. The intestine is ill-famed.

The body glycogen store is rapidly depleted and energy need is increased. Metabolic rate is increased by 40-50 per cent above the normal. Tissues protein breakdown is about 1/2 to 3/4 pounds of muscle per day. Nitrogen catabolism is three times above the normal.

Dietary Modification : A bland non-irritating diet, low in fibre content, should be given to prevent intestinal irritation. If diarrhoea is not present milk can be used , on the basis of the diet. High fluid content is essential. About 3,500 kcals, 100 gms of protein, and 3,000 ml of fluid is recommended during the febrile period.

Foods Allowed : Milk with barley water and glucose, fruit juices with glucose, strained vegetable juices, milk puddings, cereal gruels, baked fish or minced meat, vegetable purees and thin dal curries are permitted.

A soft or fluid diet is suggested. Small feedings in more intervals are better. All irritating fibres, highly flavoured and spiced food items are harmful since the intestinal tract is inflamed.

Multi-vitamin tablet supplementation is essential. High carbohydrate, high protein beverages and puddings are ideal.

A Sample Menu during Typhoid Fever

Time	*Meal*	*Menu*
6 a.m.		Milk with Complan
8 a.m.	Breakfast	Milk, Poached egg, Bread, Fruit cup.
10 a.m.	Mid-time	Cornflakes in milk
11 a.m.	Mid-time	Orange juice
12.30 Noon	Lunch	Double boiled mashed rice or soft chapathi, Mashed carrot. Dal mashed, Biscuit pudding.
2 p.m.	Mid-time	Eggnog
3 p.m.	Mid-time	Lime juice with glucose
4 p.m.		Egg and cheese sandwich, Tea
6 p.m.		Tomato juice
		Wheat gruel. Mixed vegetable puree, Soft chapathi, Pineapple cocktail.
9 p.m.	-	Complan

Tuberculosis : Tuberculosis is an infectious disease caused by the bacillus mycro bacterium tuberculosis. Usually lungs, lymph nodes and kidneys are affected.

Alimentary tract, lymph nodes of the neck, liver, spleen and bones and joints of children are more affected compared to adults.

Tuberculosis is a highly communicable disease. Congested dwelling and unhygienic living spread this infection. It takes years to manifest the symptoms after the initial attack.

Pulmonary tuberculosis is more common. Pulmonary tuberculosis is an inflamatory disease of the lung.

Symptoms : Wasting of tissues, exhaustion, persistent cough, expectoration and fever are the initial symptoms. Cough which persists for more than two weeks is the warning symptom. Loss of weight, pain in the chest, poor appetite, fatigue and blood-sputum accompany the other symptoms. The chronic phase of the disease is accompanied by low-grade fever.

The most important factor of treatment is complete rest along with drugs and diet. Antibodies are used as drugs.

Dietary Modification : A high calorie, high protein, high vitaminised and mineralised, high fluid soft diet is recommended. Easily digestible, good quality diet reduces strain on the body. Diet plays a key role in the treatment of tuberculosis.

About 500 kcals are required more during the illness. Good quality proteins of 75-80 gms help quick regeneration of serum albumin. Calcium is essential to promote healing of the tuberculous lesions. Iron is also required in high amount to increase the blood volume. Calcium, iron and phosphorus along with other minerals help the overall regeneration of cells, blood and fluids.

Vitamin supplements are also essential. Carotenoids are not converted to vitamin A very effectively. Vitamin C is also essential for many regenerative purposes. Prolonged administration of chemo-therapeutic agents in tuberculosis manifest antagonistic effect on certain B vitamins, especially on B6 folate. Interconversion of glycine and serine are also affected. Peripheral neuritis, characteristic of B6 deficiency, is common among tuberculosis patients. Supplements of these vitamins are essential.

Since most patients have very poor appetite small feedings with more intervals are recommended. Attractive, appetising meals induce appetite.

Milk and egg-based diet is better for a tuberculosis patient. Money cannot be considered as a criteria in the treatment. Liberal intake of citrus fruits and leafy vegetables and protective foods are essential in the dietary of a tuberculosis patient.

A Sample Menu for a Tuberculosis Patient

Time	*Meal*	*Menu*
6 a.m.	_	Milk
8 a.m.	Breakfast	Soft paralhas or idli, Tomato-egg curry or groundnut curry, Poached egg, Complan.
10 a.m.	Mid-time	Water melon juice, Bombay toast
12 Noon	Lunch	Soft chapathi, Dal curry, Fish molee, Rice, Curd, Fruit salad.
2 p.m.	Mid-time	Grape juice
4 p.m.	Tea	Three-layered sandwich (with cheese, scrambled egg and coriander leaves chutney).
6 p.m.	Mid-time	Pineapple milk shake.
8 p.m.	Dinner	Broken wheat gruel, Liver saute, Vegetable puree, Pumpkin chutney, Orange custard.
10 p.m.	Bed time	Proteinex

During Deficiency Diseases

Good wholesome food is essential for normal growth and development Hippocrates, the father of medicine, used food as a remedial agent many centuries ago. Now it is an established fact that food is not only essential for growth but also required for preventing certain diseases. Inadequate intake of essential nutrients and improper utilisation of them leads to deficiency diseases. Body reserves of nutrients are depleted first and normal biochemical reactions are upset later on. Slowly automatic lesions develop and manifestation of malnutrition occurs.. Functional disabilities are followed by fatal conditions in some cases. Deficiency may manifest within weeks to years. Children are more prone to develop deficiencies. If the signs of good nutrition are known it is easy to make a positive diagnosis of most nutritional deficiencies in early stages. Good nutrition is reflected not in the absence of disease alone but in proper physical, emotional and mental conditions of an individual. Well proportioned body with enough fat, proper height and weight for the age, well developed and firm muscles, smooth, clear and slightly moist skin, glossy hair which is neither too glossy nor brittle, smooth nails, clear eyes without dark circles under them, alert and pleasant facial expression, erect posture, broad chest, even shoulders, good natured attitude, sound appetite, digestion, good bowel movement and sleep are the signs of good nutrition. Well-fed people have a general feeling of well-being.

Loss of interest in and appetite for food, loss of weight, poor concentration power, insomnia, irritability, nervousness, frequent infections, sore tongue, mouth, dermatitis, and skin diseases, diarrhoea, constipation, muscular weakness, painful joints and muscles, deformities in the bone, difficulty in seeing in dim light, swollen or congested eyelids, dry eyes and poor general health and retarded growth are symptoms of malnutrition.

Common deficiency diseases are protein-energy malnutrition like kwashiorkor and marasmus, avitaminosis, ariboflavinosis and anaemia.

Protein-Energy Malnutrition : Deficiency of protein and energy during infancy is one of the most serious problems throughout the world. It leads to two clinical syndromes, kwashiorkor and marasmus. These two deficiency conditions are common among infants of lower income groups. It is a common problem of early childhood in India.

Kwashiorkor : This was first observed in 1930 in Asia and Africa. Kwashiorkor is an African word. It means, "the disease of the displaced child". It usually occurs in the first child when a second child is born. Dr. Cicely Williams reported it first from Africa. The disease is usually caused when the child is weaned from breastfeeding to foods. The foods given to a weaned child contain plenty of carbohydrates but little of proteins. Since growth is rapid and protein is essential to meet the requirement, retardation of growth occurs. Kwashiorkor is usually observed in infants between 1 and 3 years of age.

The first main symptom of kwashiorkor is lack of growth in children. Gastro-intestinal disturbances with anorexia, nausea and diarrhoea are common and enzymatic action of digestion is poor. Swelling of the body, especially on the hands, feet and face will be seen. The hair and skin show characteristic changes. Hair may be tight coloured or dispigmented to reddish yellow and fall off in patches. Skin shows patches and becomes flaky and peels off. Hyperpigmentation and dispigmentation are common.

Changes occur in the structure and functional efficiency of liver. Liver may become palpable and soft. Fatty infiltration and enlargement of the liver, fibrosis and cellular necrosis are common. Due to liver disorder protruded bellies are common. Biochemical changes in the body fluids, in the composition of blood, utilisation of amino acids, electrolyte imbalance and anaemia are common among kwashiorkor children. The child becomes apathetic and all functions of proteins are impaired. Pancreas shows atrophic changes and internal activities of the body are upset. Histological changes occur in the small intestine. The mucosa of the intestine become thin and villi is flattened; atrophy of villi is common. Enzyme activity in the intestine is diminished and disaccharides are not properly assimilated. Fat is not transported through the intestine which results in fat deposition in the cells, Triglycerides level in the blood is increased. Potassium is depleted from body fluids and muscles; magnesium deficiency is also common. Bacterial and viral infections occur in kwashiorkor children as their persistence power is low. Evidence of vitamin deficiency co-exists with protein deficiency condition.

The mortality is high in the absence of proper treatment. The rate of mortality depends upon the degree of fatty infiltration and degree of malnutrition in the child. Infections, other deficiencies, hepatic coma, low potassium level in the serum, or cardiac failure cause death. Though kwashiorkor occurs all over the country, the degree of severity is not the same in all places. It is mostly seen in the southern states of India.

Studies on protein calorie malnutrition by the National Institute of Nutrition has brought to light that the disabilities affected by it are not only on physical growth but also on brain development. Apathy, irritability, listlessness, psychomotor retardation, reduced attention and concentration, low decision-making and problem-solving capacity manifest poor brain development. Psychological development of a malnourished child is poor. Severe protein-calorie malnutrition during infancy can cause permanent and irreversible structural lesion in the central nervous system. Reduced brain size and weight decrease the brain cells. Language development is delayed and malnourished children show poor learning abilities and low scholastic achievements. Poor performance in intelligence tests is common. As the brain development is rapid at pre-school age protein malnutrition can cripple if enough of it is not given during infancy.

A Sample Diet for Kwashiorkor Child

Time	*Meal*	*Menu*
6.30 a.m.		Milk (Skimmed Milk)
8 a.m.	Breakfast	Rava porridge, Boiled groundnut
10 a.m.	Mid-time	Ragi porridge, Gingelly seed laddu

Time	*Meal*	*Menu*
12 Noon	Lunch	Dal rice or soft chapathi, Scrambed egg or egg curry, Vegetable puree, Guava.
2 p.m.	Mid-time	Tender coconut water
4 p. m.	Tea	Soyabean milk, Mixed flour biscuit
6 p.m.	Mid-time	Green soup
8 p.m.	Dinner	Soft chapathi, Fish molee
9 p.m.	Bed time	Milk

Marasmus : Marasmus is due to severe deficiency of proteins and calories in the diet. It is not due to calorie deficiency alone because marasmic children subsequently develop kwashiorkor.' In both the cases protein and calorie deficiencies are present but the degree of protein or calorie deficiency results in kwashiorkor or in marasmus. The clinical picture of marasmus is basically due to lack of calorie intake though protein inadequacy is present. Loss of body weight and failure in weight gain and gradual emaciation occurs. Body fat is depleted, muscles are wasted. The child shows the appearance of a withered old man. Ribs and bones stand out and the abdomen may be distended or sunken. The body temperature is subnormal and the child may have starvation type of diarrhoea. The marasmic child is characterised by its thin, lean and skinny appearance whereas a kwashiorkor child is flabby with oedema.

The Treatment

Kwashiorkor is common among children from low socio-economic group. Prevention and cure include measures whereby highly nutritious low-cost diets are provided for them. Protein foods based on blends of soyabeans, groundnut, cottonseed, legume flour with cereal powders and protein-enriched cereals are recommended for practical purpose. A high calorie, high protein, high vitaminised and mineralised diet with high fluid is recommended for kwashiorkor child. The daily requirement is 90 to 100 kcals per kilogramme of body weight. In this 20 per cent of calories must be from protein sources. In hospitalised cases skimmed milk powder is used for the treatment of kwashiorkor as the main source of protein. Vegetable protein mixtures from various pulses, cereals or millet combinations are evolved by the National Institute of Nutrition (NIN) for the treatment of kwashiorkor. Groundnut milk, dried beans and pulses, small fish, organ meats like liver or brain can be used liberally in the diet of a kwashiorkor child. Ragi halwa, wheat kheer, bajra pongal, idli, uppuma, sweet potato or potato porridge, gram laddu, and green vegetable soups are some of the protein-rich low-cost items. Meal plan for an infant must have some form of milk on rising and cooked cereal pulse preparation for breakfast. Soft-boiled egg or fruit juice can be given to an infant at mid-time. This can be substituted by a millet-pulse porridge and green vegetable soup. For lunch, cooked cereals, or starchy vegetables or millets can be cooked. Boiled pulses, fish or minced meat or organ meats can be included depending upon the economic status. During mid-afternoon, supplements like fish liver oil or sources of vitamins and minerals from cheap sources can be included. For dinner, cereals like suji, broken wheat or ragi can be used as porridge. And before bed-time milk from any source or its substitutes can be given. Indian Multipurpose Food (MPF), malt food, Bal-ahar and supplementary foods are the commercial protein foods developed for kwashiorkor treatment by CFTRI, NIN and AHSCW (Avinashilingam Home Science College for Women). MPF is a blend of low fat groundnut flour and bengal gram fortified with vitamins A and D, thaimine, riboflavin and calcium carbonate. This formula contains 42 per cent of protein. Three different forms of MPF are available: one seasoned with masala which can be incorporated in curries or in soups, unseasoned which can be incorporated with flours and unseasoned with milk powder which is a substitute for milk. CFTRI has conducted studies with pre-school children and they have recorded highly significant improvement in the nutritional status of the pre-school children with the use of MPF.

Malt Food: This is another product of CFTRI where a blend of cereal malt (40%) and low fat groundnuts (40%) and roasted bengal gram flour (20%) is fortified with vitamins and calcium salts. This provides 28 per cent good quality proteins and is comparatively cheap.

Bal-ahar: Bal-ahar is another product of CFTRI, a blend of whole wheat flour (70%), groundnut flour (20%) and roasted bengal gram flour (10%), fortified with calcium salts and vitamins. This contains about 20 per cent proteins. Vitamin A, riboflavin and calcium are present in appreciable amounts.

Supplementary Foods: NIN has developed supplementary foods for the treatment of protein calorie malnutrition. Supplementary food is a blend of roasted wheat flour (30%), green gram flour (20%), groundnut (8%), and sugar or jaggery (20%). This supplement provides 12.5 per cent proteins and has proved effective in the treatment of kwashiorkor.

Sri Avinashilingam Home Science College for Women is engaged in extension activities among rural people. One of its projects is to impart nutrition education to rural women. They have developed a low cost supplementary food based on maize which is known as "Kuzhandai Amudhu". It is a blend of maize flour (30%), green gram flour (20%), roasted groundnut (10%), and jaggery (20%). This supplement supplies 14.4 per cent proteins and has brought significant improvement in growth rate and nutritional status of pre-school children.

A Sample Diet for a Marasmic Child

Time	*Meal*	*Menu*
6.30 a.m.		Milk
8 a.m.	Breakfast	Sweetened mixed flour chapathi, Soft boiled egg, Plantain
9 a.m.	Mid-time	Sago porridge
10 a.m.	Mid-time	Vegetable soup

Time	Meal	Menu
12 Noon	Lunch	Soyabean pulao, Sprouted green gram raita, Fruit salad
2 p.m.	Mid-time	Ragi porridge
4 p.m.	Tea	Gingelly seed laddu, Ripe mango
6 p.m.	Mid-time	Groundnut milk, Carrot halwa
8 p.m.	Dinner	Wheat gruel, Green peas saute, Guava
9 p.m.	Bedtime	Groundnut Milk

Prevention of Protein Calorie Malnutrition : Prevalence of malnutrition is due to various causes. Ignorance about the importance of pre-school nutrition and the non-availability of low cost nutritious foods are considered important reasons for kwashiorkor and marasmus. Nutrition education on these aspects assumes special significance in the prevention of malnutrition. Food fads and faulty food habits are stumbling blocks in improving the nutritional status of pre-school children. Prolonged breastfeeding up to the age of 2 to 3 years is common in rural areas. Proper emphasis is not given on weaning or supplementary foods for pre-school children. The infant is exposed to an adult diet and deficiencies are the result. Nutrition education must be related to supplies available in local conditions and dietary habits. Customs based on traditional habits are difficult to change. Only sincere efforts from various sources can bring gradual changes.

Anaemia : Anaemia is a condition in which there is reduction in the haemoglobin content of blood. This is due to a reduction in the number of blood cells or size of the red blood cells or due to defective maturation of the red blood cells. There is continuous degeneration and building up of blood cells in our body. The normal lifespan of a red blood cell is about 120 days. Building up of red cells and their maintenance require certain nutrients. Deficiency of any of these nutrients leads to anaemia. Iron, protein, B vitamins like B 12, folic acid, vitamin C and copper deficiency can produce anaemia. Diarrhoea, sprue or pellagra and low acidity of stomach glands affect the normal absorption and utilisation of iron. Malaria, hookworm infestation and other intestinal parasites or chemical agents like coal-tar products interfere with red blood cells concentration in the blood. Exposure to X-rays or radium, bone tumours, cirrhosis of the liver, carcinoma and leukaemias interfere with red blood cells formation. Haemorrhage due to extravascular blood loss from peptic ulcer, bleeding piles, excessive menstrual flow, aesophagal varies and hernia also can produce anaemia. Infancy, adolescence, pregnancy and lactation are special phases where anaemia is common due to rapid growth. Closely spaced pregnancies and prolonged breastfeeding may also result in anaemia. If phylates, phosphates and oxalates are present in the diet in large amounts they interfere with iron absorption which results in anaemia. Generally only 10 per cent of ingested iron is absorbed because of this.

Normally 100 ml of blood contains 14 to 15 gms of haemoglobin. When the haemoglobin content is below 12.5 gms the person is considered anaemic. About half the pregnant women in our country are anaemic and one out of every four maternal deaths is due to anaemia. In India 50 to 60 per cent of children and about 80 per cent of adolescents are anaemic.

Modification of the Diet : The cause of anaemia should be discovered before treatment. Diet alone is not enough as its causes are many. A well-balanced diet with high protein, iron, vitamin C and B complex must be accompanied with ferrous sulphate supplements. If diet is used as the only treatment for anaemia restoration of normal haemoglobin level it is a slow process. Since undernutrition is the cause of anaemia which is due to prolonged poor appetite, during treatment planning of diet must be from carefully selected best sources of nutrients. Sustained diet therapy is essential to regain normal health. Those who can afford organ meats can include it as they are excellent sources of iron. Liver, kidney and bone marrow in any form are the best sources to get iron. Dried fruits like raisins, currants, dates, dried Figs, prunes and molasses, green leafy vegetables, drumsticks, green mango, solanum torvem, soyabeans, rice bran, gingelly seeds, watermelon, peaches, passion fruit and chiku fruit are excellent sources of iron. Egg is also a good source of iron and protein and can be taken by those who can afford it.

Pernicious Anaemia : Pernicious anaemia is not due to the deficiency of iron or other blood-cell-forming substances. This is caused by the lack of intrinsic factor in the stomach which is essential for-the absorption of vitamin B 12 in the intestines. As a result red blood cells are not produced in the bone marrow after the old ones die.

In pernicious anaemia the red blood cell (RBC) count is low which is about 1.5 to 2.5 million per mm of blood where the normal count is 4.5 to 5.5 million of RBC. In pernicious anaemia the RBC are big in size and so it is also known as macrocytic anaemia. Haemoglobin content is as low as 7 to 9 per cent. The patient of this type of anaemia has lemon yellow pallor. Poor digestion and low hydrochloric acid secretion reduces the appetite and results in general weakness, sore tongue and glazed alimentary tract. If neglected, it will lead to numbness in the limbs and difficulty in walking. Slowly it progresses into anorexia or spasticity.

Dietary Modifications : A well balanced diet with B 12 supplementation is essential. Supplementation of liver extracts was found very effective in the treatment of pernicious anaemia. A high protein diet of 100 to 150 gms of protein with a high calorie diet is recommended. Fat content must be reduced because of the low hydrochloric acid secretion in the stomach. Liberal intake of minerals and vitamins and supplements of iron are recommended. Since anorexia or irritation of the gastro-intestinal tract and sore throat are present a soft or liquid diet is recommended. Refer to soft diet given earlier for meal planning.

Underweight

A person who eats little for a long period looks emaciated and shows underweight. Living habitually on an inadequate diet, especially of protein, results in low body weight. When food intake is 2/3 to 3/4 of the requirement among poor people the body weight is reduced up to 25 per cent. Underweight also results from debilitating diseases like tuberculosis, diabetes, malabsorption syndrome or cancer. Infections are common among them. Basal metabolic rate, resistance to infection and voluntary activities are reduced considerably, psychological efficiency as a whole is reduced and their power for concentration and decision-making and withstanding calamities are very poor. Internal structure and functional capacity of various organs is reduced due to deficiencies of essential nutrients. Extreme tissue wasting, depletion of adipose tissues, oedema, disturbed renal function and diarrhoea are common among such persons. Working efficiency is poor and the productivity is less. Lack of nourishment makes the worker inactive and weak. An undernourished person becomes weak and cannot work continuously for a long period.

Dietary Modifications : A high calorie, high protein, high fat diet with liberal vitamin intake is recommended. Depending upon the activities, the energy requirements vary. Along with the normal requirement an additional 500 kcals per day is recommended. Instead of 1 gm of protein 1.2 gm protein/kg of body weight is recommended. Good quality protein is completely utilised by the body and as far as possible best protein sources must be liberally included in the initial stage.

Even though fat content is increased, easily digestible fats are to be included. Fried foods are not suggested in the beginning as the patient may develop diarrhoea. Apart from this, fatty foods reduce appetite and so their intake is not advisable. High carbohydrate sources must form the basis of the diet. Dried fruits, sweets, nuts, desserts, preserves like jam, jelly, cereals, non-vegetarian foods and roots are rich sources of energy and these can be liberally included in an underweight person's diet. Since the persons were used to taking small quantities of food the number of meals has to be increased. Two-hourly feeds incorporating soups, juices or sweets in between major meals improve the nutritive value of the diet. Easily digestible forms are suggested for an underweight person. Porridge with milk and honey, cutlets, desserts, potato chips, high protein drinks like milk, punch, malted milk, eggnog, fruit punch, banana stew and enriched milk drinks can be used in the meal planning. Thick soups and fruit whips with honey are easily digestible and highly nutritious items.

Regular exercises enable one to stimulate appetite. Enough fluid must be taken so as to avoid constipation. Good dietary habits and healthy living promote weight gain. If there are any diseases or parasite infestation in the body they must be treated simultaneously. Synthetic drinks, saccharine, and salty tit-bits like popcorns, soft drinks, other aerated drinks, alcohol, too much coffee or tea and smoking reduce appetite and an underweight person must avoid all these. Emotional well-being is essential to have a good appetite.

A Sample Diet for an Underweight Person

Time	*Meal*	*Menu*
6 a.m.	Bed coffee	Coffee
8 a.m.	Breakfast	Poori, Egg-tomato curry, Apple, Tea
10 a.m.	Mid-time	Rava porridge or chapathi
12 Noon	Lunch	Vegetable pulao, fish cutlet, Sprouted green gram, raita ice-cream
2 p.m.	Mid-time	Green soup
4 p.m.	Tea	Tea, Egg pakoda, Grapes
6 p.m.	Mid-time	Groundnut milk
8 p.m.	Dinner	Chapathi, Vegetable kurma
9 p.m.	Bed time	Horlicks

14

Specific Nutrition

During Pregnancy

Pregnancy is a normal physiological phase where rapid growth of foetus takes place in the mother's womb. The foetus in mother's uterus grows more rapidly than after birth. The zygote develops into a seven-pound baby within 9 months. At the time of birth, the infant is generally 9 months old. Optimum development of the infant is necessarily a function of parental diet. Inadequate maternal nutrition results in low birth weight of the infant and high depletion of mother's body reserves of nutrients. Premature death, maternal death and low vitality of the infants are due to poor nutritional status of pregnant mothers.

Before pregnancy a woman needs nutrients for growth and maintenance of her body. Good nutrition keeps her healthy. During pregnancy additional requirement for all nutrients occurs to enable the foetus to grow normally in the uterus. A full-term infant has about 300 ml of blood, 500 gms of proteins, 30 gms calcium, 15 gms phosphorus and about 300 to 400 gms of iron. Apart from these foetal reserves in the body, the pregnant mother needs nutrients for the development of the uterus, breasts, placenta, amniotic fluids and reserves for parturition. A full-term pregnant mother gains about 10 to 12 kg body weight and only an adequate diet can provide the nutrients for the normal weight gain. If the pregnant mother is underweight the infant born would be small in size and low in birth weight. Infectious diseases and infant mortality rate are common among such infants. Like underweight, overweight among pregnant mothers is not desirable. Overweight at the beginning of pregnancy or an excessive rate of weight gain during the second and third trimester results in pre-eclampsia and eclampsia. Correct weight gain during pregnancy is 1.5 kg in the first three months and 1.5 kg and a little more during the last two trimesters. Sudden changes in weight gain or weight loss are harmful.

The Complications

Nausea and Vomiting : Morning sickness like nausea and vomiting are common in early pregnancy. They may continue in some women till later stages of pregnancy. Even though the aetiology is not clear mental stress or emotional disturbance aggravate the situation. Diminished secretion of hydrochloride acid brings heartburn and gastric distress. Mild morning sickness can be controlled by consuming high carbohydrate foods such as biscuits or crackers. Small meals must be taken to help digestion. Fatty foods like sweets, fried items and strongly flavoured vegetables must be reduced, besides minimising coffee or tea.

Constipation : In the second and third trimesters constipation occurs among pregnant mothers. The amount of pressure exerted by the developing foetus on the digestive tract, lack of enough exercise and thiamine deficiency are the causes of constipation among pregnant mothers. Lack of fluid, fibre and bulk or cellulose also lead to constipation. If purgatives are used, excessive potassium is lost and this can lead to constipation. Excessive use of irritating foods, fried items and emotional distress affect the normal bowel evacuation and result in constipation. Liberal intake of fruits, wholegrain cereals, leafy vegetables, other vegetables and fluids and a happy mental attitude are suggested to avoid constipation.

Toxemia : Toxemia occurs most commonly among patients who are overweight at the time of conception and during pregnancy. Pregnant mothers with underweight at conception and who fail to gain enough weight during pregnancy also manifest it. Excessive protein, salt and vitamin C metabolism in the body cause toxemia. Poor nutritional status also contributes to toxemia of varying degrees. During toxemia oedema, hypertension, albuminuria and convulsions occur. Kidney or heart diseases can manifest symptoms of toxemia. Sodium is restricted to 200 to 800 gms depending upon the condition and just enough protein is suggested.

Anaemia : About half the number of pregnant women in our country are anaemic. One out of every four maternal deaths are due to anaemia.

Complications of pregnancy, both foetal and maternal, can take place in an anaemic mother. The maximum rate of growth in a baby occurs before birth, in the fourth month of foetal life. Maternal malnutrition, especially anaemic condition, affects the growth of the foetus. Foetus grows from 15 gms of its weight at 12th week to 3,200 gms around the 40th week. Infants of anaemic mothers are frequently born with a subnormal iron store. Still birth, premature birth, toxemia of pregnant mother and various infections and diseases of the newborn infants occur if the mother is anaemic. A pregnant woman is termed as anaemic if from 28th week onwards the haemoglobin level is less than 10 gms per 100 ml of blood. The normal haemoglobin level is 15 gms per 100 ml of blood. Even if it is above 12.5 gms per 100 ml of blood the person is not considered anaemic. Poor loss due to any cause can also result in anaemia. Apart from rich sources of proteins, iron, vitamin C, folic acid and B 12, copper and molybdenum, supplements of iron, that is, 30 mgs of elemental iron per day, after the first trimester of pregnancy prevent anaemia.

Diabetes in Pregnancy : A diabetic woman who is pregnant requires additional nutrients. So she has to adjust the insulin dosage. Glycogen depletion, hypoglycaemia, acidosis and frequent infections are the complications that occur in her. Milk secretion also fails in a diabetic mother.

Dietary Recommendations in Pregnancy **:** During pregnancy energy allowance should be increased so as to support the growth of the foetus, placenta, maternal tissues and for the increase in basal metabolic rate. During the first trimester 5 per cent BMR and during the second and third trimesters 12 per cent BMR increase takes place. For an Indian woman with 45 kgs weight the total energy lost of pregnancy is about 62,500 kcals. Some energy is deposited as fat during pregnancy for lactating period. Additional intake of 300 kcal/day during the second and third trimesters is the recommendation of the ICMR Committee in 1981. Besides, 35 gms of cereals and 10 gms of sugar or jaggery must be added to the normal balanced diet to derive the extra energy.

Protein intake must be increased for the development of the foetus and placenta and for naccessary maternal tissue formation; 14 gms of protein along with the normal requirement will satisfy the demands of protein in the second and third trimesters of pregnancy. An additional quantity of 15 gms of pulses and 100 ml of milk along with the normal requirement will furnish the extra demands of protein.

Additional requirement of fat is not necessary during pregnancy. Since the foetal organs, especially the liver and brain, contain phospholipids rich in essential fatty acids, a normal balanced diet satisfies this demand.

During pregnancy minerals like calcium, phosphorus and iron are required more. A full grown foetus has about 25 to 30 gms of calcium. Most of the calcium deposition occurs during the last two months of pregnancy. The first set of teeth begins to form in the foetus in the eighth week. But its calcification starts just before birth—0.5 gm of calcium is recommended during the second half of pregnancy. Phosphorus allowance must be equal to that of calcium.

During pregnancy about 400 mgs of iron for haemoglobin

formation and more than 240 mgs of iron for storage in the foetus are required. Loss of iron through the placenta and blood during parturition are about 90 mgs. To meet all this iron requirement during pregnancy 8 mgs of iron per day is additionally recommended. Iodine, an essential constituent of thyroxine, must be supplied in enough quantities to prevent goitre in infants and pregnant mothers.

All vitamins are required in additional quantities during the gestation period. But for most of the vitamins the exact amount needed in additional quantities is not known. Intake of 400 I.U. of vitamin D as against 200 I.U. of normal amount is recommended. If a well balanced diet is taken, enough vitamin C and riboflavin will be supplied. Thiamine requirement is related to energy consumption and 0.5 mg per 1000 kcal is enough during pregnancy also. Based on the observation that urinary excretion of metabolites of tryptophan is higher in pregnant mothers it is assumed that conversion of the amino acid into niacin is more and 2 mgs more of niacin is recommended during pregnancy to about 200 mgs and it is difficult to supply it through food sources alone. So supplements with folate is essential. About 0.5 mg of B 12 a day is recommended during pregnancy.

The requirement of various nutrients during pregnancy is given along with balanced diets. Five or six small feeds are better than three or four meals so as to avoid fullness in the stomach. Leafy vegetables, fruits, other vegetables and fluids tend to maintain normal bowel evacuation. Rich, highly spiced and fried foods, heavy desserts, rich gravies and excessive amounts of salts must be avoided not to gain excessive weight. It is better to use jaggery instead of sugar as it contains more iron.

Due to tradition and habits many food fads are prevailing in our country. In the light of nutritional knowledge many of these food fads were proved to be prevalent without any scientific basis. Many mistaken beliefs still prevent pregnant mothers from consuming very useful foodstuffs. For example, in South India papaya, which is an excellent source of vitamin A, is avoided for fear of abortion. In the same way pumpkin and jackfruit which are good sources of carotene (vitamin A) are avoided, being classified as hot foods. In certain places, the quantity of food eaten during pregnancy is cut down stating that delivery will be difficult. Wheat, jaggery, meat, fish, eggs, mangoes, tea and coffee are also tabooed as hot foods. There is not scientific basis in such beliefs and a pregnant mother can consume all foods like a normal woman. The composition of a balanced diet during pregnancy includes additional quantities such as 35 gms of cereals, 15 gms of pulses, 100 ml of milk or milk products and 10 gms of sugar or jaggery. For non-vegetarians some modification is normal.

A Sample Diet during Pregnancy

Time		*Meal*		*Menu*
Time 6.30	-	Bed coffee	-	Coffee
8 a.m.	-	Breakfast	-	Chapathi, Dal curry, Soyabean milk, Guava
10 a.m.	-	Mid-morning	-	Lime Juice
12.30 Noon	-	Lunch		Vegetable pulav, Sprouted green gram salad, Curry-leaves chutney, Lassi
2.30 p.m.	-	Mid-time		Tender coconut water
4 p.m.	-	Tea	-	Tea, Moong dal laddoos
6 p.m.			-	Amaranth soup
8 p.m.	-			Chappathi, Liver-tomato curry, Cucumber salad, Fruit cup.
9 p.m.	-		-	Milk.
This diet provides		Calories		2,600 kcals
		Proteins		62 gms.
		Calcium		1.4 gms.
		Iron		45 mgms.

Composition of Balanced Diet during Pregnancy

Items		*Quantity*
Cereals	—	475 gms
Pulses	—	55 gms
Leafy vegetables	—	100 gms
Other vegetables	—	40 gms
Root and tubers	—	50 gms
Milk and milk products	—	250 ml
Oils and fats	—	40 gms
Fruits	—	60 gms
Sugar and jaggery	—	40 gms

During Lactation

The nutritional link between the mother and the child continues even after birth. The newborn baby depends for some period solely on breast milk for its sustenance. Unfortunately, most of the modern mothers do not want to breastfeed their children because they fear that they will lose their shape and charm. But breastfeed is not only the birthright of the baby, but proper emptying of breasts reduces the chances of mastitis and even of breast cancer. Studies have shown that mothers who have never fed their children have higher rate of malignancy. Nutritionists are of the opinion that there is no food equivalent to breast milk for a newborn baby. Nature has designed it to be a complete food for the first few months of a baby's life. Breast milk immunises the baby against infection also. To secrete enough milk for the baby the mother should have nutritious foods. Nutritional needs of a lactating mother are higher than that of a pregnant mother. The quality and quantity of breast milk depends on maternal diet. In an inadequate diet the quality of mother's milk is maintained by drawing the nutrients from her body reserves and from tissues and bones. That is why the milk secreted by poor women is equal in its nutritive content to that of lactating mothers from developed countries of the world. The diets consumed by many lactating mothers in our country are very poor. A lactating mother requires more calories so as to secrete enough milk and to meet the high BMR during this period. The ICMR recommends about 550 kcal/day additionally during the first 6 months and 400 kcal/day from 6 to 12 months for a lactating mother. An average of 600 ml of milk is secreted by a lactating mother in India. About 420 kcals are supplied through this milk. The efficiency of conversion of diet calories to human milk calories is only 60 per cent.

The human milk contains 7.2 gms of milk protein and 14.4 gms of protein is required to produce so much milk protein. Therefore, 25 gms of additional protein per day is recommended for a lactating mother during the first six months of lactation. The calcium content of breast milk of Indian mothers are about 30 to 40 mgs/100 ml and to meet the additional needs 500 mgs of calcium is recommended along with the normal requirements of 500 mgs. Thus 1 gm of calcium is recommended for a lactating mother.

The concentration of iron in breast milk is about 0.72 mg/600 ml. During lactation menstruation is not common, thus about 1 mg of iron is saved. So iron is not recommended by the ICMR committee for a lactating mother. But care must be taken to provide a balanced diet to meet the normal iron requirement. Since our Indian diets are predominantly based upon cereals, the high phytate content interferes with iron absorption. Good calcium and vitamin C ratio can minimise this phytate interference but our diets are again deficient in these nutrients.

The quantity of vitamin A in 600 ml human milk is 300 mgs and to meet this requirement 300 μ gm (Microgram) of retinol or 1600 μgm carotene is recommended by the committee.

The quantity of ascrobic acid in human milk is only 15-30 mgs. ICMR committee recommended an additional 40 mgs of vitamin C per day. The thiamine content in breast milk is 60 μgms per 600 ml. Depending upon the energy requirements thiamine demand varies. The normal requirement of 0.5 mgm per 1000 kcals is applicable to lactating mother also. For riboflavin an additional recommendation of 0.3 mg/ day is enough to meet the needs of a lactating mother. The niacin requirements during lactation is 4 mgms additional to normal requirements. Increased fluid intake is recommended during lactation period to enable the normal functions in the body. There are no foods which require restriction as it is customary in various parts of India based on food fads and fallacies. A lactating mother requires adequate nutrition for the proper development of the baby.

The composition of a balanced diet during lactation is based on the characteristic of a normal person. Additional requirements must be met by making slight variations in the intake of food groups. The ICMR committee of 1981 recommended an additional intake of 60 gms of cereals, 30 mgs of pulses, 100 ml of milk, 10 gms of fat and 10 gms of sugar. These additional quantities of various foodstuffs supply about 521 kcals besides 25 gms of protein and other requirements by the body during lactation. If such a diet is consumed, a lactating mother can produce enough milk for the baby without affecting her health.

Composition of Balanced Diet for a Sedentary Lactating Mother

Foodstuff		*Quantities*
Cereals	-	500 gms
Pulses	-	70 gms
Leafy vegetables	-	100 gms
Other vegetables	-	40 gms
Roots and tubers	-	50 gms
Milk and milk products	-	250 ml
Oils and fats	-	50 gms
Fruits	-	60 gms
Sugar and jaggery	-	40 gms

During Old Age

Good nutrition throughout the life serves as a sound insurance for health for the years of old age. The process of aging brings about marked physiological changes in the body. Inadequate dentition, diminished sensitivity to taste and smell, diminished secretion of hydrochloric acid in the stomach and digestive enzymes, biliary impairment, if any, which interferes with fat digestion, irregular bowel evacuation, general ill-health, economic or emotional insecurity and unwanted feelings are some of the problems common among old people. Diseases of old age like diabetes, hypertension and other heart diseases also pose more problems to them. In modern society, with nuclear families, problems of old age are varied. In a joint family, old people are wanted and respected and they enjoy their position. But in our modern society old people often feel neglected and psychological problems created by this reflects as many ailments. Loss of appetite is a common complaint of old people.

Nutrition requirements of old change from normal adult requirements. The lowered metabolic rate reduces the caloric requirement by about 25 per cent compared with normal adults. Physical activity is also less compared to a normal person. If an old person has normal body weight adequate calories can be given. For obese people the calorie intake should be adjusted to reduce body weight whereas for underweight persons the calorie intake should be enough to bring them to normal weight. For a normal sedentary worker 2,100 kcals for males and 1,700 kcals for females are enough to maintain normal condition.

Protein deficiency is common among old people. Protein-splitting enzymes like pepsin, trypsin and erepsin are mild in their action and so protein is not digested properly. Absorption of nutrients is poor among old people due to changes in intestinal wall. Loss of appetite and difficulty in chewing and masticating food must be supplied to old people to provide 1.5 gms of protein per kg of body weight. Though pulses are rich sources of protein, they produce flatulence among old people. Cooking methods adopted for geriatric people must be like steaming or boiling, making food easily digestible. Fat digestion is difficult and delayed in old age. Moreover, cholesterol level could be high among old people and so it is better to avoid saturated fat from animal sources, coconut and palm oil. Vegetable oils reduce the blood cholesterol level and 40 to 50 gms of such fats or oils can be used.

Assimilation of minerals is poor in old people compared to a normal person. Osteoperosis and anaemia are common among elderly people. Poor absorption of minerals and hormonal imbalance, especially of androgen and oestrogen, produce osteoperosis in old people. About 0.8 to 1.00 gm of calcium and 30 to 40 mgms of iron are recommended for them. Chronic arthritis and hypoactivity of the thyroid diminishes the activity of bone marrow which results in anaemia. Generally vegetables, raw vegetables or fruits are consumed in less amounts by old people which produces signs and symptoms of various vitamin deficiencies. B complex vitamin deficiency is common and along with a good diet a multi-vitamin supplement is essential.

Fluid intake must be liberal so as to form 1 to 1.5 litres of urine daily. Since many renal diseases are common among old people proper urine output must be checked. Only proper urine formation eliminates the urea, uric acid and other metabolic by products.

Since constipation is a common complaint of this age bulk or roughage must be included in the diet. Too much of refined carbohydrate foods, sweets and juices lack bulk and produce constipation. Muscle tone of the intestine is reduced and physical activities are also less, so only roughage in the diet can stimulate the intestinal movements.

For non-vegetarians the amount of milk is reduced to 400 ml and pulses to 55 gms for males and 45 gms for females. One multi-vitamin mineral tablet is recommended for them. Individual variation is common among old people depending on their health status.

Nutrition of Workers : Requirement of various nutrients for labourers and industrial workers differ from normal adults.

Calories, thiamine and riboflavin requirements are high. Working efficiency of a person depends to a great extent on the pattern of diet consumed. To get the maximum output a labourer must have adequate diet. Manual work demands more energy and to assimilate energy sources properly B vitamins are essential. Energy requirement varies according to the climatic condition and pattern of work, that is, whether under the sun or inside a factory.

Composition of Balanced Diet for Geriatrics Over 60 Years

Food Stuffs	*Males*	*Females*
Cereals	320 gms	220 gms
Pulses	70 gms	55 gms
Green leafy vegetables	100 gms	125 gms
Other vegetables	75 gms	75 gms
Roots and tubers	75 gms	50 gms
Fruits	75 gms	50 gms
Milk	600 ml	600 ml
Fats and oils	30 gms	30 gms
Sugar and jaggery	30 gms	30 gms

Protein requirement is not increased for labourers, but if the energy requirement is not met from energy sources proteins are utilised for energy purpose. Climatic conditions again affect the protein requirements, for, instance, about 50 per cent more proteins are required in cold climate.

Vitamins must be present in adequate amount in the diet. Thiamine is essential to maintain normal appetite because deficiency of it interferes with metabolism of carbohydrate. Therefore, 0.5 mg of thiamine per 1,000 kcals is the required amount. Riboflavin and niacin are also required in good amount to enable proper utilisation of energy.

Minerals like calcium, phosphorus and iron must be the same as in the diet of a normal adult. Adequate nutrition ensures working efficiency. Undernourished persons reduce their voluntary activity. An anaemic person cannot work hard or concentrate on anything. His output is low and this yields low income. Purchasing capacity of such people is low and as a result they buy foods insufficient for the family and consume inadequate diet. Inadequate nourishment brings ill-health and this cycle is continued. Low-cost foods can be substituted for high-cost ones. But often people are not aware of the cheap nutritious sources which can nourish them well. Nutrition education is essential to select low-cost foods like roots and millets like ragi or jowar, cowgram, horsegram, soyabeans, cluster beans, groundnuts, leafy vegetables, amla, papaya and locally available vegetables and fruits.

Composition of Balanced Diet for Labourers or Industrial Workers

Food Stuffs	*Male*	*Female*
Cereals	630 gms	575 gms
Pulses	80 gms	60 gms
Green leafy vegetables	125 gms	100 gms
Other vegetables	100 gms	100 gms
Roots and tubers	100 gms	100 gms
Fruits	60 gms	60 gms
Milk	400 ml	400 ml
Fats and oils	50 gms	40 gms
Groundnuts	50 gms	50 gms

For non-vegetarians 60 gms of meat or fish or one egg can be included and pulses reduced to 55 gms and 50 gms for males and females, respectively.

During Adolescence

Adolescence is a period of rapid growth after infancy. The rate of growth reaches its peak between eleven and fourteen years for the girl and between thirteen and sixteen years for the boy. Internal activities like secretion, hormonal reactions, basal metabolism and biochemical reactions are more during this stage. Pubertal growth demands more body-building substances and basal metabolic rate is increased which demands more energy. Since the period of adolescence is accompanied with considerable stress due to physiological and psychological changes attitude towards diet is often very unhealthy. Boys are usually well-fed in adolescence as they prefer to be tall and well-built with strong muscles. Therefore, an adolescent boy is more receptive to form good dietary habits. Girls are often self-conscious of their figure and they avoid many foods labelling them as fattening. Complexion, pimples and other marks are often associated with certain foods and their consumption. Withdrawal attitude, a common problem of adolescents, is often taken on food. Weight control is another important problem with adolescent girls and they eliminate essential nutrients in this effort. Skipped meals, poor lunches, snacking in-between, munching in-between, consuming large quantities of soft drinks and salty tit-bits which reduce the appetite are the common unhealthy dietary habits observed among adolescents.

On the contrary, an adolescent girl requires all nutrients in good quantities not just for the rapid growth but also to obtain optimal storage for later requirements during pregnancy and lactation. Underweight is undersirable for them because it helps further susceptibility to infection. Studies on obstetric performance of adolescents have shown that high incidence of eclampsia, toxemia, miscarriage and premature deliveries occur among undernourished pregnant adolescent mothers.

Nutritional requirements for boys and girls differ at adolescence.

Requirement of Various Nutrients

Group	Age (years)	Calories (kacls)	Protein feW	Iron (mgm)	Retinol (gm)	β Carotene (mgm)	Thiamine (mg)	Riboflavin (Mg)	Niacin (mgm)	Vitamin C(mg)	Calcium (mgm)
Boys	10-12	2420	42.5	30.25	600	2400	1.2	1.5	16	40	.0.4-0.5
Girls	10-12	2260	42.1	30.25		"	1.1	1.4	15	40	0.4-0.5
Boys	13-15	2660	51.7	25	750	3000	1.3	1.6	18	40	0.6-0.7
Girls	13-15	2360	43.3	35	"	"	1.2	1.4	15	40	0.6-0.7
Boys	16-18	2820	53.1	25	750	3000	1.4	1.7	19	40	0.05-0.06
Girls	16-18	2200	44.0	35	750	3000	1.4	1.3	15	40	0.05-0.06

The ICMR expert group suggested the following composition of diet to derive the above recommended allowance for adolescent groups.

Composition of Balanced Diet for Adolescents

Group	Age (years)	Cereals	Pulses	Leafy vege-	Other vegetables	Roots & tubers tables	Milk (Ml)	Oil &	Sugar and jaggery fat
Boys	10-12	420 gm	45 gm	50 gm	50 gm	30 gm	250	40 gm	45 gm
Girls	10-12	380gm	45 gm	50gm	50gm	30gm	250	35 gm	45 gm
Boys	13-18	420 gm	70 gm	50 gm	50 gm	30 gm	250	40 gm	45 gm
Girls	13-18	380 gm	70 gm	100 gm	50 gm	30 gm	250	40 gm	45 gm

For School Children

Majority of our school children consume inadequate diet and so they are malnourished. School children usually skip their meals due to various reasons. Poverty, ignorance and disturbed emotional status due to maladjustment in schools are some of the factors which produce malnutrition among school children. Western countries have shown a general trend towards an increase in the average national height of the people with each succeeding generation. Better socio-economic condition and better nutrition contribute to this. But this is not true in our case. Diet surveys carried out in our country have shown that diet consumed by school children is deficient in calories, proteins, vitamin A, riboflavin, folic acid and iron. Deficiencies in the diet are both qualitative and quantitative. More than 50 per cent of our school children are anaemic. The growth rate is poor and they gain low body weight and height. Their capacity to put maximum effort for work is poor. They are unable to concentrate, their power of grasping is reduced and their learning ability is poor. Thus an undernourished child is hurdled in its physical and intellectual development. Periodical check-up of height and weight manifest if there is retarded growth.

Nutritional requirements of boys and girls are more or less the same till the first 9 years. After that there is variation in some nutrients. Recommendation of allowances of various nutrients for school children suggested by the ICMR is given below:

Recommended allowances of these nutrients can be derived from a balanced diet with the following composition:

Recommended Dietary Intake of Nutrients

Age (Years)	*Calories (kcals)*	*Proteins (gm)*	*Calcium (gm)*	*Iron (mgm)*	*Retinol (mgm)*	*β Carotene*	*B1 (mgm)*	*B2 (mg)*	*Vitamin C (mg)*
1-3 year	1220	22.0	0.4-0.5	20-25	250	1000	0.6	0.7	40 mg
4-6 "	1720	29.4	0.4-0.5	20-25	300	1200	0.9	1.0	40 mg
7-9 "	2050	35.6	0 4-0.5	20-25	400	1600	·1.0	1.2	40 mg

Foods	*Age Group* 1-3 years	4-6 years
Cereals	175 gms	270 gms
Pulses	35 gms	35 gms
Leafy vegetables	40 gms	50 gms
Other vegetables	20 gms	30 gms
Roots and tubers	10 gms	20 gms
Milk	300 ml	250 ml
Oils and fats	15 gms	25 gms
Sugar and jaggery	30 gms	40 gms

Among non-vegetarians 50 per cent of pulses can be deleted and instead 1 egg or 30 gms of meat or fish can be added.

For Pre-school Children

The growth rate declines after the child is one year old, but the foundation of good health is laid during the pre-school age. In India about 20 per cent of the total deaths occur among toddlers in the age group of 1 to 4 years. A child who has failed to grow during this crucial period may not make up the loss in growth even with an excellent diet in later life. Deficiency of vitamin A which leads even to blindness and anaemia are common disorders found in children in the age group of 1 to 5 years. About 1 to 2 per cent of pre-school children suffer from severe deficiency diseases like kwashiorkor and marasmus. Studies in India have shown that the performance of children who had earlier suffered from malnutrition, was clearly inferior to that of children who had not gone through malnutrition. Their diets in general consist of cereals, roots, tubers and vegetables. Important items like pulses, leafy vegetables, yellow vegetables, milk and milk products and other protein sources and fruits, are consumed much below their requirement. Deficiency of protein calories, vitamin A and iron are very common among this group due to their inadequate dietary habits. Non-availability of protective foods, low purchasing capacity, illiteracy and ignorance about the importance of nutrition during this period, traditional habits, food fads and fallacies, insanitary living conditions and prevalence of infectious diseases are the main causes of malnutrition. Physical and mental retardation set in and high mortality takes place among infants. It has also been shown by studies that the measurement of head circumference usually indicates that the brain volume is less among malnourished children. Malnutrition reduces memory and hearing ability and impairs intellectual functioning.

The Requirements

Energy requirement varies according to age, activities, climate and the growth pattern. Proportionately, a child requires more calories per kilogram of body weight compared to an adult person. This is mainly due to the high basal metabolic activities, extra physical activity of the child and extra energy needed for growth. The ICMR Committee (1981) suggested that the ideal weight chart must be consulted before recommending energy requirements.

Height and Weight of Indian Pre-school Children

Age Yrs	*Boy's Height cm.*	*Girl's Height cm.*	*Boy's Weight kg.*	*Girl's Weight kg.*
1-2 yrs	82.61	79.89	10.94	10.21
2-3 yrs	91.14	89.63	12.79	12.11
3-4 yrs	98.36	96.21	14.78	13.79
4-5 yrs	104.70	104.19	16.12	15.85

Energy Allowance for Children

Age Group	*Body Weight*	*Energy Requirement*
1-3 yrs	12.03 kg	1220 kcals or 5.1 MJ
4-6 yrs	18.87 kg	1720 kcals or 7.2 MJ

Protein allowances for children of 1 to 3 years is 1.83 gms/kgs or 22 gms. For 4 to 6 year old, 1.56 gms/kgs or 29 gms to ideal weight is recommended.

From 1 to 6 years calcium requirement is 0.4-0.5 gms and iron requirement is 20-25 mgs. Retinol during 1 to 3 years 250 μgm and 3 to 6 years 300 μgm is enough, β Carotene is required 1,000 μgm and 1,200 μgm respectively. Also 0.6 mgm of thiamine and 0.7 mg of riboflavin and 8 mgs of niacin are recommended for 1 to 3 years. For both groups 40 mgms of vitamin C and 100 mgms of folic acid and 200 I.U. of vitamin D are recommended. All these nutrients are required for maintaining health and well-being of the growing child. Since childhood is the age of rapid growth, proteins of high biological value must be included in the diet. Iron deficiency is common among this group, food rich in iron must be made available in the diet. Low intake of iron was found in a high percentage of 1 to 5 year group which leads to iron deficiency anaemia.

A study on pre-school children has shown that average per head intake of leafy vegetables is 4 gms against the recommendation of 40-50 gms per day. Intake of other vegetables is 14 gms instead of 30 to 50 gms. Only 7 gms of fruit is consumed by a pre-schooler as against a recommendation of 60 gms. For proteins 40 to 50 gms of pulses are recommended, but the average consumption is only 14 gms; 80 ml of milk instead of 200 ml of milk or milk products. Thus our pre-school children are exposed to an inadequate diet which is the major cause of malnutrition in them. The children often become victims of traditional beliefs and food fads and due to that many essential food items are forbidden to them. To an extent, malnutrition results from this. Cereals, pulses, other vegetables, leafy vegetables and cheap fruits are essential to provide energy, proteins and vitamins to the child. Milk can be substituted by giving other forms of milk like groundnut or soyabean milk. Composition of a balanced diet for a pre-school child is given below:

Balanced Diet for Pre-school Children

Age group	*Cereals*	*Pulses*	*Leafy vege-tables*	*Other vege-tables*	*Roots & tubers*	*Milk*	*Fats & oil*	*Sugar or jaggery*	*Fruits*	*Egg*	*Non-vegetarian Meat or fish*
1-3 years	175gm	35gm	40gm	20gm	10gm	300ml	15gm	30gm	60gm	1	30gm
3-6 years	270gm	35gm	50gm	30gm	20gm	250ml	25gm	40gm	60gm	1	30gm

If such a balanced diet is provided to the pre-school child, it will be reflected in normal growth pattern. An average of 12.4 cms height and 2.5 kgs weight is gained by a pre-school child during 1 to 2 years. The growth pattern of a pre-school child of 2 to 3 years is 8.9 cm height and 2.1 kgs weight per year. During 3 to 4 years there is a slight decline in the growth pattern, that is, 7.3 cms height and 2 kgs weight per year. Height gain of a pre-schooler of 4 to 5 years per year is only 5.6 cms and the weight is 1.8 kgs. Even though there are different factors which affect the height and weight gain of a child the proportionate rate has a pattern and marked variation in it must be taken seriously.

During Infancy

Nutrition during infancy lays the foundation for health. Growth is rapid and changes in body composition take place at this age. Chemical maturation of the body is accomplished and internal activities occur at a high speed. Basal metabolic rate is also high. Compared to an adult in terms of body weight, an infant needs all nutrients in more quantities. A healthy newborn baby doubles its birth weight by the fifth month and tribles by one year. The average birth weight of Indian infants is less than the average European infant. But the growth rate of Indian infants is on par with the developed countries in the first few months when it depends entirely on breast milk. A diet survey conducted in various parts of India shows that a lactating mother of lower socio-economic class consumes only about 1800 kcals and about 40 gms of protein which is much below to her requirement. Despite this, she is able to breastfeed her baby successfully during the first six months. Qualitatively her milk is not inferior to a well-nourished mother. But beyond three to four months, breast milk alone is not able to supply the needs of the infant. Supplementary foods are needed after three months. Sometimes breast milk is inadequate to meet the nutritional needs of the infants even up to six months. Continuous stress on the mother may result in her ill-health and reduction in the quantity of her milk. The nutrients from mother's body are withdrawn for milk production which leads to severe deficiency condition in her which in turn is reflected on the baby. Malnutrition impairs growth and development of the baby. Such babies have poor resistance to infection. Intellectual potentiality is impaired besides reduction in working efficiency in adult life. Studies conducted at the National Institute of Nutrition (1981) indicate that children from well-fed, well-to-do sections of the community are taller and heavier and their resistance power against diseases is far better.

Nutritional Requirement of the Infant : Infants in the age group of 0 to 3 months are mostly breastfed and lactating mothers of poorer section also secrete enough milk for their baby in the first three months. In our country, breastfeeding is traditionally prolonged and continues for one or two years. A well-fed mother secretes 850 ml of milk up to three months. Mothers from poorer sections secrete to an average of 600 ml/day. The energy requirements for infants of 0 to 3 months are 120 kcals/kg of body weight. If the mother secretes 600 ml of milk the infant gets 420 kcals per day.

Protein intake of healthy infants is found to be 2 gms/kg of body weight Six hundred millilitre of breast milk supplies about 7.2 gms of protein for the baby. Fat content of breast milk is 3.8 per cent and about 24.8 gms of fat is supplied by the breast milk. Fat in breast milk supplies 50 to 60 per cent of energy; 100 mgs of iron and 0.5 mgm to 0.6 mgm of calcium per kilogramme of body weight is required by the baby. Calcium builds the skeletal structure of the baby's body.

Vitamins are essential for the rapid development of the infant. Breast milk supplies 140 gms of vitamin A during the six months of life. This is not enough when the requirement is 400 mgms of retinol during 0 to 6 months and 300 kcals gms from 6 to 12 months. They utilise the reserves in the body. Vitamin A deficiency is very common in our children. In India there is plenty of sunshine which is a rich source of vitamin D and 200 I.U. of this vitamin D is sufficient to meet the requirements and 20 mgs of vitamin C is recommended for infants. In 100 ml of breast milk 15 mgms to 20 gms of thiamine is present Thus about 0.17 gms of thiamine is ingested through breast milk and the requirement is 59 mgs/ kg of body weight, requirement of riboflavin is 0.25 gms/1000 kcals. Niacin requirement for infants is not studied and 780 mgms/kg of body weight is recommended by the committee. For infants recommended requirement of folic acid is 25 mgms and B 12 is 0.72 gm.

Growth Rate of Infants

Infancy is a period of rapid growth and the growth rate is given below.

Age	*Body Length*		*Weight*	
(Months)	*Male (cm)*	*Female*	*Male (kg)*	*Female*
At birth	47.5	47	3.1	3
1	50.6	50	3.8	3.7
2	53.7	53	4.8	4.7
3	56.8	56	5.2	5.1
4	58.8	57.9	5.8	5.2
5	60.8	59.8	6.4	6.1
6	62.8	61.7	7.0	6.6
7	64.5	63.4	7.4	7.1
8	66.2	65.1	7.8	7.5
9	68.9	66.8	8.0	7.7
10	70.2	68.1	8.2	7.9
11	71.5	69.4	8.4	8.1
12	72.8	70.7	8.6	8.3

Breastfeeding : Scientific studies have shown that the watery human milk is what the human infant needs. Cow's milk or buffalo's milk has the composition fit to match the rapid growth of its calves and not for a comparatively slow growing human infant. The nutritive value of breast milk is better than buffalo's or cow's milk. During the first two days after childbirth the yellowish fluid that is secreted is known as colostrum. This is very nutritious and good for the baby as it is a good source of vitamin A and contains substances which protect the baby from diseases. But many mothers do not feed the colostrum to the baby with the belief that it is not good for the child. The average quantity of milk secreted by an Indian woman is 600 ml or equal to four glasses of milk.

From the table, it can be seen that the protein content of cow's, buffalo's and goat's milk is three times that of human milk. The casein content is also more. In the stomach, hard curd is formed in children fed on animal milk. Fat content is almost the same except in the case of buffalo's milk where it is about twice as much as that in other milks. Minerals and vitamins are almost the same in all milks.

Composition of Human, Cow's, Buffalo's and Goat's Milk (100 ml)

Nutrients	*Human*	*Cow*	*Buffalo*	*Goat*
Proteins	1.2 gm	3.30 gm	3.8 gm	3.3 gm
Fat	3.8 gm	3.7 gm	8.5 gm	4.1 gm
Calories	71 kcals	69 kcals	100 kcals	76 kcals
Lactose	7.0 gm	4.8 gm	4.4 gm	4.7 gm
Calcium	33 mg	125 mgm	210 mgm	130 mgm
Iron	0.15 µmg	0.10 µmg	0.20 µgm	0.05 µgm
Vitamin A	48 µmg	47 µgm	60 µgm	36 µgm
Thiamine	0.02 mgm	0.04 mgm	0.05 mgm	0.05 mgm
Riboflavin	0.04 mg	0.18 gm	0.10 mg	0.12 mg
Vitamin C	4 mgm	2 mgm	2.5 mgm	2 mgm

Advantages of using breast milk as an infant's food are many. No substitute has ever been developed that matches the numerous advantages of this specific baby food. It contains various elements in the correct proportion required by the baby. Human milk is a dilute fluid which is easily digestible and it is the ideal starting food for the baby. Breast milk is readily available and it is very economical. By giving any food, breast milk can be produced in a lactating mother. No time is required for its preparation and the chances of contamination are nil. Artificial feeding requires complete cleanliness and in a country like ours where sanitary conditions are poor infections are more among artificially fed babies. Colic pain and respiratory diseases are common among such children. Polyomyelitis, influenza, mumps and infectious diseases are also common among artificially fed children because breast milk contains high concentration of antibodies which give resistance against infections. Milk allergy, constipation and fullness of the stomach, gas formation and gastro-intestinal discomforts are less among breastfed infants. A mother who is not feeding her baby due to some reason subconsciously feels guilty.

The infant gets close physical relationship with the mother which provides emotional security and well being to the baby. Apart from these advantages, emptying the breasts reduces the chances of mastitis and cancer. Milk secretion is reduced if the secreted milk is not drained by suckling the baby. Only by emptying it further secretion is stimulated. Worry, tension, anxiety and emotional disturbances reduce the secretion of milk. Cleanliness of breast and nipple, care of inverted, fissured and cracked nipples are essential to ensure proper feeding. If the child is sick and is not feeding then the mother must empty the breast either manually or with the help of a breast pump. An infant must be fed at a breast for twenty minutes. An adequate diet, relaxed attitude, enough rest and willingness to breastfeed serve as the key factors to secrete enough milk by a lactating mother. Suckling position is also important. The mother should offer her whole breast to the baby rather than just the nipple, because the baby will not suck the whole milk secreted by the breast by sucking at the nipple. The feeding of the baby must be developed by every mother.

Individual variations are there in this matter. For the first few days most of the babies are reluctant to suck as they are not very hungry. From the third day onwards the infant may want to feed as many times as it is fed. This may be to get the closeness and warmth of the womb from the physical contact in the new environment. From the second week onwards most babies can be trained to follow a routine of feeding.

In diseases like tuberculosis, typhoid, severe neurosis, psychosis, septicaemia and in eclampsia breastfeeding is not advocated.

Artificial Feeding : Industrial revolution, urbanisation and life-style of modern women, fast social life and employment status of mothers are some of the causes for the decline in breastfeeding. Commercial pressures from the advertisement of marketed foods, ignorance about the advantages of breastfeeding, misconception of the mothers that breastfeeding affects the figure, and lack of self confidence among lactating mothers are other factors which promote artificial feeding. Due to certain illnesses, some mothers are unable to feed their babies and they have to depend on artificial feeding.

Much care and awareness of the formulas are the factors to be considered when artificial feeding is opted for the new born to avoid complications. Preparation of a sterile infant formula is expensive and time-consuming. Morbidity and mortality rates are more among artificially fed children because the bacteriological safety of the artificial feed is inferior. A beneficial bacteria, lactobacillus bifidus, in the intestinal flora of the breastfed infants promotes better resistance to the infant

If animal milk is used for infant feeding, adjustment of the fat content of the feed, sterilisation, dilution and addition of sugar are the factors to be considered seriously. Fat content of buffalo's milk is very high and it has to be adjusted. The animal milk has to be diluted with water after boiling it. Equal quantities of water and milk are enough for an infant of 1 to 2 months of age. Sugar at 5 per cent level is added. Gradually the quantity of water is reduced as the infant grows.

The number of feeds and dilution of milk vary according to the age of the infants. Seven feeds are enough for the first month. From second to seven months six feeds, and eight months to one year five feeds are recommended. From the third month onwards fruit juices and from the fourth month onwards cereals cooked in different forms must be introduced. From the sixth month onwards egg yolk, mashed vegetables, dals, vegetable soups and other forms of food can be introduced. This pattern is essential even for children who are breastfed.

For the first month dilution of milk with equal quantity of water may be done with the addition of 5 per cent cansugar. For instance, for the feed 400 ml milk, 200 ml water and 20 gms of sugar can be added. In the second month, 500 ml milk, 300 ml water and 30 gms of sugar are enough. From three months to 1 year 100 ml of milk is added and 100 ml of water is reduced and 10 gms of sugar is also added.

Various processed infant foods are available in the market. The nutritive value of these infant foods is given on the container. Certain nutrients like vitamin D, iron, and other minerals are fortified in some foods. Dilution of these formulas must be done. Otherwise indigestion and other gastro-intestinal disturbances may occur. If the dilution is more enough nutrients will not be present in the formula and the baby will not show the normal growth pattern. Since vitamin C is absent in processed foods it must be supplemented.

For low-income groups, cheap nutritious substitutes can be prepared for an infant from groundnut or soyabeans. Instead of diluting the expensive artificial foods into watery milk these substitutes can be prepared at home.

Groundnut Milk : Select fresh groundnut, shrunken or shrivelled nuts are harmful. Shell and roast gently for 5 to 10 minutes. Rub off the pink skins and soak one cup of white nuts in clean water for 2 hours. Drain and grind the soaked nuts to a fine paste sprinkling with water. When the paste is ready dilute it with 5 cups of water and filter through a fine cotton cloth. Boil the milk for 10 minutes and keep it aside for 8-10 hours in a closed vessel. Afterwards remove the layer of fat from the top and the liquid can be used as a substitute for milk.

Soya Bean Milk : Select fresh beans and discard discoloured or spoiled ones. Wash three times with water. For 1 cup of beans use 3 to 4 cups of water for soaking. Soak for 6 to 8 hours. Drain and throw away the water and rinse the beans with clean water. Grind them to a fine paste using 2 cups of boiling water and a pinch of baking powder of soda bicarbonate. Strain through a muslin cloth and add one more cup of boiling water. Boil this milk stirring constantly. Add 2 cardamoms to improve the flavour.

Children who are unable to tolerate animal food can be given these two types of milk. Artificial feeds must be given at body-temperature. The hole in the nipple should be just enough to avoid rapid flow of milk. If a large gulp is taken, air is swallowed along with it, which causes discomfort and regurgitation. A small hole in the nipple provides very little milk and the baby may become exhausted by sucking. Along with the feed some air is swallowed, therefore the baby must be made to burp.

Sterilisation of bottles, nipples, bottle-caps, strainer, spoons and other equipment used is essential.

Other Requirements : Liquid and solid supplements, vitamins and mineral supplements are essential to meet the nutritional requirements of the baby. Juices of fresh fruits such as oranges, tomatoes, grapes, or soup of drumstick leaves can be introduced to meet the vitamin C requirement. One teaspoon of fruit juice can be given to the baby from the third week onwards. At this stage the fruit juice must be diluted with equal quantities of boiled water. This can be increased to about three teaspoons (without dilution) by 2 to 3 months. Boiled leafy vegetables, carrots and tomatoes can be introduced from the third month. After boiling, mash and strain the vegetables. Add salt and lime juice. Mashed banana, pumpkin, egg yolk, meal soup without seasoning, porridge, double-cooked cereals and pulses, roasted pulse-cereal powders sweetened with jaggery are the other items that can be introduced by the sixth month. Ripe fruits are also good for them. Only one food must be introduced at a time, though a variety of items can be given to familiarise with new tastes. Only a small quantity of food must be given to the baby in the beginning. Do not force the baby to take more, otherwise it will reject it in course of time. If the baby vomits or shows dislike for a food do not force him to eat it. After an interval start again and if the dislike persists substitute it with another food. Provide variety in supplementary foods because infants like older people prefer it. If proper supplementation is not provided to the infants its growth is retarded. Foods rich in proteins, calories and other nutrients must be supplemented to prevent malnutrition because the baby is growing vigorously at this stage.

Deficiency of protein leads to physical and intellectual dwarfism in the baby. Lack of adequate vitamin A in the diet results in poor vision even in the case of an infant because mother's milk and baby's store of vitamin A may not be enough. ICMR reports that about 12,000 to 14,000 children become blind every year. Deficiency of vitamin A is observed as one of the important causes for it. Deficiency diseases are not the only consequence of malnutrition but they again impair the power of resistance of an infant and expose them to a number of diseases. Respiratory diseases, gastro-intestinal disturbances and fevers are the common ailments during infancy.

Some recipes and their nutritive value are given in this chapter. These can be included in the diet of an infant to improve the nutrient intake. Green gram dal, kheer, rice wheat or ragi porridge, ragi milk, halwa, chandan kheer, idli, groundnut halwa, pongal, sweet kichiri, vegetable soup and fruit juices are some of the foods that can be given to a pre-school child.

Ragi, Wheat or Rice Porridge

Ragi flour - 30 gms (2 tbsp) or any other flour.

Groundnuts - 30 gms

Jaggery - 50 gms

Water - 2 glasses

Method: Mix ragi flour in a small amount of water and make it into a paste. Roast and grind groundnuts into a paste. Add ragi flour paste to boiling water and stir continuously. Crush the jaggery and dissolve in half cup water. Strain and add it to the ragi mixture. Add groundnut paste and allow the mixture to cook for five minutes and remove from the fire.

Nutritive Value: This porridge supplies about 11.5 gms proteins and 225 kcals.

Ragi Milk Halwa

Ragi (grains)	-	100 gms
Milk	-	half cup
Jaggery	-	50 gms
Water	-	2 glasses

Method: Clean and soak ragi for 10-12 hours and grind into a paste. Dilute with water and strain the mixture through a thin cloth. Add milk and cook it on low heat. Stir to avoid lump formation. Add jaggery to the cooked milk.

Groundnut Halwa

Shelled groundnuts	-	100 gms
Jaggery	-	50 gms

Method: Soak groundnuts for 6 to 8 hours and grind into a paste. Add 20 to 25 ml of water to the paste and keep on fire. Add jaggery, allow to cook for 5 minutes and remove from the fire.

Pongal

Rice	-	20 gms (one fistful)
Dal	-	20 gms (2 tbsp)

Method: Cook dal, and a Hide salt, and mash it well with a ladle. Cook rice, add mashed dal. Add a little ghee to it Serve this with a soup prepared from greens.

Nutritive Value: 6.2 gm protein, 120 kcals (without ghee).

Kheer Pongal

Rice - 50 gms (4 tbsp, heaped)

Amaranth - 50 gms (one medium size bunch)

or any other greens

Green gram dal - 50 gms (4 tbsp)

Groundnut oil - 10 gms

Salt - to taste

Cumin - a pinch

Method: Roast rice and green gram dal and powder them. Boil amaranth, mash and strain. Mix amaranth puree with rice and dal powders and make into a paste. Add this mixture to the boiling water. Fry cumin in oil and season the pongal.

Nutritive Value: 4.0 gm protein, 100 kcals. Low Cost Recipes

Chandan Kheer

Roasted bengal gram flour - 25 gms (2 tbsp)

Milk - 200 ml (1 glass)

Sugar - 15 gms

Method: Add a little milk to the bengal gram flour to form a paste. Boil the remaining milk and add bengal gram flour paste to it. Stir continuously to avoid lumps. Allow it to cook for five minutes. Add sugar and remove from the fire.

Nutritive Value: 4.0 gms protein, 110 kcals.

Sweet Khichiri

Wheat - 45 gms (4 tbsp)

Roasted bengal gram dal - 45 gms (3 tbsp)

Jaggery - 50 gms (4 tbsp)

Method: Lightly roast wheat and bengal gram dal and powder them. Make into a thin batter. Add water to jaggery and make it into a syrup. Add jaggery syrup to the batter and allow to cook till there is no raw flavour.

Nutritive Value: 5-0 gms protein, 150 kcals.

Drumstick Leaf or Spinach Chapathi

Drumstick leaves	-	25 gms
Onion (big)	-	15 gms
Salt and water	-	enough
Wheat flour	-	50 gms
Chillies (green)	-	1

Method: Chop onion and chilli. Clean and cut leaves into pieces and cook. Mix all three to wheat flour and make it into a soft dough. Divide into balls and make chapathi and cook it.

Nutritive Vulue: 8.0 gm proteins, 196 kcals.

Value of Food

Food is basic for survival of life. It is needed for the body's growth, repair and reproduction. Food provides energy required for all life activities. Satisfaction of hunger is usually the primary criterion for adequate food intake. But, satisfaction of hunger itself is not a safe guide for selection of proper food. Also, when the types and variety of foods available for consumption are many and constantly change, a scientific knowledge of nutrients in food becomes essential. Hence, there is a need for an introduction to nutrition in a book on foods.

Good health is a major factor in our happiness and for an active life. Food is vital for building strong bodies and promoting good health. The science of nutrition helps in planning a diet, which improves growth rate, longevity and health. This is only one aspect of nutrition. In addition to material aspects, nutrition should help to promote emotional, energetic and spiritual quality, resulting in holistic health.

Finally, the role of food is not just for providing for life and health. The dynamic force of food should interact with the dynamic force of one's total being. Thus, this chapter deals with food in respect of nutrition, health and consciousness.

Quality of Food

There are different concepts of nutrition. The most commonly studied aspect is the one based on laboratory research on how the various food components of our diet are digested, absorbed and metabolized to carry out various activities of the body. It also helps to understand the various diseases which occur due to malnutrition and deficiency. The wealth of information encompassing these aspects of nutrition is many times more than that of food.

Diet : The three basic foods which constitute our diet are carbohydrates, fats and proteins. Carbohydrates and fats are considered to be energy providing foods whereas proteins are growth-promoting substances. Mineral salts and vitamins, which are required for many metabolic activities, form the minor components of the diet. For a diet to be adequate and balanced, these foodstuffs must be ingested in the correct proportions.

Carbohydrate is the fuel on which the body functions are based. Energy produced through oxidation of carbohydrates forms the primary source of energy for the body. In terms of quantity carbohydrates make up the bulk of the diet and consist of simple sugars like glucose, fructose and sucrose and starch from food grains or tubers like potato. The sugar should form only a small portion of carbohydrate intake as large amounts lead to obesity and serious health problems.

Fat is the most concentrated source of food energy, providing on a dry weight basis, more than twice the number of calories derived from protein or carbohydrate. Fat is taken in lesser quantity than carbohydrates. Food fat serves as a carrier for fat-soluble vitamins A, D, E and K. Fat is stored in the body to afford energy for later use, its high caloric density and low solubility providing superior qualities for purposes of storage. Dietary fats may be from plant or animal sources, but, healthwise, vegetable oils containing poly-unsaturated fatty acids are preferable. The deposits of fat in adipose tissue provide both insulation and protection for the body. With the exception of central nervous system, virtually all tissues of the body utilize fatty acids directly as a source of energy.

Protein in the diet is necessary to provide sources of nitrogen and amino acids to be utilized in the synthesis of body proteins and other nitrogen containing substances. The proteins of the body contribute to tissue structure and are involved in a variety of important metabolic functions. Proteins in excess of these needs serve as a source of energy. The nutritional value of a protein depends upon the composition of its amino acids. Vegetable foods generally contain small quantities of protein and the amino acids present are rarely in the proportions required by animal tissues. Therefore there is a danger of malnutrition if only one vegetable food forms the major component of the diet. However, a good vegetarian diet can be worked out which provides the complete range of protein requirements by using a wide variety of protein-containing vegetable foods. These include cereals, legumes, nuts, fruits and other vegetables. Most of the animal proteins contain a high proportion of essential amino acids in balanced amounts and are termed biologically good proteins.

The minor components of food contribute about 2 per cent of the dry weight of our diet. Of these vitamins form the accessory food factors. These are complex organic components present in very small quantities in natural food and absorbed into the body from the small intestine. They possess no energy but are essential for good health and maintain the body's normal metabolic activity. If the diet is deficient in a particular vitamin, metabolic activity is impaired. This produces a disorder symptomatic to that particular vitamin deficiency. This is known as deficiency disease. This deficiency disease can be avoided by supplementing the diet with the missing vitamin.

Mineral salts are the second important minor components of our diet. Some minerals in the form of their salts (sodium, calcium and potassium) are found in the body in large amounts while others like zinc, copper, cobalt, manganese and iron are present in small amounts. Some of these metals are part of several enzymes and complex organic molecules, which play a crucial metabolic role. Our requirement of minerals is met by the foods we eat, particularly vegetables and leafy stuff, which constitute our diet. If need be, there could be an external supplement of minerals.

Digestion : The process by which our food is broken down from complex insoluble substances into simple soluble ones is called digestion.

Digestion starts in the mouth; when food is properly chewed, there is thorough mixing of salivary gland secretion with food. The salivary enzyme— ∝-amylase—acts on the starch component of the food breaking it into shorter components - dextrins. When food enters the stomach its contents become acidic due to gastric secretion and starch digestion due to enzyme ceases. Further digestion of starch into sugar takes place in the small intestine. The mucosa of the stomach possesses many tubular glands, which are lined with different types of cells such as chief cells and parietal cells. Chief cells secrete the inactive enzyme pepsinogen and prorennin while parietal cells secrete a 0.05% solution of HCl which makes the pH of the stomach contents 1-2.5, ideal for the optimum activity of the stomach enzymes. The acid promotes the conversion of pepsinogen to pepsin which hydrolyzes protein into smaller polypeptides. Hydrochloric acid converts prorennin to rennin which in turn coagulates caseinogen, the soluble protein of milk, into the insoluble calcium salt of casein. The calcium salt is then digested by pepsin.

Relatively little digestion of fats occurs in the stomach because the pH of the stomach is too low for gastric lipase to be active. In the lower regions of the stomach, triacylglycerols (fats) are mixed with proteins, carbohydrates, gastric juice and other substances. Partial degradation of this mixture and churning action of the stomach result in the formation of chyme. This results in the elevation of pH, which allows some gastric lipase activity to occur. Chyme then enters the duodenum where it is mixed with pancreatic juice, which contains bile salts, pancreatic lipase and esterase. Pancreatic lipase ultimately breaks down triacylgrycerols to fatty acids and glycerol.

The pancreas is a large gland whose cells called acini produce a variety of digestive enzymes that are poured into the duodenum via the pancreatic duct. They include amylase to convert amylose to maltose, lipase to convert fats to fatty acids and glycerol, trypsinogen, which when converted to trypsin by enterokinase, digests proteins into smaller polypeptides, chymotrypsinogen which is converted to chymotrypsin to digest proteins to amino acids, carboxypeptidases to convert peptides to amino acids, and nucleases to convert nucleic acids to nucleotides.

Absorption : Digestion reduces food to a solution of fatty acids, glycerol, glucose, fructose, nucleotides and amino acids. If these small, soluble molecules are to be of any use to the cells of the body, they must be moved out of the intestine into the blood stream. The process of moving nutrients and water from the intestine to the blood constitutes absorption.

Since the small intestine is the place where nutrient and most water absorption takes place, we should expect it to have a large exposed surface area. This is exactly the case. The small intestine is quite long and is packed into the abdominal cavity as a series of coils. Besides, the surface of the small intestine also contains folds and enormous numbers of fingerlike process called Villi. Additionally, each villus is covered with epithelial cells, and the plasma membrane of fingerlike projections called microvilli, it further enhances the absorptive surface area. The residues of food that cannot be digested or absorbed leave the small intestine and pass through the ileo-colonic valve into the large intestine. There, water and vitamins are absorbed, .and waste materials are compacted into faces.

The absorbed nutrients do not directly go into systematic circulation. Instead, everything is channeled into the portal vein, which goes to the liver where it breaks up into tiny capillaries. The liver cells then process the absorbed food for proper use when they pass into the blood stream through another vein, venacava. The liver also stores absorbed and processed food for release into blood stream when required.

The study of nutrition based on the biochemical make-up of the diet, the action of digestive juices on it, the role of the pancreas, liver, etc., has given us valuable information on various aspects of nutrition. The information available is voluminous. Foods, in addition to nutritionally important components, contain a lot of other substances in small quantities, which have significant pharmacological activity. Also cooking and food additives affect the nutritional value of food. The composition of food also varies depending on conditions of production and processing. Their effect varies from person to person who eats it. Although, the information available on nutrition is voluminous, it is responsible for some contradictions one observes in the literature.

Consciousness about Health

Knowledge of nutrition helps man to know the types and quantities of different foods to be taken in our diet to maintain good health. According to ancient Indian concepts, health based on just the diet is *Arogya*—a state of no disease with which the physician is primarily concerned. According to the World Health Organization(WHO), the term "health" means more than the presence or absence of symptoms and has a more comprehensive concept of a multidimensional, global well being.

Dimensions of Health : Growth of psychological and social sciences has shown that illness is conditioned by psychological, social and cultural factors. Epidemiological diseases are due to social and cultural factors, while psychosomatic diseases are due to conditions of mind. While the psychosocial concepts of health are important, they are not enough for the total well-being of man. For, as Dr. Brisht points out, "if the components of health are restricted only to physical, mental and social parameters, then a pack of wolves who are physically strong, mentally alert and socially well-knit would be ideally healthy". If this is so, a group of human beings would be no better than a pack of wolves.

Man is a multidimensional being and he has a spiritual perspective too that transcends other modalities of life. In his case the definition of health should be enlarged to cover spiritual well-being in addition to physical, psychological and social well-being. The Sanskrit word for health is *"Swasth"*, which means "footed in the self true health exists only when man's consciousness is fixed in spiritual self, the "*swa*".

Most persons believe that philosophy, religion, ethics and morality constitute spiritual health. These are only approaches to spiritual truth and not the spirit itself. When we go beyond these misconceptions and understand the spiritual reality by identification, we discover that there is an unity of experience that cuts across the barriers of time and space. Therefore, spiritual health conveys a special concept of a holistic and integral viewpoint of health. The WHO, in its programme of health for all, has recognized the spiritual dimensions of health.

Spiritual Health : Spiritual health evokes different images to different persons. To the materialistic Western mind it is paranormal healing, to the Eastern mind it is a boon or miracle of grace that heals our suffering and pain. To the materialist spiritual health is either a hoax or faith healing, while to —a time rationalist it is moral and ethical values in life which help man become a better race. To some others the word "spiritual" is a supreme something or someone whom none has known or can know.

According to Vedas and Upanishads (Indian scriptures), the spiritual state is a reality, which cannot be described but experienced. Seekers of consciousness have come in contact with spiritual reality and their life has been moulded by its influence. They have discovered in it something quite other than our customary notions of moral, ethical and religious values. Spiritual knowledge is a state of knowledge of that, the ultimate reality; it is revealed in a few, veiled in others, and present in all.

The seers who have experienced and lived spiritual life affirm that "The spirit is other than the mind". It is unity and oneness while the mind is duality and division. It is peace and bliss, harmony and truth, while the mind dwells in pain, pleasure and indifference. The mind also fumbles through error and ignorance. The spiritual state of health cannot be defined. It is best communicated and understood in the silence and stillness of our being. It is the highest perfection man is capable of through self-evolution.

This higher and greater consciousness is not tangible to the mass of humanity as yet. The next cycle of humanity will see the evolutionary emergence of this spiritual dimension. The resurgence of interest in Yoga, the debate over the possibility of consciousness independent of material reality, the turn towards global life, the liberalization of spiritual pursuits, the growing need for man for freedom, love and oneness, inclusion of the spiritual dimensions in the field of psychology, education, health and the findings in modern physics, are some areas indicative of such phenomena.

Those who have realized spiritual heights affirm that it is possible for man to enter and live in it and with a greater consciousness and power. If we attain that state, the disorders and conflicts that afflict humanity can be solved and it will release us from the yoke of suffering and death, and impart harmony and peace we so much lack now as a species. It is this that justifies and even makes it necessary to include the spiritual dimension as a factor with regard to health. This factor, being a source and origin of all, will also include lesser terms of our existence - mental, social and even physical. The spiritual dimension is all comprehensive, the simplest and the most fundamental. It should be sought after by man who is missing peace.

Science and Spirituality : Science is concerned with matter. In its quest to understand matter science has acquired incredible powers and harnessed it for the purpose of improving man's outer life. In the process, life has been reduced to a mechanical formula and man has been reduced to a machine among other machines.

Spirituality is the study of self and consciousness based on tapping the hidden powers of life and mind. Spirit or consciousness runs as a common thread through all phenomena. It is not an exclusive dimension that exists in isolation without any hold on the creature that inhabits it. The spiritual dimension includes the material and can intervene subtly to alter the laws and processes of the material universe and change the course of purely material and biological processes. Thus spirituality not only helps in attaining spiritual dimension but also it subtly intervenes to alter the laws and processes of the material universe.

Science seeks the truth of matter reality. Scientific methods and equipment can measure gross events. Scientific experiments can be seen, verified and reproduced. Scientific observations and inferences can be codified, resulting in physical laws.

Spirituality seeks after the truth of spirit, which is quite an other reality. Spiritual dimensions are subtler truth, which cannot be measured by conventional equipment. Subtler levels can only be experienced. One must reach a level of experience, then go to the next level and on and on till reaching an awakened state. Here, life and mind are open systems and keep growing and evolving, which upset old experiences.

Thus, science and spirituality are proceeding on their own lines of enquiry in search of a common goal. In the sincerity of their search, they will meet and when they meet they will realize that spiritual and material reality are two phases of one reality. The scientist would learn that "One Force" gives birth to the many. The spiritual scientist would discover that matter is created by a condensation of the spirit of One Reality that gives birth to various forms, phenomena and processes. This will result in the integration of human consciousness from a fragmented one, when one experiences bliss.

Evolution of Consciousness : Man's life is riddled with disease, death and infirmity. His attempts to conquer them will remain precarious at his own level of evolution. At best, he may arrive at a healthy equilibrium with his environment. All the stress and strain that besieges him is a call to evolve to a state of consciousness more perfect than his.

Man's problem of want, greed and lust and desire are due to his sense of self or individuality. His false sense of ego-self (I-ness) has to be shed off and replaced by true "I", the individual soul in him. This evolution of consciousness results in his feeling of peace, fullness and joy, with their immediate results of progress, health and fitness in the physical, quietness and goodwill in the vital, clear understanding and a general feeling of security and satisfaction. It will open the heart to a deep, pure and calm capacity to love without possessiveness and turbulent attachment. These will help one to be calm and balanced, free from fear, things which help in healthy living and even cure one of diseases.

It is possible for consciousness to evolve further, when man will be immune from all types of diseases and even death. But, this type of consciousness is possible only for a few. Contact with such evolved persons will help others to awaken, the sleeping soul in them, better than any other means.

16

Desirable Food

Quality is the ultimate criterion of the desirability of any food product. The overall quality of a food depends on the nutritional and other hidden attributes, and sensory quality as assessed by means of human sensory organs. The absence of nutritional qualities and possible presence of hazardous microbes, environmental contaminants, food toxins and chemical additives cannot be easily judged by the consumer. Governments in many countries protect the interest of the consumer regarding nutritional and hidden attributes by stringent controls to assure good food quality and enactment of food laws regarding inspection, grading, packaging and labelling of foods. Qualities of foods are evaluated by sensory organs—eye, nose and mouth—or by the use of instruments.

Judging the Quality

Sensory evaluation consists of judging the quality of food by a panel of judges. The evaluation deals with measuring, analyzing and interpreting the qualities of food as they are perceived by the senses of sight, taste, touch and hearing. By the sense of sight, the size, shape and colour of foods and other characteristics, such as transparency, opaqueness, turbidity, dullness and gloss, could be perceived. Colours of foods contribute immeasurably to one's appreciation of them. In addition, colour is associated with other attributes, e.g., the ripeness of fruits is judged by colour. The strength of coffee and tea is judged, in part, by the colour of the beverage.

Other sensory organs, the nose and mouth, are utilized to obtain information on flavour. Flavour embraces the senses of taste, smell and a composite sensation known as mouth-feel.

Sensory evaluation may be designed to reflect common preference, to maintain the quality of food at a given standard, for the assessment of process variation, cost reduction, product improvement, new market development and market analysis.

Selection of Panel of Judges : Actually, one extremely discriminating, painstaking and unbiased individual would suffice for tasting. However, human judgement is individual and is not always consistent. Physical conditions of the individual, psychological factors and environmental factors may affect one's judgement. Further, one individual may not be able to discriminate different aspects of the food quality. For these reasons, for sensory evaluation, a panel of judges is used. Members of the panel should be carefully selected and trained to find out difference in specific quality characteristics between different stimuli and also direction and/or intensity of difference. The panelists should be of sound health and average sensitivity and conscientious individuals. The number of members in the trained panel should be small, varying from 5 to 10. The semi-trained panel should consist of 25 to 30 members. The findings in the case of the untrained panel should be based at least on 100 independent judgements.

Preparation of Samples : Careful sampling of the food is necessary for sensory evaluation. A well-mixed homogeneous sample, if possible, is desirable. With non-homogeneous materials, samples should be taken from the same area. Samples to be tested should be prepared by identical methods. All samples in a series should be at the same temperature. The number of samples used in any one session depends on the sensory nature of the test product and the evaluation method used.

Types of Tests : Different sensory tests are employed for food evaluation. The tests are grouped into four types; they are difference (discrimination) tests, rating (quantitative differences) tests, sensitivity tests and descriptive tests. The selection of a particular test method will depend on the defined objective of the test, accuracy desired and personnel available for conducting evaluation.

Difference Tests : Difference tests are used to determine if there is any difference between or among samples. The three basic types of differences tested are simple difference, directional and quantitative difference, and quality preference difference. The methods of difference testing commonly used are the paired comparison, duo-trio and triangle (triad) tests. : In paired comparison test two samples, one standard and the other experimental, are presented to the panelists to determine if the samples are different and the directional difference in a specific characteristic. The duo-trio test employs three samples, two identical and one different. The panelists are first given the reference sample and then the other two samples are given successively in random order and asked to match one of them with the first. The triangle test also employs three samples, two identical and one different. All the three samples are presented simultaneously to the panelists who are asked to determine which of the three is the odd sample.

Rating Tests : These tests are difference tests with a quantitative aspect through direction and degree of judgements using suitable defined scales or scores. A number of methods are employed for this purpose. In a ranking test, judges are asked to rank a series of samples in the increasing or decreasing order of a specified characteristic, such as flavour, odour, colour or texture. A single sample (monadic) test is used for testing foods that have an after-taste or flavour carryover which precludes the testing of a second sample in the same session.

In two sample difference tests, the panelist is served with four pairs of samples. In two pairs, the test sample is a duplicate of the reference sample. In the other two pairs, the test sample is the test variable. The panelist is asked to judge each pair independently as to the degree of difference between the test sample and standard on a scale indicating no difference to large difference.

When more than one test variable is to be evaluated, multiple sample difference test is employed. Each panelist is served 3-6 samples depending upon the number of test variables. One sample is a known standard. The panelist compares the test sample with the known standard. One test sample is a duplicate of the standard. The difference of the test sample from the standard according to the scale—none, slight, moderate and large—is evaluated.

A hedonic rating test is used to measure the degree of pleasurable and unpleasurable experience of the food product on a scale of 9 points from "like extremely" to "dislike extremely".

The numerical scoring test is used to evaluate a particular characteristic of one or more samples indicating the rating as excellent, good, fair and poor.

Sensitivity-threshold Tests : These tests measure the ability of the individual to smell, taste or feel specific characteristics in food or beverages. The tests are most commonly used in selecting panel members for evaluating, and with materials such as spices for assessing the intensity of odour or flavour.

Descriptive Tests : These tests help identify the perceptual characteristics of a product and express them on an agreed scale. The panelists record the impact of all quality attributes in a total perspective but not a single attribute judgement with precision, for statistical analysis. The tests include flavour profile tests to describe the aroma and flavour intensity characteristics of food and textural profile tests to describe the sensory manifestation of structure of inner make-up of foods, comprising concepts of texture, body and consistency of foods.

Judging : The environment is an important factor in judging food. There should not be any distraction so that the judges can concentrate. Judgements should be made independently and it is preferable to have panel booths and no communication between panel members should be allowed. The best- time of the day for sensory testing is an hour after any normal meal, i.e., mid-morning or mid-afternoon, when the judges are neither too well fed nor too hungry. The panel members should not smoke, chew pan or supari or take intoxicant for at least half an hour before the test. Use of odoriferous substances (cosmetics) should be avoided. The panelists should be provided with room temperature water for rinsing between samples.

Results : The results of evaluation are recorded in suitable evaluation cards prepared for different-type methods. The data are tabulated, averaged and analyzed for the answer to the question posed in the experiment. This method may not be sufficiently trustworthy in many cases for it to be stated with confidence that the results obtained are significant. For a correct interpretation of results, their statistical analysis is necessary.

The Evolution

The evaluation of food quality does not rely mainly on human sensory organs. Objective methods have also been developed. These methods use instruments or a standard method to evaluate food quality by physical and chemical methods. The results obtained by these methods are reproducible, can be permanently recorded and are less susceptible to errors than the sensory methods of evaluation. Results obtained from the objective methods of evaluation should correlate with those obtained from sensory evaluation to ensure consumer acceptance. Objective evaluation includes chemical, physicochemical, microbial and physical methods of analysis.

Chemical methods include the determination of nutritive value of foods before and after cooking, products of food decomposition and adulterants in food. For details of the method, one has to refer to manuals on food analysis, such as the publication of the Association of Official Analytical Chemists (AOAC). Physico-chemical methods include determinations, such as the hydrogen ion concentration by the use of a pH meter, sugar concentration and the degree of hydrogenation of fats by a refractometer, and a qualitative analysis of sugar solution with a polarimeter. Some properties of foods which depend on the structure or the physical arrangements of their components, such as whipped cream, or meat, vegetable and fruit tissues, are examined by microscopic methods.

The most widely employed objective methods are the measurements of physical properties by the use of instruments. Measurements of the appearance and volume of foods are of importance, particularly in the evaluation of baked products. A record of size, shape and grain (cell structure and distribution) of such foods can be recorded by photography and the volume determined by suitable methods.

Measurement of Colour **:** The importance of colour in food, the natural food colours, the changes they undergo during cooking, processing and storage are worth consideration. Natural and synthetic colours are also added to foods to bring the produce to the generally accepted standard. Therefore, the colour of food is measured to identify its properties.

A number of instruments are used for colour measurement. A simple method is to match the colour of the food with coloured chips or coloured glass. Disc colourimetry is another method used. Different coloured discs' are spun on a stage so that the colours merge into one colour without flickering. The test sample is placed adjacent to the spinning disc and the colours are matched. Tintometers are simple instruments used to determine the colour and its depth in foods.

For a more reliable measurement of colour, spectrophotometers are used. In the case of clear or transparent solutions, spectrophotometric measurements give quantitative results. As most foods are opaque in nature, reflectance spectrophotometry or, more commonly, tristimulus colourimetry is used. In a tristimulus system, colour is specified by three attributes: dominant wavelength, brightness and purity, according to CIE system (Commission Internationale de L' Eclairage). These three attributes refer respectively to the actual colour, the luminosity and the strength of colour. Several colourimeters are available for the evaluation of these attributes or complete specification of colour.

Measurement of Texture : The texture of food is an important factor in its acceptance. The textural properties include the mechanical properties of hardness, cohesiveness, adhesiveness, chewiness, crispness, gumminess, viscosity and elasticity (springiness). A number of instrumental methods are available to evaluate the texture of various foods.

The tenderness of meat is an important quality for consumer acceptability. One aspect of tenderness of meat is tested by measurement of structure of meat with a penetrometer. This measurement gives an idea of how easy or difficult it is for the teeth to bite into a piece of meat. A more commonly used device to measure tenderness is an apparatus (Warner-Bratzler shear) which measures the force needed to cut the meat in simple shear, usually across the fibres, and estimate the force necessary to chew the meat.

The textures of fruits and vegetables are evaluated by a number of methods. A puncture testing is used to evaluate the firmness of fruits. It measures the amount of force required to penetrate the sample to a specific depth. A shear press is used to study the tenderness of fruits and vegetables. This consists of a rectangular box with evenly spaced slits in the bottom. A series of blades is moved through a sample of food. As the blades move the food is compressed, sheared and extruded through the openings in the box.

Some characteristics of foods depend upon their rheological properties. Rheology is the science of flow and deformation of materials, both liquids and solids, and has three aspects: viscosity, elasticity and plasticity.

Viscosity or consistency is an important factor in influencing the quality of a large number of food products. The acceptability of foods like salad cream, tomato products, jams, jellies, mayonnaise, syrups and fruit pulps, depends upon their consistency. Measurement of viscosity is also important in the processing of foods. A number of instruments are available for the measurement of viscosity and the type of instrument used depends on the nature of food.

Solids do not Flow : However, some solids can be deformed by force and they recover when the force is removed. This is elasticity. Gels like those of pectin, gelatin and starch, baked custard and rennet curd are examples of elastic solids. There are a number of objective tests to determine the firmness of gels. A material that is plastic resists flow until a force is applied; but unlike elastic flow, plastic flow is not reversible.

Texture of dough and batters determines the quality of the finished product. The consistency of batters is determined by a line-spread apparatus which indicates the nature of dispersion of incorporated air. The consistency and stability of doughs are measured with a farinograph which measures the force required to turn mixer blades at a constant speed during mixing of the dough. A micrograph also gives information similar to that of farinograph.

Textures of baked products such as pastries, cookies and crackers are evaluated by shortometer. The instrument measures the force required to break the product. A compressimeter is used to evaluate firmness of bread crumb or softness of a baked product. The force required to break through (shearability) a sample of a baked product is also obtained using Warner-Bratzler shear.

Texture as perceived by human beings is a composite of characteristics. To arrive at a textural profile, different instruments have to be used. New instruments have been developed which could evaluate more than one characteristic constituting the texture of a food.

Non-nutritional Constituents and Food Safety : A diverse group of Non-nutritional chemicals find their way into foods. Their presence in foods represents real or potential health risks of different characters and magnitudes to persons consuming them. The undesirable constituents that affect the safety of foods include toxicants naturally occurring in foods, toxins resulting from microbial growth, environmental contaminants—such as those arising from processing and accidental contaminants—and chemical additives.

Naturally Occurring Toxicants : Certain plant and animal products contain natural constituents that are toxic. When foods containing them are consumed in sufficient quantities, the toxins present may prove to be hazardous.

Toxicants in Plant Foods : Plants are capable of synthesizing a multitude of chemicals that cause toxic reactions when consumed by men or animals. Pulses contain a number of toxic substances, such as protease inhibitors, lathyrogens and flavism agents, cyanogens, haemagglutinins, and saponins. Some of these toxins are also present in other foods, e.g., protease inhibitors in cereals and potatoes. Saponins are present in spinach and asparagus. Goitrogens (which cause hypothyroidism and thyroid enlargement due to thioglucosides) are present in cabbage and related species, in rapeseed and mustard. Practically all foods contain proteins which may act as allergens in sensitive individuals. Some varieties of mushrooms are poisonous. Oxalic acid, a constituent of rhubarb, spinach and beet, may cause oxalic poisoning in certain individuals.

Toxicants in Animal Foods : Tissues of marine forms of animals contain toxic chemicals and cause adverse responses when eaten. About 500 species of marine fish are known to be poisonous (ichthyotoxism) when eaten and many of these are among edible varieties. The toxic agents arise from blue-green algae and are then passed directly to herbivorous fish and indirectly to carnivorous species. Poisonous syndromes from their ingestion are variable in character and are usually designated by the kind of fish involved.

Shellfish have concentrated toxins from plankton constituting their food supply. The ingestion of shellfish (clams and mussels) results in paralytic shellfish poisoning. The toxic agent has been isolated. It is not destroyed by heating.

Microbial Toxins : Some micro-organisms promote desirable changes in foods under controlled conditions. Use of yeasts in making breads and alcoholic beverages, and molds and bacteria in making cheese and fermented dairy products, are examples of beneficial effects of micro-organisms. However, they also cause harmful effects and are involved in most cases of food spoilage.

Mycotoxins : Mold growth on foods, especially if they are moist, is a common observation. Some molds, during their growth, produce toxic substances of various kinds. These substances are referred to as mycotoxins and the poisonous effect on men or animals as mycotoxicoses. Mycotoxins remain in the food long after the mold producing them has died and can therefore be present in foods that are not visibly moldy. Further, many mycotoxins, but not all, are stable and survive the usual conditions of cooking or processing. Mycotoxin contaminated foods when eaten are thus hazardous to man. Foodgrains, especially bajra, rye and jowar, get infected with the parasitic ergot fungus, *Claviceps purpurea.* Ergotism, a toxicosis, results from eating grain contaminated with this fungus. Eating moldy grains also results in alimentary toxic aleukia (ATA), a mycotoxicosis.

Aflatoxins : Mycotoxins produced by some molds, *Aspergillus flavis* or *A. parasiticus,* are known as aflatoxins. *A. spergillus* develop in many foods, particularly groundnuts and cottonseed, and their cakes and flour. Aflatoxins have been much studied. There are 14 chemically related toxins and one of them, aflatoxin B, is most frequently found in food and is the most potent carcinogen known. Liver cancer due to aflatoxin ranks high in our country.

Bacterial Toxins : Just as the growth of spoilage molds can introduce toxic substances into foods, the growth of certain bacteria can also result in production of toxic substances. These include *Clostridium botulinum, Staphylococcus aureus* and *Bacillus cereus.* These produce sufficient toxin in the food to cause illness in a susceptible host. In addition to these, *Bacillus lichiniformis* and *Bacillus subtilis* are organisms for which evidence for toxin production is beginning to accumulate.

The disease caused by the toxins of *C. botulinum* is known as botulism. The toxins are produced after an incubation period of 18-36 hours. They act on the nervous system and are potent poisons. A concentration of less than 1.0 μg is fatal for man; death occurs in 1 or 2 days. If one survives the effect of the toxin, convalescence is slow and takes 6-8 months. The toxins produce in human beings disturbances of vision and difficulties with speaking and swallowing as the mucous membranes of mouth, tongue and pharynx usually become dry. Progressive weakness and respiratory failure set in.

The botulism toxins are proteins. Six serologically distinct toxins designated as A, B, C, D, E and F are known. The protein is produced as a single polypeptide chain and when released from the bacterial cell is cleaved by a protease producing two fragments—∝ and β. The toxin is probably associated with a haemagglutinin and thereby protected from proteolysis and denaturation in the gut. The toxin acts by inhibiting the release of acetylcholine from cholinergic nerve endings. The neurotoxin absorbed from the gut binds to nerve endings through fragment β while the a-fragment is responsible for neurotoxic effects.

The toxins causing botulism are thermolabile; they lose their activity on heating for 30 min at 80°C. The cause of botulism in man is inadequately heated or cured foods. Canned foods, low in acid, could be hazardous if they have not been heated sufficiently to kill the spores of the organism which might be present.

Staphylococcal food poisoning is perhaps the most commonly experienced form of food borne disease, but it is much less serious than botulism. To be pathogenic to man, the organism must be present in sufficient quantity, the food must support toxin production and an incubation period of 2-6 hours is required. The toxic period will last for 12-24 hours and results in nausea, vomiting, diarrhoea and abdominal pain. Severe cases will result in collapse and dehydration. However, there will be no fever.

S. aureus toxins are also proteins, single-chained and globular. At least seven serologically distinct toxins are recognized. Although termed entero-toxins, they are probably neurotoxins.

They are absorbed from the gut and activate receptors on the abdominal viscera, the stimulus reaching the vomiting centre.

The toxin of *Bacillus cereus* is produced after an incubation period of 8-16 hours and it is active for 12-24 hours. Abdominal pain, diarrhoea, vomiting and nausea are the features of the toxin. Two or more toxins are involved in this food poisoning, one causing diarrhoea and another inducing vomiting.

Bacterial Food Poisoning : Over 50 genera of bacteria have been associated with food spoilage, food poisoning, food-borne diseases or general contamination. In general, Gram-negative, non-aciduric, nutritionally non-fastidious bacteria are commonly associated with the spoilage of moist proteinaceous foods, related aciduric genera with acid fruit products and lactic acid bacteria with foods rich in nutrients and fermentable carbohydrates.

Food poisoning bacteria grow in a food and infect the persons eating it. They form populations sufficiently large to colonize the gut of a susceptible individual. This situation obtains with *Salmonella* spp, *Vibrio parahaemolyticus, Escherichia coli, Yersinia enterocolitica, Clostridium perfringens* and *Compylobacter jejuni.* With these organisms, a casual relationship between a specific micro-organism and a specific disease exists.

Salmonella are ubiquitous, but they are more numerous in foods, such as pork, poultry and eggs, and products containing them. The illness caused by the organism is known as salmonellosis. As the multiplication of the organism in the intestine after ingestion of the food takes time, the illness starts 12-36 hours after ingestion and continues from 1-7 days. Diarrhoea, abdominal pain, vomiting and fever are caused by this type of poisoning. Infants are more susceptible to this infection than adults. Acids and temperature tend to destroy the micro-organism.

Clostridium perfringens grows in the alimentary canal producing the poison, some 8-12 hours after the ingestion of contaminated food. The symptoms of illness are diarrhoea, abdominal pain, nausea but rarely vomiting, and no fever. The toxin is a protein which is the structural component of the spore and acts on the membranes of the cells of the gut disturbing the flow of Na^+ and Cl^- ions. The spores of the organism can withstand heating at 100°C for one hour, but there are marked variations between strains.

Contaminants arising from Processing : These include residues that become part of food as a result of processing, handling and distribution of food. Some of them are the following.

Fumigants are used to sterilize food under conditions in which steam heat is impractical. Ethylene oxide is a commonly used fumigant. This and other epoxides react with food components to produce toxic products or destroy essential nutrients. Ethylene oxide reacts with inorganic chlorides to form ethylene chlorohydrin which is toxic.

Solvents are used for the extraction of oil from oilseeds. Solvents like trichloroethylene that was formerly, used as a solvent reacts with the substance being processed, with the production of a toxic product, although the chemical used in processing it is itself nontoxic.

During processing of foods a number of changes can be induced in their lipids. On prolonged heating, oxidative and polymerization reactions take place and these bring down the nutritional efficiency of the processed product.

Smoking of meat and fish for preservation and flavouring is an old practice. Such foods get contaminated with polycyclic aromatic hydrocarbons (benzopyrine, for example), many of which are carcinogenic. In areas where smoked fish is consumed in plenty the incidence of stomach cancer is high. Smoke from woods also contain many other classes of compounds such as phenols, acids, carbonyls and alcohols most of which have toxicological activity.

Metal Contaminants : Metals are one of the many unintentional contaminants of foods. They find their way into foods through air, water, soil, industrial pollution and many other routes. Metals, when present beyond small quantities, are toxic. Mercury, cadmium, lead, tin, etc., are the toxic metals present in foods.

Mercury : Toxicological effects of mercury depend on the chemical form involved. Elemental mercury and inorganic salts of mercury are much less toxic than organic mercurials. Methyl mercury is very poisonous and practically all the methyl mercury in the diet comes through fish taken from water contaminated by the industrial use of mercury. Mass poisoning due to mercury has been reported in Japan in areas where the fish consumed were caught from mercury-contaminated waters.

Cadmium : Cadmium is becoming a major environmental pollutant as the metal is extensively used in industries. The metal is readily absorbed from air, water and food, and is built up in the body. Ingested cadmium is stored in the kidney in the form of a metal-protein complex. Long-term exposure results in renal tubular damage, liver dysfunction and testicular damage.

Lead : The human system absorbs lead not only from foods but also from water and leaded dust in the air. Lead contamination of food is due to water conveyed through lead pipes, contact with machines, equipment, packing, etc., containing lead, and lead containing sprays and dusts used as pesticides of fruits and vegetables. Lead, absorbed by the human system, brings about changes in the kidney and arteries that tend to shorten life.

Other Metals : Metals may enter foods from certain utensils. Enamel-ware of poor quality contributes antimony and galvanized utensils zinc, which are toxic. A major source of tin contamination of foods is tin plate. A variety of containers with tin plate are made for storing all types of processed foods. Canned foods, if acidic, and foods stored in tins after opening, change in colour or may develop a metallic flavour that is unpalatable. Small quantities of metal are dissolved when foods are cooked in aluminium utensils but this does not impart harmful properties to foods. Copper is an essential trace element required by the human body but copper-contaminated foods are toxic.

Other Contaminants from Food Processing : These include lubricants, boiling water additives, packing material, etc. Mineral oils are used as lubricants for the extrusion of foods and rapid economic production of bread by permitting it to come clearly out of the baking pan. Chemicals are added to boiler feed water to prevent scale formation as a result of hardness of water. When steam from the boiler is used in food processing, small amounts of added chemicals may be carried into the food. To strengthen paper used for food packaging, resins are used, which might migrate to the food.

In addition to the contaminants discussed above, food will contain a number of other contaminants. Further, a number of chemicals are intentionally added to foods to accomplish improvements in nutritional value, maintenance of freshness, creation of desirable properties or aid in processing.

Adulteration of Food

Adulteration of food consists of substituting it wholly or in part by any cheaper or inferior substance or of removing any of its constituents, wholly or in part, which affects adversely the nature, substance or quality of the food. According to the Indian Prevention of Food Adulteration Act (PFA) 1954, any ingredient which, when present in food, is injurious to health is an adulterant. Thus, according to the PFA definition, many of the food contaminants discussed in the previous section are adulterants and come under the purview of food adulteration.

Adulteration of foods was practised even in ancient times. It was not a serious problem then because business was on a small scale and the transactions involved a large measure of personal accountability. Later, with the increased centralization of food processing and distribution, and corresponding decline in personal accountability, intentional adulteration of food increased. Even in the early nineteenth century, many adulterants were used in articles like pepper, essential oils, vinegar, beverages (coffee, tea, beer, wines), butter, bread, etc. In recent years adulteration of foods has become a serious problem the world over. In western countries there is a rising concern over the safety of the food supply and many remedial actions, both voluntary and enforced, have been taken.

The percentage of adulterated food sold in various parts of

India is 30 to 35 per cent. Unfortunately, in our country, there are still no strong consumer associations to give proper education to the public at large about the various methods of food adulteration and ways to detect it. Food adulteration, apart from cheating the consumers, often results in disorders or diseases. Some of the foods commonly adulterated in India and the adulterants encountered in them are the following.

Pulses are an important component of the Indian diet. Pulses like masoor, black gram and chana, other as gram, split pulses (dals) or gram flour, are mixed with the corresponding forms of khesari pulse. Consumption of khesari dal for a longtime produces lathyrism, which results in paralysis of the lower limbs.

Some seeds, barks, leaves and other matter are dressed up to look like genuine foodstuffs for marketing as genuine products or to adulterate the pure ones. For example, roasted tamarind and date seeds are ground into coffee powder, and exhausted tea leaves or coloured sawdust are mixed into fresh tea. Exhausted bark or seeds of coffee, spices, etc., are dried, suitably coloured and substituted for the fresh commodity. Powdered bran and sawdust may be present in wheat flour and ground spices. Strips of jute or foreign plant material may be suitably dyed to be sold as saffron. Easily obtainable seeds are substituted for cumin, cardamom, black pepper, mustard seeds, etc.

Edible oils and fats are adulterated with cheap edible and non-edible oils. Argemone seeds are obtained from *Argemone mexicana* which grows widely in the country. The black seeds resemble mustard and are used to mix with mustard seeds. Argemone oil itself, extracted from the seeds, is used to adulterate oils such as coconut, sesame and groundnut. Argemone oil is poisonous and its use results in dropsy in human beings. Orthotricresyl phosphate is a colourless industrial chemical freely soluble in oils but if soluble in water. This is used to adulterate some oils. The chemical can cause permanent damage to the nervous system. Oils and fats are also adulterated with petroleum products causing gastrointestinal disturbances. Other common adulterants are animal fats in vanaspati and vanaspati in ghee.

Stones, sand, marble and earth are usually found mixed in foodgrains and pulses and their flours. Talc and chalk powder are used to adulterate wheat flour, arrowroot powder, panir and confectionery. Starch is used as a filler in milk, milk products and confectionery. Starch is also found in ground turmeric, coriander, mixed spices, etc. Addition of excess common salt to powdered spices, such as curry powder, is a common practice. Water is a common diluent of milk, curd, etc. It is also added to non-alcoholic beverages in more than the recommended quantities. Methyl alcohol is an adulterant of alcoholic beverages. This has resulted in a number of serious liquor tragedies in this country.

The most frequently used food adulterant in India is colouring matter. Colour is used in many foods such as milk products, confectionery (including Indian sweetmeats), soft drinks, alcoholic beverages, tea and spices. Colours are also added to foods such as egg preparations, bakery products, fruit products and others. More than 70 per cent of the colour containing marketed samples of foods are found to contain non-permitted colourants like the coal-tar dyes and mineral pigments like lead chromate and red or yellow earth. Use of foods containing non-permitted colourants results in various health hazards.

Check and Control

The governments in many countries play an important role in ensuring food quality. National official standards are set to safeguard the consumer's health and ensure fair food trade practices. In 1963, the FAO and WHO established a Commission for setting of international food standards.

Codex Alimentarius **:** The Codex Alimentarius are international standards set by FAO/W.HO for all the principal foods, whether processed, semi-processed or raw, for distribution to the common man. It also includes standards in respect of food hygiene, food additives, pesticide residues, contaminants, labelling and presentation, and methods of analysis and sampling. A Codex, Standard may be accepted by a country in its entirety or with more stringent requirements for trade and distribution of the food within its territory. A country which accepts Codex Standards cannot hinder the distribution in its territory of imported foods which conform to the standards.

Indian Standards : In India, food standards have been prescribed based on the International Codex Alimentarius with suitable modifications to suit the country's conditions. The most important standards are those set by the Indian Standards Institution (ISI).

The ISI is responsible for preparing and promoting general adoption of standards at national and international levels. The institution has an Agriculture and Food Products Division Council and a number of sectional committees dealing with various commodities. The standards are formulated and revised from time to time after eliciting the opinion of interested parties and based on the recommendations of a technical committee. Standards are available for a number of foods and food products like foodgrains and foodgrain products, bakery and confectionery products, processed and fresh fruits and vegetables, protein-rich food products, spices and stimulant foods like tea, coffee and cocoa. The institution has also published specifications on alcoholic and carbonated beverages, meat products and fish and fisheries products.

Chemicals used in the manufacture of food products to maintain their nutritional quality, enhance keeping quality and stability, etc., are subject to ISI standards. Before a chemical is permitted to be added, it is ensured that the substance is toxicologically safe, is added in safe dose and is of the required purity.

Hygienic quality of food is very important. Unless the factory producing the food is governed by the strict hygienic code in respect of layout, plant and personnel, the food produced cannot be considered safe, however nutritious it may be. Therefore, ISI has prepared codes for sanitary conditions in the food processing, bakery, soft drinks, ice cream, fruit and vegetable canning industries.

ISI has also worked out standards for sensory evaluation of foods. It safeguards the food trade interest of India, by maintaining effective liaison with organizations like the International Organization for Standardization and Codex Alimentarius Commission.

The Indian Standards Institution operates a certification marking scheme under which manufacturers are licensed to use the ISI mark on goods produced by them in conformity with the relevant standards. The ISI mark on products has been very helpful to consumers, organized purchasers, exporters and export inspection authorities. Food products covered under the ISI Certificate mark scheme are bakery and confectionery products, cereals, pulses and their products, dairy and allied products, beverages and food additives.

In addition to ISI standards, a number of other steps have been taken by the Government of India to control the quality of foods. Some of them are the following.

The Agricultural Produce (Grading and Marketing) Act provides for the grading and marketing of agricultural and other products. The Agmark Standards, incorporate grades, 1, 2, 3 and 4, or special, good, fair and ordinary, based on the physical and chemical characteristics, intrinsic as well as acquired, during processing or otherwise. The Agmark gives the consumer an assurance of quality according to the standards laid down. The grading system makes better buying and selling of agricultural produce.

The Preventing of Food Adulteration Act, with its various amendments, provides for the prevention of adulteration of food. The Director General of Health Services on behalf of the Central Government or the Chief Officer in charge of Health Administration in a state operates PFA rules under the Act.

The Vegetable Oil Control Order stipulates that any vegetable oil product, unless it conforms to the standards of quality and offers requirements for vanaspati or bakery shortening or margarine, shall not be manufactured, stocked or sold. There is also an order to regulate the production, distribution and quality of solvent extracted vegetable oils and vegetable oil products.

The Fruit Products Order (FPO) lays down minimum standards relating to the quality of various fruits and vegetables. The order specifies standards of sanitation and hygiene to be followed in the factories and gives directions regarding packing, marking and labelling of containers.

The Meat Products Order provisions are meant to control production, quality and distribution of raw and processed meat.

There are thus numerous organizations in the country to control the quality of food, its production and distribution. Sometimes confusion occurs among consumers and manufacturers regarding the multiplicity of food standards, such as ISI standard, PFA standard and Agmark standard for the same product. Hence, it is felt that there is a need to have a single organization to ensure food quality control, whether it is checking for food adulteration or ensuring quality control for home consumption or export.

17

Food Preparation

Some foods like fruits, vegetables and nuts are eaten raw. It is good that they are consumed raw as in the uncooked condition they retain most of their nutritive value. However, most foods are cooked before they are accepted. Cooking of food is the use of heat to bring about desirable changes in foods being consumed. The source of heat may be the result of combustion of wood, coal, gas or oil; by electric heating elements contained in hot plates or electric ovens; or by a microwave cooker.

Cooking Food

Cooking of food produces improvement in flavour, texture, and appearance, and this makes the food more palatable and easily digestible. Most foods in the raw state contain harmful micro-organisms and they are destroyed during cooking.

Improvement of Food Quality : Cooking improves the natural flavour of food, e.g., the flavour of meat is developed and enhanced by heating; the flavour of bread develops in the crust during baking; coffee flavour is formed during the roasting of green coffee, and so on. If a blend of flavours is required, several foods could be cooked together to bring about this. If the object is to change the flavour of a food, cooking helps achieve this by addition of required flavouring material. Cooking could also destroy the flavour of a food. In such a case, if the original flavour of a food is to be retained, there should be minimum cooking. Overcooking results in the vitalization of flavour substances and a less desired product may be obtained. Colour and texture also influence flavour. Cooking helps develop the desired colour and texture in foods.

Destruction of Micro-organisms : Micro-organisms are ubiquitous in their distribution; they are found everywhere in every environment, and adapt themselves to almost every growth condition. They make their presence known in many ways. Their action may be beneficial as in the production of cheese, pickles, leavening of bread, etc., or harmful as in food spoilage.

The latter type of micro-organisms are not normally present as food contaminants. When present they cause infections or produce toxins. Infective types of bacteria, such as *Salmonella* and *Shigella,* multiply in the intestinal tract and cause disease through the infection of the host. In contrast, bacteria like *Staphylococcus aureus* and *Clostridium botulinum* produce the toxins present in the food at the time of consumption and are the direct causes of illness. Food storage under conditions that prevent bacterial growth do not provide safety against infective pathogens but do so against toxinogenic food poisons.

Molds also produce toxins. The mold *Aspergillus flavus* produces a toxin (aflatoxin) which, when present in food, is a health hazard. There are many other molds producing toxins referred to as mycotoxins. One of the most important methods of protection of food against harmful micro-organisms is by the application of heat. Cooking food to the required temperature for a required length of time can destroy all harmful micro-organisms in foods.

Various Methods

Heat may be transferred to the food by conduction, convection, radiation or by the energy of microwaves (electronic heat transfer).

Conduction is the method of transfer of heat by contact. Convection is the transfer of heat as a result of the flow of a liquid or gas travelling from the hotter to a less hot part of an oven or saucepan. Radiation is the emission of heat in the form of waves from hot objects. Microwaves are a form of electromagnetic radiations similar to radio, TV, radar, light and infrared waves.

Conduction : In conduction, heat flows from the source to the material absorbing it. Certain materials are better conductors of heat than others. Copper utensils are the best conductors; aluminium ones conduct heat more slowly, and steel ones still more slowly. Glass is a very much less efficient conductor of heat than any of the metals. For efficient conduction to take place from a hot surface to another surface, such as the bottom of a saucepan, it is important that there is as large an area of contact as possible. Hence, the bottoms of pans should be flat and thick.

Convection : When a liquid or air is heated, the portions nearest to the heat become warm and less dense. They rise and are replaced by the denser material, i.e., convection currents flow from a more dense to less dense areas. The convection currents usually flow in a vertical direction and they are hindered by solid materials. Roasting is mainly accomplished by convection. The heat source at the bottom of the oven heats the air which rises and is continuously replaced by cold air. These convection currents create uniform temperature in the centre of the oven where the food is kept, resulting in roasting.

Radiation : Radiation waves travel at the same speed as light rays. Like light rays they are absorbed by dull black or rough surfaces and reflected by smooth, white or metallic surfaces. Radiation waves travel through gases, clear liquids or glass without heating them, or through vacuum. In cooking, when heat radiations reach the food, only the surface is heated by them. They do not penetrate the food. The rest of the food is cooked mostly by conduction and also to some extent by convection. Radiation heat is used in broiling. Toasting of bread is essentially by radiation heat.

Microwave Heating : Microwaves are absorbed and penetrate the food. The energy of these electromagnetic radiations excite the water molecules (in food) which bear a positive electrical charge in one portioa and a negative charge at another position of the molecule (dipole). When the electric field of the microwave interacts with the water dipole, the water molecules begin to vibrate very rapidly in food. This vibration produces friction that creates heat within the food, thereby cooking it. The excitation of water molecules occurs as far within the food as the microwaves are able to penetrate. This is different from heating by convection methods which transmit heat from the edges of the vessel to the centre. Heating of food beyond the depth of penetration of the microwaves occurs as a result of the conduction and/or convection of the heat created by microwaves.

Media of Cooking

Cooking can be carried out in various media or no media at all. Air, water, steam and fat, or combinations of these, are used as cooking media. Microwave heating involves generation of heat within the food; it is not a cooking medium.

Cooking in Air Grilling : roasting and baking take place in air. Grilling consists of placing the food below or above a red-hot surface. When under the heater, the food is heated by radiation only. This results in the browning of many foods. Then the heat is more slowly conducted through the surfaces of the food downwards. As heating is mostly superficial, gritted foods are usually reversed or rotated in the oven. If the food is above the heater, heat is transmitted to the food through convection currents, as well as radiations with consequent increased efficiency.

Roasting and baking are essentially the same. They are carried out in an oven between temperatures of 120° and 260°C. Generally, the term roasting is applied to meat cooking, while baking is used for breads, cakes and biscuits. The food is cooked partially by dry heat and partially moist heat, if the food is high in moisture content. In baking, the oven atmosphere should be moist initially so that the moisture condenses on the cold surface. This helps in heat transfer and plays a part in the formation of crust. Roasting and baking involve heat transfer from the heat source in the oven by radiation, conduction and convection. Heat is transferred directly onto the container of the food through which it is conducted to the food. Convection currents of air help keep the temperature of the oven fairly uniform. Rough and black surfaces absorbing more radiated heat are more efficient for baking than the bright shiny ones.

Broiling is the cooking of food by exposing it to direct heat. In this case, cooking takes place by conduction through direct contact of food with the hot broiler. Some radiation cooking also takes place in broiling.

Cooking in Water : Boiling, simmering or stewing involves cooking in water. In these cases the medium transferring heat is water. Water receives heat by conduction through the sides of the utensil in which the food is cooked and passes on the heat by convection currents which equalize the temperature and become very vigorous when boiling commences. Water is a poor conductor of heat and its heat capacity is high, i.e., it requires more heat than any other liquid of the same weight to raise the temperature. The boiling point of water is 100°C and it is altered at high altitudes and in presence of electrolytes. Simmering and poaching are methods of cooking of food by immersing in a hot liquid maintained at a temperature just below the boiling point.

Cooking in Steam : Steam is the medium of cooking in steaming, "waterless" cooking and pressure cooking. Cooking by these methods involves moist heat. In steaming, food is cooked by steam from added water, whilst in waterless cooking the steam originates from the food itself. Cooking food wrapped in aluminium foil or in a plastic bag is a form of waterless cooking. In this case, there is the advantage of preventing the transmission of flavour from or to the sealed food. Pressure cooking is a device to reduce the cooking time by increasing the pressure so that the boiling point of water is automatically raised. While water boils at 100°C at normal atmospheric pressure, it boils at 121°C at a pressure of 1.07 kg/cm^2 which is the pressure at which food is cooked in a kitchen pressure cooker. In cooking by steam, the food is heated as a result of steam condensing on the food, and the release of the large quantity of heat (latent heat) contained in the steam. This continues until the heated food reaches the same temperature as steam.

Cooking in Fat : Fat is used as a medium for cooking in sauteing, shallow fat frying (pan frying) and deep fat frying. Sauteing is the cooking of food in a slightly greased pan. Only thin pieces of food (dosas, for example) are cooked this way. This prevents food from sticking to the pan. The heat is transferred to the food mainly by conduction. The food is to be turned from one side to the other to complete the cooking. In shallow fat frying, food is cooked in a larger amount of fat, but not enough to cover it. Heat is transferred to the food partially by conduction by contact with the heated pan and partially by the convection currents of the food. This prevents local burning of food by convectioning away the intense heat of the frying pan. As in sauteing, even in this case, the food must normally be turned over to ensure some degree of uniform cooking. Both sauteing and pan frying are really a type of baking.

Deep fat frying is similar to boiling. Food is cooked by vigorous convection currents and cooking is uniform on all sides of the food. As fat can be heated to a much higher temperature than the boiling point of water, cooking can be rapidly completed in deep fat frying. In most foods, this high temperature results in rapid drying-out of the surface, and the production of a hard, crisp surface, usually brown, and the absorption of a fair amount of fat, which raises the calorific value of the food substantially. Fats should not be heated to the smoking point as they decompose at that point to fatty acids and glycerol, followed by the decomposition of glycerol to acrolein, which causes irritation to the eyes and nose.

Foods may also be prepared by a combination of media. Preparation of *uppuma*, for example, involves the use of a combination of fat and water media. Some components (onions) of the preparation are first browned in a small quantify of fat followed by the cooking of semolina in water.

Microwave Cooking

Microwave cooking, which was first recognized as valuable for cooking food in 1947, is becoming more and more popular because it is a convenient and very quick method of cooking food. Microwaves do not require any medium for transfer of heat in cooking. They are generated by an electric instrument called magnetron. Microwaves have a high frequency of 2,450 megacycles (or 2,450 million times) per second. The microwaves can be absorbed, transmitted or reflected when they impinge on substances. They pass through paper, china, glass and some plastics without absorption, and are reflected by metals and absorbed by food. When food is kept in the cavity of a microwave oven for cooking, microwaves generated by the magnetron strike the food and the metal walls of the oven. Microwaves that strike the metal wall are reflected and bounce back so that they disperse through the oven. This is important for accomplishing a uniform heating of food. Microwaves penetrate food to a depth of 2.5 to 7.5 cm. Up to this limit of penetration of the microwaves, the food gets heated and cooked. Thus, food will heat up inside and outside at the same time. When the thickness of food is large, microwaves will heat it up throughout at the same time to the depth of their penetration and the portion of food beyond it will be heated more slowly by conduction. Food, for cooking in a microwave oven, should be kept in containers that transmit the microwaves and should not absorb or reflect them. This is achieved by-using paper containers, such as paper plates or cups, or utensils made of plastic, glass or chinaware, which do not contain metallic substances.

Advantages of Microwave Cooking : The most important advantage of microwave cooking is the speed with which cooking may be accomplished resulting in a considerable saving of time in cooking. Microwave cooking is ten times faster than cooking by the conventional methods; a cake cooks in just five minutes. The length of time of cooking will be increased if the quantity of food to be cooked is increased. Microwave heating also saves time in heating refrigerated or frozen foods; the latter can be defrosted in minutes instead of hours. Another advantage of this method of cooking is that only the food is heated during cooking. The oven does not get heated and even the utensils do not become hot, except when the cooking period is relatively long and some heat is conducted from the food to the container. The flavour and texture of prepared food do not change when reheated by microwaves. This is another advantage of this type of cooking. Electrical energy required for microwave cooking is less than that required by the traditional method.

Limitations of Microwave Cooking : There are some limitations to microwave cooking. As the process of cooking does not rely on the conduction or convection of the material being heated, it is normally possible to heat the whole of the food simultaneously. Due to the short period of time of cooking, the food does not become brown on the surface as many foods do when they are roasted or baked in a conventional oven. Baked products without a brown surface do not have appeal. To overcome the problem created by lack of browning a microwave oven is combined with a browning unit. Another disadvantage of microwave cooking is that it cannot be employed for simmering or stewing for tenderizing foods, as also for deep-fat frying. Also, the short cooking time may not give a chance for the blending of various flavours to develop as in the conventional methods of cooking.

New Trends

When food is subjected to heat many changes occur; there is some destruction of proteins, lipids and vitamins, which is detrimental to the nutritional value of food. However, there are also some beneficial changes. Cooking is required if we have to obtain the maximum nutritive value of some foods and maintain a safe and wholesome food supply. Heat treatment is also one of the most common and effective methods of food preservation and may be used alone or in combination with other preservation techniques. Some of the changes that take place in the constituents of food during cooking are discussed below.

Changes in Proteins : The principal effect of heat on protein is de-naturation. This results in the destruction of micro-organisms and inactivation of microbial and natural enzymes within the food. Cooking also destroys the toxic proteins and peptides, enzyme inhibitors, antivitamins and other natural toxicants in food, which can seriously affect their nutritive value. Legumes contain trypsin inhibitors, haemagglutinins and other toxic substances which affect the digestibility and availability of sulphur-containing amino acids. These are destroyed by heat. Approximately 40 per cent of the growth-depressing effect of uncooked soyabeans is due to the presence of trypsin inhibitors. Of the remaining proteins of soyabeans digestibility increases after cooking. Cereal grains also contain trypsin inhibitors and natural toxicants. Heat destroys these antimetabolites in rice, wheat and oats, but has little effect in other cereals.

Cooking can also result in the interaction of protein with nonprotein components of the food system; there can be interaction of protein with carbohydrate or lipid oxidation products'. There can also be interprotein and intraprotein reactions in the presence or absence of oxygen. These changes in cooking result in nutritional unavailability of proteins.

There is significant loss of lysine and the sulphur-containing amino acid cysteine after heating proteins. On prolonged heating, tryptophan, methionine and the basic amino acids are also lost. Charring and the presence of off-odours during cooking is due to destruction of amino acids and proteins. These changes affect the palatability of the final product.

Interaction between the free amino groups of proteins with reducing sugars or carbonyl groups formed by lipid oxidation results in non-enzymatic browning (Maillard browning). This reaction is of importance because it is responsible for many of the specific tastes, aromas and colour of foods. In this reaction, the amino group of the essential amino acid lysine reacts with carbonyl groups of sugar and fatty-acid oxidation compounds, which results in a decrease in the nutritive value of proteins.

Changes in Carbohydrates : Monosaccharides, oligo and polysaccharides undergo many transformations when cooked in an aqueous medium. The sugars are subjected to degradation and epimerization and, of over 100 compounds that are formed by such transformations, hydroxymethyl furfural is the most important compound. This compound and furfural are also products of non-enzymic browning reactions. But these compounds have no adverse effects.

Starch molecules which are the main source of calories in many diets, when heated in an aqueous or moist environment, swell and rupture, and this permits greater enzymatic digestion by enzymes like amylases. Cooking thus increases the digestibility of carbohydrates. Starch, when subjected to dry heat at a temperature of 200°C or higher, breaks down resulting in the formation of dextrin and volatile compounds like furfural and hydroxymethyl furfural.

Changes in Lipids: Lipids undergo hydrolytic, oxidative, polymeric or other degradative changes which modify not only the physical properties of the lipid but also their biological properties when heated. The hydrolytic and oxidative changes result in rancidity. Hydrolytic rancidity is catalyzed in food at high temperature and pressure in an aqueous medium in the presence of acids, alkalis and lipolytic enzymes (Upases). Hydrolytic rancidity by itself does not bring about any significant change in the nutritive value of the food. However, the objectionable flavour imparted by free fatty acids lowers the consumption of food.

Oxidative rancidity is responsible for more losses in the quality and nutritive value of lipids than any other change. This rancidity results in the formation of hydroperoxides as primary products owing to the attack of oxygen on the unsaturated centres of lipids. The products of oxidation exhibit strong unpleasant flavours even when present in extremely low amounts. The oxidation of a fat at high temperature, in addition to volatile and non-volatile compounds associated with lipid oxidation at normal temperature, gives isomerization products (trans- and conjugated double bond products), cyclic compounds, dimers and polymers. While lipids oxidized at normal temperatures exhibit no toxicity, thermally oxidized lipids have shown various detrimental effects. But the lipid or food system would be unpalatable long before the concentration of the toxic compound reached a hazardous level.

In addition to the effect on the biological properties of lipids, thermal effects bring about physical and chemical changes also. In sauteing and shallow fat frying, the quantity of oil used is small, cooking time is short and there is generally no reuse of fat or oil and thus there is little concern over the nutritional effects of lipids absorbed from such cooking. In contrast, there has been a great deal of concern over deep fat fried foods. If the deep fat frying is continuous, oxidative changes are small because the fat absorbed by the food is constantly replaced. In discontinuous deep fat frying, as is common in homes, there is liberation of fatty acids due to the addition of water to the oil from the food, decreased unsaturation and increase in peroxides, conjugated double bonds and polymers. Such fats absorbed by foods could be toxic when consumed.

Changes in Vitamins and Minerals : These are lost primarily by leaching, oxidation of the water-soluble nutrients and thermal destruction.

The loss of water-soluble vitamins ranges from 0 to 60 per cent as a result of leaching and thermal destruction. In addition to losses by water and heat, ascorbic acid is lost by oxidation due to exposure to air of food during cooking. Vitamin A and carotene are water insoluble and, as such, are not lost as a result of leaching and their destruction due to oxidation is very slight. Frying and roasting cause their loss up to 40-60 per cent. Minerals also are lost on account of leaching and their losses are smaller (0 to 35 per cent).

Changes in Colour : Colour factors in foods, such as anthocyanins, carotenoids, chlorophylls, myoglobin, etc., are affected by heat. In addition to heat, the acidity or alkalinity of the cooking medium, oxygen and presence or absence of metals, also contribute to colour changes when heated. In some cases, the colour changes that take place in foods on cooking are desirable (as in baking) while in some other cases the changes may be undesirable (as in the prolonged cooking of cabbage). The cooking condition should be so organized as to obtain the desired colour qualities in the cooked food.

Art of Cooking

For every human being, the food is essential and nourishes the body. It is defined as anything eaten or drunk that can be absorbed by the body to be used as an energy source, building, regulating or protective material. Food can be defined as anything solid or liquid, which when swallowed, digested and assimilated in the body keeps it well. Food is a prerequisite of nutrition. Nutrition is defined as food at work in the body. In other words, food being processed and used for various functions in the body.

The Functions

1. Food provides materials for tissue building, growth and body repair mainly through proteins and minerals, eg., proteins and minerals.
2. Food provides energy to the body through nutrients like carbohydrates and fats (lipids), eg., carbohydrates, fats.
3. Protective foods are essential for safeguarding against the diseases, eg., Vitamins, minerals.
4. Regulatory foods are needed for the normal working of the body which includes heart beating, body temperature maintenance, muscle construction, blood clotting, waste products removal from the body and control of water balance.
5. Food also serves the social function. Special foods are served in public gatherings, ceremonies and religious functions, eg., water, roughage.

Various Groups : A balanced diet is one that contains different types of foods in such quantities and proportions from which the need of calories, minerals, vitamins and other nutrients is adequately met. These foods are divided into various groups as follows:

Group I : It includes cereals, millets, roots and tubers. All these primarily supply energy or calories, eg. rice, wheat, jowar, maize, bajra, ragi and tomato, potato, sweet-potato, colocasia, yam. These are an important source of thiamine, niacin and iron.

Group II : The food stuffs in this group are primarily sources of protein, eg. Dals, grains, peas, beans, groundnuts, cashewnuts, almonds, coconut, milk, curd, buttermilk, paneer, mava, eggs, fish, mutton, chicken, pork and other flesh foods. Milk and milk products are important sources of calcium and riboflavin. Meat, fish and eggs rank first for their protein, iron and niacin content.

Group III : These food stuffs supply energy or calories, ·g., vegetable oils, vanaspati ghee, butter, cream, sugar, aggery. This group constitutes about 1/6th of the energy value of he diet. Cooking oils include mustard oil, coconut oil, til oil, groundnut oil, palm oil and sunflower oil supply essential fatty acids.

Group IV : These are mainly suppliers of minerals and vitamins. This includes protective vegetables and fruits.

(a) Green leafy vegetables, palak, methi, gogu, drumstick, coriander, fenugreek and arvi leaves, kulfa and similar greens supply vitamin B_2, folic acid, calcium, iron, fibre and carotenoids.

(b) Yellow or orange fruits and vegetables - papaya, mango, carrots, yellow pumpkin provide carotenoids.

(c) Fruits and vegetables rich in vitamin C - amla, guava, lemon, orange, phalsa.

These are the only important sources of ascorbic acid, contribute half of the vitamin A requirement, supply 1/5th of the iron required.

Group V : Other vegetables and fruits are included in this group. These provide variety in taste and texture and furnish roughage in the diet. eg. fruits, stems, leaves and flowers of plants, lady's finger, brinjal, bitter gourds and other gourds, cabbage, cauliflower, drumstick supply carotenoids, folic acid, calcium and fibre in the diet. Various fruits included in this group are bananas, melons, grapes, apples, sapotas, berries, pears, plantain, lichis, pomogranate etc.

Various Methods

Food preparation is an important step in meeting the nutritional needs of the family. It is not enough that food be nutritious, it has to be pleasing in appearance and taste so that it is eaten.

Principles of Cooking

1. All foods must be cooked in a way that 'keeps the flavour in'.
2. Sometimes the flavour of the food is 'drawn out' into the gravy or broth.
3. The preservation of the maximum nutritive value can be ensured by using correct methods of cooking, suited to the particular foods.

The process of subjecting foods to the action of heat is termed as cooking. Food can be cooked by various methods to make it edible.

Roasting : Food is brought into direct contact with the hea source. The food is periodically coated with fat and turned ove the fire from time to time to cook it evenly. It can be done on live coals, under a grill, in the tandoor or any other oven. Temperature to be maintained is 350° C to 375° C. The term roasting is applied to meat cooking. It is of three types.

(a) *Spit roasting:* The food to be cooked is brought in contact with direct flame in front of a clear bright fire. The food is basted over with fat and is also turned regularly to ensure even cooking and browning, eg. Barbecued meat.

(b) *Oven roasting:* This is cooked in a closed oven with the aid of fat. The food is put into a very hot oven for 5 to 10 minutes and the temperature is lowered to allow the joint to be cooked. Cooking in a moderate oven for a longer time produces a better cooked joint than cooking at high temperature for a shorter period as the meat retains its moisture and flavour.

(c) *Pot roasting:* This method is used to cook small joints and birds if no oven is available, but a thick heavy pan is essential. Enough fat is melted to cover the bottom of the pan. When the fat is hot the joint is browned. It is then lifted out and 2 or 3 skewers are kept at the bottom on which the joint is placed. This is to prevent the joint from sticking to the pan. The joints should just touch the fat. The pan is then covered tightly with a well fitting lid and cooked over a very low fire. Prepared root vegetables and potatoes can also be cooked round the meat.

Broiling or Grilling: The food is placed on a metal grill directly over or below the source of heat either gas or electricity. Under the heater, the food is heated by radiation only. This results in browning of various foods. Then the heat is more slowly conducted through the surfaces of the food downwards. If the food is above the heater, heat is transmitted to the food through convection currents, as well as radiations with consequent increased efficiency. This method is usually used for tender cuts of meat, poultry, etc. and when foods need to be browned as made crisp on the surface, eg. pizzas, sausages, bacon, etc. When food is cooked uncovered on heated metal or a frying pan, it is known as pan-broiling.

Baking: It requires an oven or tandoor as any equipment in which hot air circulates around the food placed in the action of dry heat is combined with the steam generated from the food during cooking. Foods baked are generally brown and crisp on the top and soft and porous in the centres, eg. cakes, breads, puddings, vegetables, biscuits, pastries, potatoes, meat dishes in sauce etc. Temperature maintained in this is 120° C to 160° C. Baking involves heat transfer from the heat source in the oven by radiation, conduction and convection.

Frying: In frying the food is cooked in hot fat. Fat has very much higher boiling point than water. Frying can be done by different ways:

(a) *Sauteing :* This method involves cooking food in just enough fat or oil to coat/base of the pan in which the cooking is done eg. Dosa. The food is tossed occasionally or turned over to enable the pieces to come in contact with the oil or fat and evenly cooked and prevents food from sticking to the pan. The heat is transferred to the food mainly by conduction.

(b) *Shallow frying :* Sufficient quantity of fat is used in the pan and food is turned to cook both sides equally as it is done for paratha, omelette, pancake, and tikki. Heat is transferred to the food partially by conduction and partially by convection currents.

(c) *Deep frying :* It is done in a deep saucepan or kadai that contains excess quantity of fat or oil to immerse the food fried. Potato chips, bonda, pakoras and puris are deep fat fried preparations. For satisfactory results, food should be fried in fats and oils heated to 320° C. Fat can be heated to a much higher temperature than the boiling point of water, so cooking is rapidly completed. In most foods, this high temperature results in a hard, crisp surface, usually brown and the absorption of a fair amount of fat which raises the calorific value of the food substantially.

(d) *Fricasseeing :* It is cooking in a small amount of fat and then serving with sauce.

Moist/Wet Heat Methods

1. *Boiling:* Cooking foods in water that is bubbling constantly over the food in a pan. The temperature of the water is 100° C when it boils, eg. potatoes, eggs, sweet potatoes, rice, etc.
2. *Simmering:* It is done at 85° to 90° C temperature when foods are cooked in water or liquid which is not bubbling vigorously as in boiling, it is simmering. The very tiny bubbles coming to the surface and breaking. This method takes longer to cook food than boiling eg. cuts of meat used for stews or stock preparation.
3. *Blanching:* In this method of cooking, the food is usually dipped in boiling water for 5 seconds to 2 mn, depending on the texture of the food. The purpose of this method is to remove peels of fruits, vegetables, nuts, etc. easily

without changing their texture too much. The process of subjecting foods to boiling temperature for short period is known as blanching.

4. *Steaming:* It requires food to be placed in a vessel in which steam can enter and cook the food. The steam is generated by boiling water in a pan and another pan is placed in water. The second pan contains the food to be cooked, e.g. Idlis, khaman, dhokla and other fermented products. This food is easily digestable, nutritious and full of flavour. While in waterless cooking the steam originates from the food itself. Cooking food wrapped in an aluminium foil or in a plastic bag is a form of waterless cooking.

5. *Pressure Cooking:* This is a method of cooking food by steam under pressure. While water boils at 110° C at normal atmospheric pressure, it boils at 121° C at a pressure of 1.07 kg/cm^2, which is the pressure at which food is cooked in a kitchen pressure cooker (food is cooked at 110°-112° C). It is a quicker method than pan steaming generally done in pressure cooker. The storter cooking time enhances nutrient retention and palatability eg. curries, soups, broths, stews, etc.

6. *Poaching:* This method involves cooking in a small amount of liquid at a temperature just below the boiling point (simmering). Foods generally poached are eggs, fish, fruits, etc.

7. *Stewing:* This is a gentle method of cooking in a pan with a tight fitting lid, using small quantities and the other half in the liquid is cooked at simmering temperature (98° C). It is usually used for cooking meat, dais, etc.

Other Methods

Braising: This is a combined method of roasting and stewing. It is cooking over direct heat or in an oven in a small amount of liquid at a low temperature with the pan tightly covered.

Solar Cooking: It is a method of cooking food by converting the solar energy into heat energy. Solar cooker is placed at such an angle that the mirror reflects the sun's rays into the food placed in the container. The containers are blackened to absorb the maximum of the sun's heat.

Infra-red Radiation or Microwave Cookery : The food to be cooked is placed in an electronic oven where it is exposed to the penetration of microwaves produced by a magnetron tube. The microwaves cause agitation of the molecules within the food so that heat is generated. The microwaves can be absorbed, transmitted or reflected and they can pass through paper, china and glass. Cooking time is shortened to ten times less than may be needed by conventional methods.

Preservation of Food : Food spoilage is brought by the action of enzymes present in foods or due to the action of micro-organisms such as mold, yeast and bacteria or due to infestation with insects and worms. The environment unfavourable to the action of enzymes or to the growth of micro-organism is the main objective of food preservation. Preservation of food also helps in increasing the shelf life of foods, making seasonal food available through out the year, adding variety to the diet, and improving the nutrition. Preservation is defined as the state in which any food may be retained over a period of time without being contaminated by pathogenic organisms or chemicals and without losing optimum qualities of colour, texture, flavour and nutritive value.

The different methods of food preservation (household and commercial) are of two types:

(a) *Bactericidal Methods:* Bactericidal method are those which destroy bacteria. These include applying heat by cooking, canning, sterilization, irradiation and preservation.

(b) *Bacteriostatic Methods:* Bacteriostatic method are those in which the growth of bacteria, yeasts and moulds is retarded by dehydration, freezing, treatment with antibiotics, salting and pickling.

Bactericidal Methods

Heating: Food is commonly preserved through the application of high temperatures. A temperature considerably above that of the body may result in either a pasteurized by being held at a temperature from 60° C to 66° C for thirty to forty minutes, during this time most of the organisms, although not all, are killed. This method is used for temporary preservation of milk and for preservation of fruit juices and other fruit products of delicate flavour.

Canning: It is the preservation of food in sealed containers, after the application of heat, through steam under pressure. If the effectiveness of pasteurization and sterilization is to extend over a period of time of practical significance, the material thus treated must be protected from fresh contamination by micro-organisms. The first foods preserved by canning were sealed in glass.

Drying: Removal of moisture is of benefit in preserving food. Drying alters greatly the character of the food and requires some time for preparation both before and after the process. Meat and fish have been dried for centuries. Other foods that are preserved through dehydration method are figs, apples, prunes/plums and raisins.

Sun drying is a common method of food preservation. Dried foods include papdi, papads, macaroni, bari, potato wafers and so on. Fruits like apricots, bananas, dates, figs, grapes, raw mango, peaches, pears, pomegranate seeds are also preserved by sun drying.

Smoking: Foods can also be dried by exposing them to smoke by burning some special kinds of wood. in this method, while the heat from the smoke helps in removal of moisture, exposure to smoke imparts a characteristic flavour to the food. Fish and meat are the foods usually preserved by this method.

Mechanical Drying: Dehydrators, rollers dryers and spray dryers are the mechanical devices used for drying food. Solid foods such as papads, vegetables such as green peas, onions, potatoes are spread in thin layers on metal trays inserted in the dehydrator and then dried by heat. Food in the form of a fine dry powder can be obtained by using either roller drying or spray drying. In roller drying, the finely ground wet suspension of the food is spread as a thin layer on a revolving drum which is heated. The resultant dry powder is then scraped off with a blunt knife and packed. In the spray drying process the food in the form of a liquid or a finely ground suspension is pumped through fine jets and falls as a spray into a chamber through which hot air is circulated. The fine droplets of the liquid quickly lose their moisture by evaporation and fall on the floor of the chamber as a fine powder.

Sterilization by Cooking: Sterilization by cooking is a method of preserving foods by preventing the growth of micro-organisms through the application of high temperatures. Boiling temperature (212° F or 100° C) if maintained for a sufficiently long period of time, helps the heat to completely penetrate the foods and kill the bacteria.

Pasteurization: Pasteurization may be brought about by the holding process in which milk is heated to at least 62° C (143° F) and kept at that temperature for at least 30 minutes; or by the high temperature short time method in which milk is heated to 71° C (160° F) and kept at that temperature for at least 15 seconds.

Milk may be sterilized either by boiling for a period of time or by the application of heat as in the preparation of evaporated milk. Sterilization depends on the colour of milk and gives it a slightly caramelized flavour, while pasteurization does not change the colour or flavour of milk.

Preservation of Foods by Irradiation: In this process, gamma rays or high speed electrons are used to destroy micro-organisms. These radiations are termed as ionising radiations.

Low level irradiation presents the germination potatoes, onions and carrots. Metabolic processes can be controlled by this treatment in foods thus delaying their ripening. Pork and beef can be made free of tapeworms and trichenella by irradiation. Heavy losses in the granary due to insect infestation can be checked by irradiation..

Bacteriostatic Methods

Refrigeration: Micro-organisms, although not readily destroyed by severe cold, and much less active at low temperatures i.e. 0° C to 5° C, refrigeration is widely used both in homes and in commercial plants, as a means of maintaining the low temperature found satisfactory in the storage of perishable foods. Fresh milk, meat and similar foods are kept just above the freezing point. Certain fruits and vegetables also keep better when cold.

Wrapping certain fruits and vegetables in paper or cellophane, or coating them with wax, improves the keeping quality. Pears and apples of high quality to be kept for winter use and oranges, lemons and grapefruit are often wrapped. (The fruit or the paper in which it is wrapped may be treated to retard mould formation.) Green peppers, tomatoes, oranges and other citrus fruits, cucumbers and cantaloupes are among the foods whose keeping quality is improved when they are coated with wax.

Freezing: Freezing, (-18° C to -40° C) like cold storage, does not destroy the micro-organisms and enzymes present in the foods. Foods can be quick frozen in about 90 min or less by placing them in contact with the coil through which the refrigerant flows, by blast freezing in which cold air is blown across the food and by dipping in liquid nitrogen.

Scalding to destroy the enzymes is essential for successful preservation of almost all vegetables by this method. Hence, vegetables to be used fresh and crisp in salads cannot be preserved by freezing. Fish, poultry and game, as well as beef, veal, pork and lamb are preserved by freezing.

Freeze-drying: During this process the frozen food is placed under vacuum to remove the water, and it is then packaged in the presence of an inert gas such as nitrogen. The advantage of this method is that the product retains its original volume and shape and rehydrates easily. Products which have been subjected to freeze drying are coffee, beef, pork, chicken, soups and several food mixtures. Products of freeze-drying have a long shelf life, possess a light weight and can be stored and refrigerated, but they are considered inferior to frozen or canned foods.

Dehydro-freezing: This process is a combination of partial dehydration and freezing. The vegetables and fruits which are subjected to dehydrofreezing are first heated in order to lose about half their water content, and then frozen. Later, when the food is cooked water is added to reconstitute it.

Chemical Preservation: Certain chemicals like benzoic acid or sodium benzoate and sulphurdioxide are helpful in preserving foods either by retarding or preventing the growth of micro-organisms. Sodium benzoate upto a concentration of 0.1 % is used for all coloured fruits and vegetables. Potassium metabisulphite is used as a source of sulphur-dioxide and is used only for colourless fruits like apple, lichi, and raw mango. Meats may be cured with smoke that contains phenols.

Sugar, a common home preservative, is often used in such quantities as to increase the concentration of the food and make it an unfavourable medium for the organisms. Salt and acid, in the form of vinegar or lemon juice, are other substances added for their preservative action. Frequently, the fermentation process is used to produce, within the food itself, acetic or lactic acid that exerts the same preservative action as is obtained by the addition of vinegar. Salt is used as an aid in the preservation of vegetables by fermentation. It aids both in drawing out the juices and in delaying the action of certain spoilage agents. Formerly, spices were often used in such quantities as to have a definite preservative effect.

Oils and spices alongwith salt and sugar provide a medium that resists the activity of the micro-organisms in food. Spices such as chillies, fenugreek, mustard and pepper are used in pickling. Certain preservative such as borax, boric acid, sulfites, and formaldehyde, once sold as canning powders, are now considered injurious to human beings, and their use is usually prohibited.

Preserving and Pickling: Preserving and pickling are methods of preservation frequently employed. Long before canning was known as a means of preserving foods, the use of preservatives was practised. Salting of foods was an early method of preservation. Salt is a valuable preservative, both as an antiseptic and as an agent for removing water. Placing foods in brine of certain concentration promotes fermentation and the foods develop an agreeable flavour. It is a good method of preserving vegetables and fruits like tamarind, raw mango, amla, fish and meat. Sugar in large amount is likewise a favourite preservative because the high concentration of sugar solution exerts a high osmotic pressure and withdraws water from the micro-organisms, thereby preventing their growth. It is the one used in making preserves, jams, jellies and marmalades.

Dehydration: Dehydration of foods to prevent spoilage does not necessarily mean complete removal of water, but it does mean concentration to such a point that the liquid is denser than the body fluid of the organisms. When the liquid outside the cell wall is more dense than that inside, the liquid within tends to be removed from the cell and the body processes are delayed or prevented. Hence, although the moisture is present, it may not be available to the organism which might cause spoilage. Scalding to destroy the enzymes is highly beneficial in prolonging the storage life of dehydrated vegetables. A variety of dehydrated food products available in the market are dehydrated soups, pre-cooked peas and cereals.

Antibiotics in Food Preservation: Very often antibiotics are used in the feed of animals or in treating them. Sometimes cows and poultry are fed on antibiotics. The Food and Drug Administration, specifies that milk from such cows should not be used for human consumption for at least three days following the treatment of the animal with the antibiotic.

Crops are sometimes sprayed with antibiotics. Since no residues of antibiotics are present in the foods eaten, there is no hazard to the health of the consumer. When fish and poultry are treated with antibiotics, their shelf life increases two to three times, because of the reduced growth of the micro-organisms. Similarly, antibiotics are used in the ice-crush used for packing raw fish and shellfish. The cooking of fish and poultry destroys the antibiotic residues, rendering them harmless for human consumption.

Food Analysis : Food has been a basic part of our existence. The study of food science involves understanding the nature, composition and behaviour of food materials under varying conditions of storage, processing and use. Many physical and chemical reactions occur due to the interaction with the medium of cooking, and the environmental conditions such as heat, cold, light and air to which they are subjected during cooking.

Cooking: Foods like fruits, vegetables and nuts are eaten raw but most of the foods are cooked to bring about desirable changes. The process of subjecting foods to the action of heat is termed as cooking.

Preliminary Preparations: It means the tasks done before the final preparation of food which includes cleaning, peeling and stringing, cutting and grating, sieving, soaking, processing, coating, blanching, marinating, sprouting, fermenting, grinding, drying and filtering.

Cleaning: Many food products like vegetables, fruits etc. may have portions to be discarded, eg., Withered or discoloured leaves in cabbage and green leafy vegetables.

Other aspect of cleaning is washing that is applicable to fruits, vegetables, cereals, pulses and non-vegetarian foods. Washing fruits render them dirt free, insecticides, sprays, and chemical free. Washing in warm water helps to kill the worms worms in cauliflower. Washing flesh food products helps to remove blood, dirt and unwanted impurities. Washing cereals or dhals help to remove husk, mud and any other unwanted matter but may cause the loss of B complex vitamins especially, thiamine.

Peeling and Stringing: Both these methods involve the removal of non edible or fibrous portion of fruits or vegetables, eg. Peeling of banana, potato, bottle gourd, stringing of beans. Peeling brings about loss of nutrients present under the surface of food, hence the product should be boiled or blanched and then peeled, eg., Vitamin C in potatoes.

Cutting and Grating: This is dividing the food into smaller pieces, thus helping in easy cooking. Various terms used under this are:

- *Cut* : to divide into pieces or to shape with knife
- *Chop* : to cut into no specified shape
- *Mine* : to chop very fine
- *Dice* : to cut into small uniform cubes
- *Slice* : to cut into uniform slices

Cutting and grating is done to make the food easily consumable and spoiled portion of the food can be discarded. But if it cut into small pieces, there is a greater loss of nutrients.

Sieving: It is done to remove coarse fibres, dirt, stones and insects. eg. sieving flour with baking powder for cake preparation.

Soaking: It is done in water either plain or salted with sodium chloride or sodium bicarbonate to hasten the process of cooking.

Processing: It includes all the things to get food ready for cooking and serving by enhancing the flavour of the product. The various processes included under this are:

- *Mix :* to combine ingredients in such a way that the parts of each ingredient are evenly dispersed in the total product.
- *Blend :* to mix two or more ingredients so completely that they lose their separate identities. Ingredients in ice creams and milk shake blend so well that individual ingredients cannot be seen.
- *Bind :* to cause a mixture of two or more ingredients to cohere as a homogenous product. Binding agents like starches and eggs are used in making custards. Another example is dough making.
- *Beat :* to move an instrument back and forth to blend ingredients together to achieve a smooth texture.
- *Whip :* to beat with a rapid lifting motion to incorporate air into a food e.g. eggs.
- *Fold :* to mix a whipped ingredient lightly with an other ingredient by gently turning one over the other with a flat implement eg. egg white in souffle preparation.

- *Mashing :* crushing the food product to a smooth structure eg. mashing vegetables in cutlet preparation.
- *Stuffing :* Introducing or filling a food stuff eg. stufing mashed potatoes in parathas.
- *Coating :* It refers to covering a food with layer of crumbs, flour or other fine substances before cooking it. The different ways of coating are:
- *Dredging :* Passing food through a fine dry or powdery substance in order to coat it Substances often used are flour, powdered almonds and bread crumbs.
- *Breading :* Three steps are involved. The product is first dredged in flour, then dipped in egg mixture liquids then in crumbs.
- *Battering :* This is dipping the food product in batter. Batter is a semi liquid. It usually consists of an egg liquid mixture thickened with flour to achieve a smooth consistency. Bengal gram flour or rice flour can also be used for this purpose.

Blanching: This is plunging food into boiling liquid and immersing in cold water. This destroys enzymes present in food hence used as preparation or preservation. Foods normally blanched are tomatoes, potatoes, almonds, carrots and beans.

Marinating : It is soaking a food in a marinade to add flavour or to tenderize it or both. A marinade is any liquid made up for purpose of marinating. Vegetables marinated are brinjal, onions, radish, bittergourd, potatoes and chillies. Meat marinade made up of oil, flavour builders and acid.

Sprouting or Germination: All kinds of grams like green gram, bengal gram, peas and cereals like ragi and wheat are generally sprouted to increase the digestibility and water soluble vitamins.

Fermentation: It is process of breaking down of complex matter into simpler ones with the aid of enzymes and bacteria. This can be done under aerobic or anaerobic conditions. Fermented foods are more nutritious than their unfermented counterparts. eg. Idli, bread and dhokla.

Grinding: This includes both wet and dry grinding to enhance the taste and flavour. Wet grinding includes the grinding idli, dosa batter and preparations of chutneys. Dry grinding is grinding spices for masala powders and wheat for wheat flour.

Drying: It is the removal of moisture from food products and prolong the shelf life of the food. Cereals, pulses and spices that are normally used are dried products only. Food stuffs generally dried are mango and gongura for pickles.

Filtering: This process is generally done to remove dirt, unwanted particles or to remove moisture from food stuff. In the preparation of cottage cheese or paneer, whey water is extracted. Food stuffs filtered are coffee, tea, rice, soups, fruit juices and tamarind water.

Roasting: This process should be grouped under actual cooking methods but certain recipes, however, demand roasting as prepreparation. eg. rava and vermicelli.

Cereals and Cereal Products : The word cereal is derived from ceres, the Roman goddess of grain. The principal cereal crops are rice, wheat, maize or corn, jowar, ragi and bajra. 80% of dry matter of cereals is carbohydrate, mainly the starch. Cereals contain 6 to 12% protein and provides more than 50% of the daily protein requirement and lipid content is 1-2%. About 95% of minerals are the phosphates and sulphates of potassium, magnesium and calcium. Whole grain cereals are an important source of B vitamins in our diet. There are various by - products of cereals especially wheat includes whole wheat flour which contains the finely ground bran, germ and endosperm of the whole kernel. In maida the bran and germ are separated. Semolina is coarsely ground endosperm. Macaroni products are also called pasta or alimentary pastes include macaroni, spaghetti, vermicelli and noodles. Macaroni is a tube form, spagetti may be either tube or rod, vermicelli is a tiny rod and noodles are flat strips. Malted wheat is prepared by steeping grains in cold water for 36 hours, allowed for germination and making flour after drying thoroughly. Amylase Rich Food (ARF) is germinated cereal flours which are extremely rich in the enzyme alpha-amylase. Glutamic acid is derived from wheat which is a salt like product generally used to bring out the flavour of other foods or seasonings. Wheat bran prevents constipation and may lower the risk of colon cancer.

Rice products include milled rice and parboiled rice i.e. soaking paddy in water for a short time followed by heating once or twice in steam and drying before miling. Other products are rice starch granules which are quite small and are embedded in a protein matrix and it is used in puddings, ice creams and custard powder. Rice bran is normally finely granulated light tan in colour and it has bland flavour and can be used in preparation like bread, snacks, cookies and biscuits. Rice bran oil is rich in vitamin E. Parched rice is a crisp product with a greyish to brilliant white colour and is sold either salted or unsalted. Puffed rice, flaked rice and aromatic rice are other rice products.

Millets are hardy plants capable of growing in areas where there is low rain fall and poor irrigation facilities. Maize and sorghum are major millet crops and bajra is a pearl millet while ragi is a finger millet.

Maize products are degerminated flour which consists mostly of the endosperm, corn germ oil which can be refined to produce a high quality vegetable oil for cooking; popcorn is a method of starch cookery; and corn starch which is very inexpensive.

Jowar, ragi and bajra are usually milled and made into flour for consumption purpose. Ragi is more suitable for malting which forms a high calorie-density weaning food with excellent nutritional qualities. Bajra is also suitable for malt preparation.

Pulses: Pulses are the edible fruits or seeds of pod bearing plants belonging to the family of leguminous. Major pulses important in our diet are red gram dhal, bengal gram dhal, black gram dhal, green gram dhal and masoor dhal. Some are used as whole grams. Cow pea, rajmah and dry peas also come under leguminous family. Pulses give 340 calories per 100 g. and are important sources of protein (17 to 25 gms/100 gms) i.e. chiefly globulins. Pulses contain 55 to 60% starch, 1.5% lipids. They contain calcium, magnesium, zinc, iron, potassium and phosphorus. Legume seeds are excellent sources of B complex vitamins particularly thiamine, folic acid and pantothenic acid.

Legumes are generally milled to remove the outer husk by wet or dry process. Whole grams which have hard outer covering need soaking prior to cooking. Whole legumes can be germinated by soaking overnight, draining water completely and tying in a loosely woven cotton cloth for a day or two and sprinkling water twice or thrice a day. By this method, digestibility increases, cooking time decreases and improves availability of nutrients.

Nuts and Oil Seeds: Nuts are seeds or fruits consisting of an edible fat containing kernel and surrounded by a hard or a brittle shell. Nuts are also rich in protein and contain a high level of fat. Groundnuts are particularly rich in thiamine and nicotinic acid.

The meal obtained after extraction of the oil from the seed is richer in protein than the seed itself as fat is removed. Oil seed cake is mostly used for cattle feed. But now improved method of extraction and careful handling of cake have helped production of edible grade de-oiled meal which is used for the development of various products like multi purpose food that are used in feeding programmes.

Coconut is not a nut but rather a stone fruit. Coconut water is a refreshing drink. The white flesh is rich in calories. From grated wet coconut kernel, good quality oil as well as protein and carbohydrate can be extracted to prepare coconut honey. The white flesh, when dried called copra has a high content of oil.

Groundnut is also known as peanut and monkey nut. The chief product is the oil, which can be used either as cooking oil or for making margarine and soap. The secondary product is the residue or cake left after the expression of the oil which is purified and used in supplementary mix. Ground nut kernels are ground to a smooth paste and made into milk which is used as supplement to the diets of pre-school and school children. Peanut butter also is prepared.

Soyabean contains about 40% protein and also upto 20% fat. The main problems with soyabean are that it has an undesirable beany odour, has a poor cooking quality and has haemagglutinins and contains trypsin inhibiting factor. These are rendered inactive by suitable heat processing. Apart from being used as oil, soya bean is used in sausages, biscuits, breakfast foods and other cereal products. Soya protein is an important constituent in some infant foods and milk substitutes. Soyabean milk is also extracted. Tofu is made out of soyabean which is a substitute for cottage cheese in cookery.

Milk and Milk Products: Milk is a complex mixture of lipids, carbohydrates, proteins and many other organic and inorganic compounds. Milk fat or butter fat is of great economical and nutritive value. The flavour of milk is due to milk fat. Milk is a true emulsion of oil-in-water. Milk fat is a mixture of several different glycerides. Casein is a milk protein which constitutes 80% of the total nitrogen in milk. Other than this, lactalbumin, lactoglobulin, lactoferrin, serum albumin and serum trasferrin are present which are together called whey proteins. The chief carbohydrate present in milk is lactose or milk sugar is a disaccharide. Milk has , good quality protein, easily digestible fat and significant amount of calcium.

Milk is not only used as such but many nonfermented and fermented products are used in cookery. Skimmed milk is made by removing fat through centrifugation method and is fortified with vitamins A and D. If 50-60% of the water is evaporated from milk, it is called vaporated milk. Sweetened condensed milk is made from pasteurized milk that is concentrated and sweetened with sucrose. Dry milk can be made with whole or skimmed milk. Milk powder can be dehydrated to about 97% by spray drying and vacuum drying. Khoa is a compact mass of very small uniformly sized granules formed due to the coagulation of milk proteins by vigorous boiling. Basundi is prepared by concentrating milk to half of its original volume by open pan concentration and adding sugar and other condiments. Ultra high temperature processed milk (UHT milk) is prepared by heating milk at temperatures higher than those used for pasteurisation for 2-6 seconds. Rabri is a prepared, concentrated and sweetened product comprising of several layers of clotted cream. Channa is a major heat and acid coagulated product used in preparation of rasagollas, sandesh and rasmalai. Ice cream is a frozen dairy product consisting of whole milk, skim milk, cream, butter, condensed milk products or dried milk products.

Standardised milk has 4.5% fat and 8.5% SNF. Toned milk is prepared by mixing milk reconstituted from skim milk powder with buffalo milk containing 7 % fat. Double toned milk is prepared by admixture of cow's or buffalo milk with fresh skimmed milk and has 9% SNF and not less than 1.5% fat. The other types of milk are recombined milk, sterilised milk, filled milk and flavoured milk. Fermented milk products are cream, butter, cheese (made of casein) and curd.

Eggs : Eggs are rich source of all nutrients except ascorbic acid. It contains 12-14% proteins which are well balanced with respect to all the essential amino acids. Egg is one of the richest sources of lecithin-a phospholipid which forms a part of the structure of every cell wall in the body. Calcium, zinc and sulphur are the minerals present in egg. It is a rich source of vitamin A, riboflavin, folic acid and B.

Flesh Foods : The term refers to muscle of warm blooded four legged animals. The chief ones being cattle, sheep and pigs. Organ meats include liver, kidney, heart, thymus and pancreas, brain and sausages which are made of ground or minced meat. Meat contains 15-20% protein of outstanding nutritive value. Fish protein has higher biological value than meat protein. The fat content varies from 5 to 40% with the type, breed and age of the animal. Carbohydrates are found in very small quantities in meat. The mineral elements occur either as separate ions or in a variety of compounds within muscle. Meat is an excellent source of some of the vitamins of the B complex and a good source of iron and phosphorus.

Poultry includes chickens, ducks, geese, turkeys and pigeons. Poultry meat has a high protein content about 25%. Chicken fat is more unsaturated than that of red meat. Poultry flesh is a good source of B vitamins and minerals.

Fish contains around 20% protein which has a high biological value. Fish contains less amount of fat compared to meat and poultry. It is rich in calcium. Fish liver oils are excellent sources of fat soluble vitamins.

Vegetables and Fruits : Vegetables are plants or parts of plants that are used as food. They are called protective foods as they are rich in minerals and vitamins. Green leafy vegetables are good sources of beta-carotene and folic acid. Roots and tubers give more calories compared to green leafy vegetables. They are fairly good sources of vitamin C. Other vegetables contain high amount of moisture, poor in all nutrients and contribute to the fibre content of the diet.

Fruits are produced from flowers and they are the ripened ovary or ovaries of a plant together with adjacent tissues. Fruits are very poor sources of protein and fat; contain high amount of moisture; poor sources of iron but good sources of carotenes and vitamin C.

Sugar and Related Products : Sugar and jaggery increase the palatability of food. Sugar provides only energy to the body, with less protein, minerals and vitamins. Sugar related products are corn syrup-contains 75% carbohydrate and 25% water; molasses - residue that remains after sucrose crystals have been removed from the concentrated juices of sugar cane; maple syrup made by evaporation of the sap of the sugar to a concentration not more than 35% water; honey-contains 17% water and carbohydrates like fructose, glucose, maltose and sucrose with small amounts of minerals, vitamins and enzymes; jaggery- obtained from sugar cane and it is rich in iron.

Fats and Oils : Fats that have a relatively high melting point and are solid at room temperature are called fats, whereas those that have lower melting points and are liquid at room temperature are called oils. These are concentrated sources of energy, excellent sources of fat soluble vitamins A, D, E and K; and provide essential fatty acids.

Spices : Aromatic food substances which enhance flavour are classified into spices, herbs and seasonings. Spices are dried roots, barks or seeds used whole, crushed or powdered. Herbs are usually the fresh leaves, stems or flowers of herbaceous plants. Seasonings are the bulbous group almost invariably used fresh like onion, garlic and shallots. Ani seed or somfu is used to conteract flatulence, asafoetida - as antimicrobial agent; bay leaves -flavouring agents for pulav, soups, meat preparations and fish; cardamom-favouring agent for sweet preparations; chillies-used in making chutneys, pickles and as seasoning agent; cinnamon-used for spicing sauces and pickles; clove-has anti mutagenic effect; coriander seed- used in flatulence, vomiting and intestinal disorders; cumin seeds - used as stimulant and carminative agent; fenugreek seeds - aid in maintaining the blood glucose levels in non-insulin dependent diabetes; garlic-used to treat various digestive disorders, as antifungal agent, reduces fat content in blood and reduce blood pressure; ginger- reduces inflammation and pain in joints; kokam and mango powder - sour agent in cookery; mint leaves-anomatic culinary herb with pepper mint oil used for flavouring gum, confectionery, tooth paste etc. and when fresh used for salad dressing and garnishing. Mustard seeds are rich in sulphur and used for seasoning of various preparations. Nutmeg has antimicrobial property and nutmeg and mace are used as flavouring agents in meat and fish dishes, pickles and preserves.

Onion is used as a flavouring agent in food preparations and has antibacterial properties, lower blood cholesterol and lipid levels and useful in preventing heart diseases. Pepper is used along with hot milk for throat infections and as garam masala. Poppy seeds are used as thickening agents in preparation of gravies. Saffron is used mainly for its yellow colour and has a pleasant aroma, essential oil crocin and colouring principle crocerin used in various sweet dishes, soups and sauces; used as a sedative and used for eye infections. Tamarind is used as souring agent in chutneys, chat, pickles and as thickening agent in gravies. Turmeric is a colouring agent used in curries which has a colouring substance curcumin. It is used to relieve sore throat, cough, cold and against flatulence. Vanilla imparts flavour and is used in ice creams, custards, puddings and cakes. Monosodium glutamate (MSG) is popularly known as Ajinomoto used as a flavouring agent.

Beverages and Appetisers : A beverage is any material used as drink for the purpose of relieving thirst and introducing fluid to the body, nourishing the body and stimulating or soothing the individual. Refreshing beverages are plain water, carbonated beverages not containing fruit juices, fruit juices, iced tea and butter milk with salt and lime juice. While nourishing beverages are different types of milk and milk products like butter milk, milk shakes, eggs, fruit juice, glucose and lemonade. Stimulating beverage includes egg nogs made with whisky, brandy, coffee; coffee or tea; cocoa or chocolate beverage. Soothing beverages are warm milk and hot tea. Soups, fruit juice and alcoholic drinks in limited quantity are appetizers. Alcoholic beverages include toddy, beer and wine.

Processing of Food

Preservation and processing begin when the soil is prepared for planting. Fruit processing is continuous from the time fruit leaves the growing plant till it is securely protected from microorganisms or macroorganisms. Harvesting, sorting, washing, peeling, preparation, heating, refrigeration, dehydration, concentrating, treating with chemicals and packing are steps in the chain of processing events. Amchur, dried chillies, ginger, kokum; apple juice, canned peaches, pears, canned mushroom, squashes, nectars, jams, jellies, marmalades are some examples for vegetable and fruit processed products. These products have limited demand due to their excessive costs, lack of traditional tastes and lack of their availability in remote areas.

The fundamental principle of preserving foods by heat is known as 'processing'. It consists basically in the application of heat in varying degrees to the food in closed containers, for a sufficiently long time to sterilize the contents before these are hermetically sealed. The method of processing varies from food to food.

The term processing as used in canning industry refers to heating or cooling of canned foods to inactivate bacteria. Processing consists in determining just the temperature as well as the extent of cooking that would suffice to eliminate all possibilities of bacterial growth. Almost all fruits can be processed satisfactorly at a temperature of 100° C. Vegetables require to be processed at higher temperatures of about 115° C to 121° C. The temperature and time of processing vary with the size of the can - the larger the can, the greater the processing time and vice-versa.

Processing Methods: There are generally three types of cookers used for canning of fruits. These are: open cookers, continuous non-agitating cookers, and continuous agitating cookers.

Open Cookers: These are very simple in construction and consist essentially of wooden tubs or galvanized iron tanks of any desired capacity. The sealed cans are placed in crates of galvanized iron and immersed in the tank containing boiling water, which is kept boiling by letting in jets of steam through perforated pipes placed underneath the false bottom of the tank.

Continuous Non-agitating Cookers : In these cookers, the cans travel in boiling water in crates carried by overhead conveyors in a single file on continuously moving belt.

Continuous Agitating Cookers: These cookers are of various designs and are generally used in big production units. The sealed cans move in the non-agitating cookers, but are at the same time rotated by special mechanical devices to agitate the contents of the cans. By this technique, the processing time is reduced considerably.

Different operations involved in processing of any kind of fruit are washing, grading, peeling and coring, blanching, canning, filling, exhausting, sterilizing, and cooling while for vegetables washing, preheating, peeling if needed like for potatoes, inspection and trimming, size grading, filling into the cans, sealing and processing and cooling the heat-processed cans.

Sorting and Grading: After preliminary sorting, the fruits and vegetables are graded. This is necessary to obtain a pack of uniform quality as regards size, colour etc. It is done by hand or with the help of grading machines.

Washing: The graded fruits and vegetables are washed with water in different ways, such as soaking or agitating in water, washing with cold or hot water sprays etc.

Peeling, Coring and Pitting: The washed fruits and vegetables are prepared for canning by peeling, coring, blanching etc. Fruits and vegetables are peeled in a variety of ways : (1) by hand or with knife, (2) by machine, (3) by heat treatment and (4) by lye solution i.e. caustic soda solution.

Blanching: Treatment of fruits and vegetables with boiling water or steam for short periods, followed by cooling prior to canning, is called 'blanching'.

Can Filling: The cans are washed with water or subjected to a steam jet to remove any adhering dust or foreign matter.

Syruping or Brining: The cans are filled with hot sugar syrup for fruits and with hot brine for vegetables. The syrup or brine should be added to the can at a temperature of 79° C to 82° C, leaving suitable head space.

Lidding or Clinching: Lid is partially seamed to the can by a single first roller action of a double seamer. The lid remains sufficiently loose to permit the escape of dissolved as well as free air from the contents and also the vapour formed during the exhaust process.

Exhausting: Before sealing the cans finally, it is necessary to remove practically all air from the contents which is called 'exhausting'. Containers are exhausted either by heat treatment or by mechanical means.

Sealing: After exhausting, the cans are sealed by special closing machines known as double seamers.

The processing time for different kinds of fruits and vegetables has to be relatively increased with further increase in the altitude. As the altitude above sea level increases, the pressure required to maintain the specified processing temperature would also increase. The pH value has a great influence upon the destruction of micro-organism. The lower the pH, the greater is the ease with which a product can be processed or sterilised. Similarly any increase in the temperature, after closing of the can, develops pressure inside the can. After processing, the cans are cooled rapidly to stop the cooking process, especially in cans at the centre of large stacks where they may remain hot for several hours. Cooling is done by (a) immersing or passing the hot cans in tanks containing cold water (b) spraying with jets of cold water (c) turning in cold water into the pressure cooker in the case of canned vegetables or (d) exposing the cans to air in small lots when water supply is scarce. Once cooling is done, batches of finished cans should be finally tested for leak or imperfect seals by tapping the can top with a short steel rod. A clear ringing sound indicates a perfect seal, while a dull and hollow sound implies a leaky or imperfectly sealed can. The other method used for testing the vacuum inside the cans is using a vacuum tester which is portable and handy.

After the cans are tested for defects, they are then labelled by hand or by machine, and packed in strong wooden cases or corrugated cardboard cartons, in standard packing. Till they are dispatched, they should be stored in a cool and dry place.

18

Safety from Deterioration

Foods gradually undergo deterioration or spoilage from the time they are harvested, slaughtered or manufactured. Some foods spoil rapidly; others keep for longer but limited periods. The useful storage life of some fruits, leafy vegetables and animal foods is less than 1-2 days at 21°C. The deteriorative changes in some foods is so rapid as to render them virtually useless in a matter of hours. These result in physiological, chemical and biological changes in food rendering them unfit for human consumption.

Preservation

A number of causes are responsible for food deterioration. These include micro-organisms (bacteria, yeasts and molds); activities of enzymes present in food; insects, parasites and rodents; temperature (heat and cold); moisture; oxygen, light and time. These factors are not isolated in nature. At any one time, many forms of deterioration may take place depending upon the food and environmental conditions. The deterioration owing to individual causes is discussed below.

Microbial Spoilage Bacteria, yeasts and molds spoil food after harvesting, during handling, processing and storage. But not all micro-organisms cause food spoilage; e.g., the use of lactic acid producing bacteria in the making of cheese and fermented dairy products, and yeasts as leavening agents and for the production of wine and beer has already been discussed. However, except the micro-organisms that are specially cultivated under controlled conditions for their beneficial effects, others that multiply on or in foods are frequently the major causes of food deterioration. They are found everywhere; they, however, are not generally found within healthy living tissues, but are always present to invade the flesh of animals and plants when there is a break in their skin or if the skin is weakened by disease or death.

Bacteria are minute unicellular plant-like micro-organisms. The length of a bacterial cell is about 1 μm and somewhat smaller than this in diameter. Bacteria are classified according to the shape of their cells. Cocci are spherical in shape, bacilli are elongated cylindrical forms and, spirilla and vibrios are spiral. They can penetrate the smallest opening; many can pass through the natural pores of an eggshell. Bacterial spores are seed-like and they are more resistant to most processing conditions than yeast or mold spores. Bacteria, with few exceptions, cannot grow in media as acid as those in which yeasts and molds thrive. They multiply by cell division. Under favourable conditions bacteria can double their number every 30 min. Some bacteria cannot tolerate oxygen (anaerobes) and some require oxygen for growth (aerobes). Some can grow in an atmosphere devoid of oxygen but manage also in air (facultative anaerobes).

Yeasts are unicellular plants (fungi) widely distributed in nature and they grow well in a slightly acid medium in the presence of sugar and water. They are found in fruits, cereals and other foods containing sugar. They are also found in soil, air, on the skins and in the intestines of animals. They are somewhat larger than bacteria. The individual cell length is of about 10 μm and the diameter is about a third of this size. Most yeasts are spherical or ellipsoidal. They have been used for centuries for leavening of bread and to bring about the fermentation of fruit juices. They can be harmful to foods if they bring about undesired fermentations.

Molds are multicellular, filamentous fungi having a fuzzy or cottony appearance when they grow in foods. They are larger than yeasts which they resemble in their nutritional requirements. They are strictly aerobes and require oxygen for growth and multiplication. They tend to grow more slowly than bacteria. Molds frequently thrive under conditions of acidity or of osmotic pressures that are inhibitory to most bacteria. This explains why they are frequently found growing on the surface of jams and jellies. Molds require less free moisture for growth than yeasts and bacteria. The absence of bright light and presence of stagnant air favour their rapid development.

Bacteria, yeasts and molds multiply best between 16° and 38°C. Some grow even at 0°C and others at a temperature as high as 100°C. They alter food constituents. Some can hydrolyze starch and other complex organic matter like cellulose, lignin and pectin; others can hydrolyze Jipids and produce rancidity; still others digest proteins and produce putrid and ammonia-like odours. They can also bring about decolonization of foods, produce acids, gases or toxins. Thus, bacteria, yeasts and molds are the most important agents in causing the deterioration of foods.

Bacterial spoilage of foods could be of two types: due to food infection or intoxication. The former type of spoilage is on account of organisms present in the food at the time of consumption which then grow in the host and cause disease, while the latter type is due to toxins produced by bacteria prior to consumption which cause disease upon ingestion. The toxin of *C. botulinum* is produced only in an aerobic condition, such as found in canned products and meats in airtight packages. In a frozen stage, *C. botulinum* survives but does not grow. Hence, frozen foods do not present the hazard of botulism.

Food Enzymes : Enzymes present in plant and animal foods continue to be present and are even intensified after harvest and slaughter. They are responsible for facilitating many changes during storage, such as the changes in colour, texture and flavour noted in fresh produce after it has been harvested. Some of these changes, such as the continued ripening of tomatoes after they are picked and natural tenderizing of meat on ageing, are desirable. But these changes can proceed too far resulting in food deterioration if not halted at the appropriate time. The enzymes responsible for deteriorative changes are to be inactivated by a suitable method at the appropriate time to prevent food deterioration.

Insects, Parasites and Rodents : Insects are particularly destructive so far as cereal grains, fruits and vegetables are concerned. The loss of food due to insect destruction varies from 5 to 50 per cent depending upon the care taken in the field and storage. Insect eggs may persist in the foods even after processing as, for example, in flour. It is virtually impossible to produce and transport grains and other food commodities completely devoid of insects and insect pests. Therefore, a certain level of insect contamination in such foods is inevitable but it should be kept to a minimum by controlling the level of insect infestation. Insects in grains, dried fruits and spices are generally controlled by fumigation with fumigants like methyl bromide, ethylene oxide and propylene oxide. Apart from the loss due to the food eaten, insects cause greater damage due to the bruises and cuts they make in foods exposing them to microbial attack resulting in total decay.

Parasitic food spoilage occurs in some foods. Hogs eat uncooked food wastes. The parasitic nematode penetrates the hog's intestine and finds its way into pork. The live worms can infect man if the pork is not thoroughly cooked. A parasite worm belonging to the genus *Anisakis* is found in fish. If such fish is eaten raw it can infect man. Another common parasitic contamination of foods is *Entamoeba histolytica* responsible for amoebic dysentery. This organism contaminates foods when raw human excrement is used as fertilizer for crops. Infected water and poor hygiene also spread the parasite. Cooking kills most of these parasites.

Rodents contribute substantially to food shortages in countries where they are not controlled. Rats live up to 3 years and may have 3-8 litters. Apart from the fact that they consume large quantities of food, they contaminate food. Rodent's urine and droppings harbour several kinds of disease producing bacteria, and rats spread such human diseases as typhus fever, plague, typhoid fever, etc.

Temperature : Heat and cold, apart from their role in food preservation, contribute to food deterioration if not controlled. The rate of chemical reaction doubles itself for every 10°C rise in temperature. Excessive heat brings about protein denaturation, destroys vitamins, breaks emulsions and dries out food by removing moisture. Uncontrolled cold also will deteriorate food. The freezing and thawing of fruits and vegetables destroy their structure. Skin rupture leaves the food susceptible to microbial infection. If milk is frozen, fat will separate and milk protein will be denatured causing it to curdle. Several fruits and vegetables are damaged even at the temperature of refrigeration (4°C). The deterioration includes off-colour development, surface biting and various forms of decay. Bananas, tomatoes, lemons and squash should be maintained above 10°C for maximum quality retention.

Moisture : Presence or absence of excess moisture in food leads to food spoilage. Moisture is required for chemical reactions and microbial growth. Foods with a high percentage of water deteriorate fast. Perishable foods have a high water content. Leafy vegetables, young shoots, juicy fruits, meats and milk deteriorate rapidly. Even if the moisture content is not uniform throughout the food, it exerts its influence. Surface moisture changes due to changes in relative humidity can cause lumping and caking, surface defects, crystallization and stickiness in foods. Condensation of even small amounts of moisture can result in the multiplication of bacteria and molds. This condensation need not come from outside. Fruits and vege tables can give off moisture from respiration and transpiration even when packed in a moisture-free package. This moisture trapped within the package is enough for the micro-organisms to grow. Even non-living foods in moisture-proof packages can give up moisture and change relative humidity in the enclosed space, which can result in microbial growth. Control of moisture in foods is thus very important from the point of view of their preservation.

Oxygen, Light and Time : Air and oxygen bring about a number of destructive changes in food components such as destruction of food colour, flavour, vitamins A and C and other food constituents. Oxygen is necessary for the growth of molds. Oxygen is therefore to be excluded from food in the course of processing, by deaeration, vacuum packing, or flushing containers with nitrogen or carbon dioxide and, in some case by the use of oxygen-absorbing chemicals.

Light destroys vitamins B-2, A and C. It also deteriorates many food colours. Not all wavelengths of natural or artificial light are absorbed by food constituents or are equally destructive. Surface discolourations of meat pigments are different under natural and fluorescent lights. Foods may be protected from light by impervious packing or keeping them in containers that screen out specific wavelengths.

All the food deteriorative factors considered so far are time-dependent. The larger the time, the greater the destructive influences. All foods, fresh or processed, have their qualities at a peak at some time after they are obtained. For best quality, they should be consumed before deterioration sets in. Deterioration with time takes place with most foods except certain foods like cheese, wine and other fermented foods which improve with ageing up to a point.

Food Safety in the Home : Despite the fact that food is free from harmful levels of micro-organisms when it is brought home, there is still a danger of food spoilage due to the causes discussed above. In drder to avoid it in the home, standards of hygiene should be maintained in all aspects of food preservation. Personal hygiene and kitchen sanitation practice should be maintained. Foods should be appropriately stored. The temperature range favourable for growth of micro-organisms should be avoided.

Foods should be kept at a temperature colder than 4°C. Hot foods should be cooled as quickly as possible to the point where they can be placed in the refrigerator.

Processing

The holding of food supplies from periods of plenty for supply during seasons of little or no production is one of the most fundamental problems tackled by man and also animals. For thousands of years, man has extensively practised food preservation. It was necessary to ensure a year-round food supply. Storing of food has become increasingly important today in the progress of economic life. Without the hoarding of food, life as we know today would be impossible.

The earliest methods used for food preservation were smoking, drying and salting. The use of ice and snow to preserve perishable foods was known to early man. Fermentation of agricultural produce also was known from early times. Barley, rice and fruit juices were used for alcoholic beverages. Fermented soyabean products have been used in the East from 2000 BC. Modern methods of food preservation have developed through the centuries on the basis of practices employed in the past. Industrial processing of food started on a small scale in the 19th century, and during this century there have been tremendous developments.

The underlying principle of all preservation techniques, whether carried out in the home or commercially, is to restrict food spoilage so that food can be used safely in a palatable form at a later time. Preservation methods are designed to inhibit the growth of organisms, the removal of organisms and killing the organisms. Food preservation should also arrest the biochemical breakdown of tissues and the transformation of its cell contents. This is achieved by heat, cold, drying, fermentation, radiation and chemicals. Food deterioration also is brought about by any one of these techniques. The technique employed should be such that micro-organisms are killed or inhibited and biochemical attacks lowered and the food is still left unaltered.

Preservation and Processing by Heat : Of the various methods of food preservation, heat finds very wide applications. The application of heat to food is so universal that "processing" and "heating" are considered as synonymous. This underlines the importance of heat in bringing about physical, chemical and biological modifications in foods. The purpose of heat treatment in food preservation is to kill the micro-organisms and inactivate the enzymes that become active in the subsequent storage of packed food. Various methods have been developed to achieve this purpose without bringing about other undesirable effects in foods.

Effect of Heat on Micro-organisms : Most bacteria, yeasts and molds show a growth optimum between 16°-38°C (mesophiles). Such organisms, in general, do not grow below 5°C and above 45°C. Some organisms grow in the range of 66°-82°C (thermophiles). Most bacteria are killed in the range of 82°-93°C. However, bacterial spores and certain other heat-resistant forms can withstand prolonged exposure to 100°C. Some organisms endure this temperature for 5½ hours. However, they last only minutes at 120°C and are destroyed in moist heat at 100°C in about 15 min. The thermal death of micro-organisms in dry air is due to oxidation. Therefore, a high temperature is required for their destruction. In wet heat, cell death is due to coagulation consisting of reactions between proteins and water; this is also accelerated by raised temperatures.

The complete destruction of microogranisms is known as sterilization. This is achieved when organisms are exposed at 121°C to wet heat for 15 min. This can be accomplished in a pressure cooker or autoclave on a small scale or, on a commercial scale, in pressure retorts. It should be remembered, however, that for storage a food need not be completely sterile. In many cases it would be enough if it is "commercially sterile" (appertized), i.e., foods may contain a very small number of resistant bacterial spores, but these will not normally multiply in the food during storage. For most foods, a theoretical reduction to $1/10^{12}$ of the original population is considered satisfactory. Canned foods which are commercially sterile have a shelf-life of two years or more.

Since the heat required for complete sterilization of food also adversely affects the properties of foods, the heat treatment given should be just enough to destroy the pathogenic organisms and toxins, and ensure desired storage life. Thus, to preserve foods by heat with safety, a knowledge of the time-temperature combination required to inactivate the most heat resistant pathogen in a particular food, and the heat penetration characteristics of the particular food including the can or container if the the food is packed, is required.

Thermal Death Time (TDT) Curve : An interesting aspect of the thermal death of micro-organisms (this applies to bacterial spores also) is that, at a given lethal temperature, the death rate is proportional to the number of micro-organisms still living. This is referred to as the logarithmic order of death, which means that under constant thermal conditions the same percentage of microbial population, will be destroyed in a given time interval, regardless of the size of the surviving population. Thus, if 90 per cent of an original microbial population is killed in the first minute, 90 per cent of the remaining will be killed in the second minute and so on. The logarithmic death rate curve for an organism provides the death rate of the organism in a specific medium or food at a specific temperature. From the death-rate curves at different temperatures, a death-time Curve is obtained. A thermal death-time curve for a specific organism in a spfecific medium or food provides data on the destruction time for a defined population of that organism at different temperatures.

A thermal death-time curve indicates that greater the initial microbial population in a food, the greater is the heat treatment required for its destruction. This strongly emphasizes the importance of good sanitation in food industries, even though heat is a destructive force for micro-organisms. In food preservation by heat, in addition to heat destruction of micro-organisms as indicated by the thermal death-time curve, a number of other factors influence microbial population. The acid pH of the food, for example, will increase the killing of organisms by heat. Foods high in acid (having a pH of 4.6 or less), such as tomatoes or orange juice, need not be heated severely because the acid increases the killing power of heat. With acid foods, in many cases, temperature at or below 100°C for a few minutes constitutes adequate heat treatment. Certain spices and food chemicals act synergistically with heat in killing micro-organisms and so reduce the heat treatment that must be used. As will be discussed subsequently, many other food constituents have an opposite effect on heat sensitivity of micro-organisms and protect them against heat. Thus, thermal death-time curves, to be valid, should be established for the specific food for which a heat process is being applied. To provide a substantial margin of safety it is better to work out the heat treatment by assuming that the food contains a heat-resistant spore and its population is large.

Environmental Factors : The data obtained from thermal death-time curves indicate the time and temperature required to destroy the micro-organisms. For proper preservation of food, every pdrticle of food (within the container if the food is canned) has to reach the lethal temperature for the required time. That is, heat should penetrate into the mass of food or throughout the can. Thus, the extent of heating depends upon the size and shape of the food or can andlalso on the nature and consistency of food. This involves the heat transfer into the food by conduction or convection. Convection heating is far more rapid than conduction heating and so a liquid food reaches the required temperature more rapidly than a food containing free liquid and solid, which in turn is heated more rapidly than a solid food.

When heat is applied from outside the food nearest to the container (can) surface will reach the sterilization temperature sooner than the food in the centre of the can. The point in the can or mass of food which is last to reach the final heating temperature is known as "cold point". To ensure necessary sterilization of food, heating must be continued till the time the cold point attains the lethal temperature and remains at that temperature for the required interval. Since the time required for penetration of heat throughout the food varies depending upon the type of sterilizing unit used, size and shape of food container and the composition of food, it is obvious that the required heat treatment will be different for each specific case. This has to be determined to complete the sterilization requirement of food.

The required lethal effect at the cold point of the food can be achieved by various time-temperature exposures. For example, destruction of *Clostridium botulinum* in a low-acid medium is complete in 2.78 min. at 121°C or 10 min. at 116°C. Also, the temperature rise during heat penetration accomplishes some degree of microbial destruction. Cooling of sterile food is not instantaneous and some additional microbial destruction takes place during the cooling period. These factors are to be taken into consideration in evaluating the temperature and time required for food preservation by heat.

Several constituents of food protect micro-organisms to various degrees against heat. Sugar in high concentration decreases their susceptibility to heat. Thus, canned fruit in a sugar syrup requires a higher temperature or longer time for sterilization than the same fruit without sugar. Fats and oils decrease the penetration of wet heat into the cells of micro-organisms and heating becomes more like dry heat. Food constituents, in addition to the above types of direct protection of micro-organisms, also contribute indirectly to the penetration of heat. Fats are poorer conductors of heat than water. Food consistency determines whether conduction or convection heating will take place. If starch is added as a thickener to a food, it may result in the conversion of the convection heat system to a conduction system thus slowing down heat penetration within the container or mass of food and this too will protect micro-organisms.

Canning : The basic process of canning consists of placing food in a sealable container, closing, heating and cooling. This method of food preservation has been in use since early 1800s though the understanding of the process came much later. Large quantities of foods are canned for preservation. In advanced countries canned foods form a significant part of the diet of the people. Most fruits and vegetables, a wide variety of meats and meat products, fish products, soups and many other items are all canned. A typical canning process includes the following steps:

1. Receiving, cleaning, grading and inspecting of raw commodity.
2. Blanching to inactivate enzymes.
3. Placing in the container with added brine or syrup and deaeration of the product.
4. Heating in a retort, under 1.05 kg/cm^2 pressure using steam for metal cans or pressurized water for glass containers.
5. Partial cooling under pressure in the retort.
6. Additional cooling by water sprays or in a cooling tank.
7. Labelling, racking and distributing.

First, the raw commodity is inspected for any treatment required before canning. Many of them require special treatment, such as washing, trimming, shelling, size grading and so on. In commercial canning, most of these operations are carried out mechanically. The food may then be blanched to reduce surface contamination and inactivate enzymes. The blanched food is placed in the containers. Brine (1.1 to 1.6 per cent salt concentration) is added in the case of vegetables, meat and fish, and syrup in the case of fruits. In some cases, only water is added. Oils are commonly added to fish products.

The containers generally preferred for most heat-processed foods are tin cans. Glass jars are easy to clean, corrosion free and transparent, but they have the disadvantage of requiring more processing time than cans of the same size. There is also the problem of breakage. As heating time is roughly proportional to volume of the container, larger containers must be heated for a longer time and food canned in such containers will be of lower quality than those placed in smaller containers.

Heating time can be reduced by placing the food in a flexible, relatively thin pouch instead of a can or jar. It has been shown that foods processed in this manner are of comparable quality to frozen foods. The pouches can be heated for serving by simply placing them in hot water, and damage in distribution would be significantly less than with can or glass jar. Pouch canning is gradually gaining importance.

The container with the food is ready for deaeration. This can be done by heating the filled cans in steam or hot water or the use of a vacuum closing machine when the air is sucked out by a pump and the lid is sealed on while vacuum is maintained. Air and gas removal is necessary to prevent the bulging of the can due to internal pressure, oxidation of the contents and inside corrosion of the tin plate.

The sealed containers are subjected to heating in a retort, a chamber in which canned foods are processed. Several types of retorts are used. Still retorts are the simplest type in which the cans remain still while they are being heated. In this case, the heating time to bring the cold point to the sterilizing temperature is relatively long. The time taken for sterilization can be markedly reduced by using agitating retorts. The cans are agitated during the heating process. The mixing inside the container helps the conduction and convection processes so that heating is achieved in significantly less time and food quality is improved. Whether still or agitating retorts are used, the high temperature required for sterilization is commonly obtained from steam under pressure. The heating may be batchwise or continuous. The heated containers are partially cooled under pressure in the retorts to decrease the internal pressure of the container. Next, the containers are cooled in water or under a spray. Finally, they are labelled and packed for distribution.

Aseptic Canning : In normal canning, heat transfer from the outside of the container to the inside will require many minutes or even hours depending upon the container size to reach the sterilization temperature. The time of sterilization can be shortened to seconds or even fraction of a second in aseptic canning. The basic principle of this method is that food is pumped continuously through a plate-type or tubular heat exchanger which heats it very quickly to a high temperature, holding it at that temperature for the time required and then cooling. Food temperature employed may be as high as 150°C and sterilization takes place in 1 or 2 s. Such a rapid sterilization at high temperature is referred to as ultra-high-temperature sterilization. The sterile food is quickly cooled, placed in aseptic containers and the lids are sealed while in a sterile environment. The food canned aseptically retains the nutrients and the sensory attributes will be good.

With acid foods, foods sterilized as in aseptic canning, while still hot, can be filled into clean but not necessarily aseptic containers. The heat of the food and some holding time before cooling the closed container renders the containers commercially sterile. This type of canning is known as "hot pack" or "hot fill".

With low-acid food (above pH 4.6) the conventional hot pack processing is not possible. In such cases, *"flash 18"* process (pressure canning) is employed. Low-acid foods are heated above 100°C under pressure for sterilty. If food at that temperature is poured into containers for sealing at atmospheric pressure, there will be violent boiling. This is eliminated by carrying out the canning process in a chamber under a pressure of 1.05 to 1.40 kg/cm^2. Thus, low acid foods can be presterilized by high temperature for a short time. They are then transferred to cans in a pressurized room and heated for an appropriate number of minutes so that commercial sterility of non-sterile cans are obtained and finally the cans are sealed and cooled.

Pasteurization : When foods are heated in containers or by other methods to a temperature below the boiling point of water for a definite period, the process is known as pasteurization. This process serves two objectives: it destroys pathogenic organisms associated with the food and extends the product's shelf-life by decreasing the microbial population and inactivating some enzymes. The choice of temperature and time of pasteurization will be influenced by the consideration of the purpose of the process and the chemical and physical composition of food. Thus, milk is pasteurized at 62.8°C for 30 min. to inactivate pathogens and whole egg (mixture of yolk and white) at 64.4°C for 2-5 min. to control the dissemination of *Salmonella* spp. With sweetened condensed milk, a mild heat treatment is acceptable because of the moderate heat resistance of yeasts, the only organisms that could grow under conditions imposed by sugar concentration. Pasteurization is also employed in the case of beer, wines, fruit juices and certain other foods mostly to increase shelf-life.

Pasteurized products are not sterile. They contain vegetative organisms and spores still capable of growth. Many pasteurized foods must be stored under refrigeration. Pasteurized milk under refrigeration can be stored for a week or more in good condition. However, at room temperature pasteurized milk may be spoilt in a day. High-temperature short-time treatment

(HTST) using a temperature of 130°C and above for short times, i.e., a few seconds to 6 min. are used to obtain a germ-free stage.

Blanching: Blanching is a heat treatment like pasteurization. The term is usually used in conjunction with vegetable processing, where the goals are to inactivate degradative enzymes and deaerate the product before further processing rather than kill micro-organisms. If omitted, off-flavour, vitamin losses and colour changes occur in the frozen storage. Blanching is usually performed by dipping the products in boiling water for two to three minutes.

Preservation and Processing by Cold : As stated earlier, preservation of food by freezing and cold storage was known to ancient people. Tribes and nations in the temperate and cooler climates froze their harvest, thawed it when necessary and consumed it. Frozen foods were even transported to short distances to consuming centres. With the development of mechanical refrigeration systems, cold preservation of food, food processing, storage and distribution have become widespread. Refrigeration has also influenced agricultural practices. It has become possible to transport perishable foods for long distances from production to consumption centres and make available seasonal foods at all times of the year.

Effect of CoW on Micro-organisms : While most bacteria, yeasts and molds grow best at temperatures of 16° to 38°C, some micro-organisms continue to grow even at low temperatures. These are known as psychrophilic (cryophilic) organisms. These grow even at 0°C, the freezing point of water. However, lowering the temperature of foods and food products de creases the growth rate of micro-organisms and the growth and multiplicity completely stop when water freezes. In some foods water does not freeze even at -10°C or lower temperatures because of the lower freezing point due to dissolved salts, sugars and other substances. The retardation of microbial and biochemical activities at low temperatures is the basis of preservation of food by cold. Cold temperature treatment, including severe freezing, only reduces the microbial activities and population but does not kill all bacteria. Foods frozen, even for two years or more, when removed from cold storage have shown bacterial activity when thawed.

Types of Cold Preservation : Cold preservation of food may be categorized into two groups: refrigeration and freezing. Household and commercial refrigerators usually run at 4.4°-7.2°C. Commercial refrigeration (cold or chill storage) may use a slightly lower temperature, depending upon the nature of food refrigerated. Freezing refers to foods maintained in a frozen condition. For good freezing a temperature of -18°C or below is required. Chill storage will preserve perishable foods for days or weeks depending upon the food. Frozen storage (deep freezing) will preserve foods for months or even years.

Refrigeration has certain advantages over freezing. It takes less energy to cool a food to just above its freezing point than to freeze it. Refrigeration storage requires less insulation and refrigeration capacity, and refrigerated products do not suffer from texture and flavour losses caused by freezing. Finally, refrigerated products do not have to be thawed before use—a process that may take as much as 48 hours with large frozen foods.

Further distinction between refrigeration and freezing temperatures relates to microbial activity. Most spoilage organisms grow above 10°C. Some food poisoning organisms grow slowly up to 3.3°C. Cryophilic organisms grow slowly from -4.4°C to -9.4°C provided the food is not frozen. These organisms, however, do not produce toxins or disease but cause food deterioration. There is no growth of organisms below -9.4°C though there may not be a total destruction at that temperature.

Chill Storage : Chill storage is useful as the principal method of preservation and as an adjunct to other methods of preservation. The shelf-life of food is directly linked with the microbial rate of growth as influenced by temperature. Storage at - 1° and - 4°C can provide stability, particularly in the presence of food preservative or modified atmosphere.

Production of Low Temperature : Chill storage requires controlled low temperature. This is achieved by taking heat away from the storage area. Heat is transferred from the storage area by the principle of latent heat of vaporization. If the state is changed from liquid to gas or from gas to liquid without affecting its temperature an amount of heat must be added or removed. Liquids like ammonia and freon (Cl_2F_2) are used as refrigerants. Liquid refrigerant is circulated through an expansion valve or capillary tube and then through a heat exchanger, called an evaporator, within the storage area. In passing through the capillary tube, the refrigerant goes from a relatively high pressure to a relatively low one, causing the liquid refrigerant to evaporate and thus reducing the temperature of the liquid-gas phase of the refrigerant. In the evaporator, the remaining liquid evaporates absorbing heat from the storage area. The temperature of the vaporization of the refrigerant is some 5°-6°C below the storage temperature. A compressor then pumps the refrigerant from the low-pressure cold condition to a high-pressure hot one. The hot gas Clows through a condenser where heat is extracted from the refrigerant and transforms it back to a room temperature, high-pressure liquid ready to flow again to the expansion or capillary tube. Air, water or a combination of air and evaporating water is used to cool the condenser.

For the construction of commercial chill storage rooms, the "refrigeration load" is to be taken into consideration. This is the quantity of heat that must be removed from the product and the storage area in order to go from an initial temperature to the selected final temperature and then maintain this temperature for a specific time. This depends on the storage area and other factors that may generate heat within the storage area or influence the removal of heat from the area. These include the light and electrical installations, number of people working, how often the doors which permit entrance of warm air are opened and the amount and nature of the food product stored in the refrigerated area. Also, the specific heat of food and the rate of respiration of such foods as fruits and vegetables have a bearing on the extent of refrigeration required. The heats produced from the respiration of fruits and vegetables vary considerably. Products like green beans, peas, spinach, sweet corn and strawberries have a high respiration rate even at 0°C.

Air Circulation and Humidity : The heat produced due to respiration in the vicinity of the food surface in cold storage is to be transferred towards the refrigerator. This is achieved by air circulation. The humidity of the circulated air is to be controlled. If it is too moist, moisture will condense on the cold food and molds will grow on food surfaces at the common refrigeration temperature. On the other hand, if the air is too dry there will be desiccation of food. The optimum relative humidity of the circulated air depends upon the moisture content of the foods and the ease with which they dry out. Most foods store best at a refrigeration temperature when the relative humidity of air is between 80 and 95 per cent. Dry and granular foods store well at about 50 per cent relative humidity.

When foods are to be chill stored for a long time they are protected by packing to prevent loss of moisture. Plastic sacks or moisture-resistant coating are used for this purpose. Cheese ripened for a long time in cold storage are wax coated. Loss of moisture from stored eggs is prevented by dipping the eggs in some oil, to seal the minute pores of the eggshell. If packing is not possible as in the case of tenderizing beef by ageing in cool rooms, ultraviolet light is employed to retard mold growth.

Modified Atmosphere : Continued chill storage, and biochemical changes of fruits and vegetables even under chill storage result in overripening, softening and general loss in quality. These changes take place at the normal chemical composition of air (78 per cent nitrogen, 21 per cent oxygen and 0.03 per cent carbon dioxide) and they can be arrested by using refrigeration in conjunction with "modified atmosphere" or "controlled atmosphere". By raising the carbon dioxide and lowering the oxygen levels, foods can be stored for an extended period of time. In a modified atmosphere of 3 per cent oxygen and 3 per cent carbon dioxide, apples can be preserved in good condition for about a year at 2.8°C and 87 per cent relative humidity. For each food there is an optimal storage temperature, relative humidity, oxygen level and carbon dioxide level which delay ripening process. Modified atmosphere cold storage in gas-tight containers has enabled shipment of even highly perishable foods like lettuce over long distances. Ramification of controlled atmosphere can have other desirable effects on cold-stored food. For example, the presence of diphenyl vapours can inhibit mold growth in citrus foods, and use of ethylenegas can speed up the ripening and colour development of citrus fruits and bananas.

Deep Freezing : Tremendous advances have been made in freezing food for preservation, storage and distribution. Many foods can be frozen for twelve months or more without major changes in size, shape, texture, colour and flavour. Frozen foods have thus attained wide acceptance by the public. At present, no form of food preservation is as well suited to provide maximum convenience as freezing. Complete meals on individual plates can be frozen and are ready for use with a single thawing-heated operation. An unlimited number of items may now be frozen in their final serving forms.

Changes During Freezing and Thawing : Uncontrolled freezing of food can result in the disruption of texture, breaking up of emulsion, denaturation of protein and many other physical and chemical changes. Substances like sugar, salt and proteins dissolved in water lower the freezing point of water, Thus, when food is kept at a freezing temperature, where the temperature is considerably below the freezing point of water, the water component freezes first and leaves the dissolved solids in a more concentrated solution which requires a still lower temperature to freeze it. Thus, different foods with varying levels of water as well as the amount and nature of dissolved substances will have different freezing points and under a given freezing condition will require different times to reach a solidly frozen state.

When food containing water is placed in a freezer it does not freeze uniformly. The portion of food nearest to the container freezes first and the first ice crystals are pure water. As water Continues to be frozen, the concentration of dissolved solids increases and finally a central core of highly concentrated unfrozen liquid remains. If the temperature is sufficiently low this central core also freezes solid ultimately. In the case of solid foods like a piece of meat at about -4°C, they appear to be solidly frozen but they still contain about 3 per cent water in an unfrozen condition. Even at -18°C not all of the water is completely frozen.

Small quantities of unfrozen water in frozen foods result in the deterioration of food with respect to texture, colour, flavour and other properties. The high concentration of dissolved substances in the remaining water can cause effects of various kinds. The dissolved substances may precipitate or crystallize imparting a gritty, sandy texture to the food; if they remain in solution, the high salt concentration or drop in pH (if the solutes are acidic) might result in protein denaturation. The disturbances in anionic and cationic concentration can disturb colloidal substances, and finally the concentration effects can cause the dehydration of adjacent tissues resulting in loss of tissue turgor. Other effects of unfrozen water are the possibilities of the growth of psychrophilic micro-organisms and the greater action of enzymes.

Formation of ice crystals during freezing can affect the texture of many frozen foods. There is water within and between the cells of food. When water freezes rapidly it forms minute ice crystals and clusters of crystals. In slow freezing, water within and between cells freezes causing physical rupture and separation of cells. If freezing is rapid, the minute crystals formed are only within the cells but not between the cells and physical damage of the cell is less severe. Rapid cooling also minimizes concentration effects by decreasing the time of contact of solutes with food tissues during the transition from the unfrozen to the fully frozen state. For these reasons, rapid freezing is desirable for better product quality.

From the point of view of quality and economic aspects, it is best to freeze foods to -18°C or lower and maintain them at that temperature during storage and transport. In order to achieve the best advantage of rapid freezing, many foods are frozen to temperature somewhat below -26°C but this increases the cost. A freezing temperature of -18°C is very safe from attack by micro-organisms as no pathogenic organisms grow below about 3.3°C and spoilage organisms below about -9.4°C. At -9.4°C, most foods retain considerable frozen water and long storage at this temperature can result in the enzymatic deterioration of food. Even at -18°C some enzymes retain activity. However the rates of reactions they catalyze will be extremely slow. In the case of fruits and vegetables, the enzyme activity even at -18°C is sufficient to bring about spoilage. In these cases, the enzymes are inactivated by blanching before freezing. Properly packed foods frozen and stored at -18°C have high-quality storage life of the order of 12 months and longer.

The kind of damages that occur to food during slow freezing also occur during thawing. Repeated freezing and thawing is therefore very detrimental to the quality of food. Even a fluctuation of 3°C in freezing temperature above and below -18°C at which the food is frozen and stored can damage many foods. Upon refreezing, water melted from small ice crystals tends to bathe unmelted crystals causing them to grow in size. Also, if thawing of frozen foods is slow there is loss of quality due to concentration effects. In slow thawing, there is more time for food constituents to be in contact with concentrated solution thus intensifying their damaging effect. Quick thawing is also desirable from the point of keeping the microbial population in check. Large volumes of frozen food can take from 20-60 hours for thawing. Since bacteria survive the thawing process, long periods and rise in tempera-. ture of products will be opportunate for bacterial multiplication. Use of microwave heating reduces the thawing time.

Methods of Food Freezing : There are three basic methods of freezing in commercial use. These are freezing in air, freezing by indirect contact with a refrigerant and freezing by direct contact with the freezing medium. Air freezing may be by the use of still air ("sharp freezing") or an air blast.

Indirect contact freezing consists of keeping food or food packages on a surface cooled by refrigerant. In direct-contact freezing, the food or package is submerged in a cold liquid or the cold liquid is sprayed on the food or package.

Air freezing: Still-air freezing is the oldest and least expensive method of freezing. This is the type of freezing carried out in home freezers. In this method, food packs are placed in the freezer in such a way that air can circulate between the packages. The freezer is maintained in the range of -23° to -29°C. There is some air movement due to convection and in some cases gentle air movement may also be promoted.

In air-blast freezing, food packages are carried on an open mesh belt through a tunnel through which air at temperatures of -29°C to -46°C is forced at velocities of 10 to 15 m/s over, under or through the product. Under these conditions, a food packet that takes 72 hours to freeze in still-air can be frozen in about 12—18 hours. A drawback of air-blast freezing is the dehydration of food in an unwrapped condition, which is known as freezer burn. This occurs due to ice changing directly to water vapour molecules without going through the liquid state. Freezer burn results in discolouration, changes in texture and off-flavour. Freezer burn can be minimized by prechilling food with air at high humidity at about -4°C and the prechil-led food is then moved into the colder zone where it is quickly frozen.

Indirect Contact Freezing : Solid foods in consumer size flat packets are placed on hallow metal plates chilled by circulating refrigerant, so that the food is in direct contact with the cold metal wall but in indirect contact with the refrigerant. The efficiency of freezing depends upon the extent of contact between the plates and the food. For this reason, the packages should be well filled or slightly overfilled to make good pressure contact with the plates. The freezing of liquids and purees by indirect freezing is carried out by pumping them through tubes on the outside of which the refrigeration flows. Through appropriate mechanical devices the frozen food is scrapped to keep the mass in motion thus enabling the continuous bringing of new portions of food into contact with the cold wall. In this method freezing occurs in a matter of seconds.

Immersion Freezing : Immersion freezing has a number of advantages. There is intimate contact between the food or package and the refrigerant. This is particularly important in freezing irregularly shaped food pieces and immersion freezing minimizes the contact of food with air during freezing, which is desirable for foods sensitive to oxidation.

The refrigerants used for immersion freezing should be non-toxic, pure, clear, free from taste, odour, colour or bleaching action Low-freezing-point liquids'cooled by indirect contact with another refrigerant or cryogenic liquids like liquid nitrogen, carbon dioxide or freon, are used as refrigerants.

The low-freezing-point liquids used are solutions of sugar, salt or glycerol. A temperature as low as -21°C can be reached with a 23 per cent sodium chloride or 62 per cent sucrose solution. With a 67 per cent glycerol-water solution, one could go down to -47°C.

Cryogenic liquids are liquefied gases of extremely low boiling point, such as liquid nitrogen (BP, -196°C), liquid carbon dioxide (BP, -79°C) and freon 12 (BP, -30°C). The most commonly used cryogenic liquid is liquid nitrogen. Its low boiling point helps very quick freezing of even large food pieces and it can give a quality unattainable by other non-cryogenic freezing methods.

Further, since the cold temperature results from evaporation of liquid nitrogen, freezing by liquid nitrogen does not require a primary refrigerant to cool this medium, and liquid nitrogen is non-toxic and inert to food constituents. The operating cost of liquid-nitrogen freezing, however, is high. With liquid nitrogen it is possible to freeze food down to -196°C, but it is seldom frozen to a temperature below -46°C. Generally, liquid-nitrogen freezing produces less dehydration loss during freezing and less drip loss during thawing than other freezing methods.

Freezing with liquid carbon dioxide is carried out in a manner similar to freezing with liquid nitrogen. Some foods frozen with this refrigerant are equal in quality to those by liquid-nitrogen freezing. In such cases, use of liquid carbon dioxide for freezing is very economical. Of late, freon freezing is coming into use. The installation and operational costs of freon freezing are high but this can be overcome by the efficient recovery of the freon which becomes vapour on contact with food, for reuse.

Packaging for Freezing : Choice of packaging material is of special concern in the manufacture of high-quality frozen foods. The material should be moisture-proof and impermeable to oxygen and flavour compounds both at freezing temperature and after thawing. It should be resistant to chemical attack from the constituents of foods. Most foods expand on freezing. Therefore, the packaging material in which the food is frozen should have good mechanical strength, have a degree of flexibility and should not be completely filled. Many packaging materials such as cans, metal foils, waxed papers, plastic-coated cardboards and plastic foils, cellophane, parchment paper, etc., are all satisfactory for frozen foods. Glass is not generally satisfactory for frozen foods due to the possibility of breakage from expansion and thermal shocks.

Drying : Food preservation by drying is one of the methods practised from ancient times. Drying is the method nature resorts to preserve foods. Grains in the field dry sufficiently on the stalk by exposure to the sun, which requires no further drying for preservation. This is also true of legumes, innumerable seeds and some spices. The observation of natural drying was adopted by early man to dry fruits, fish and meat by exposing them to the sun. Sun drying is still in use in many parts of the world for preserving certain foods, such as fruits and nuts. However, it is limited by the fact that it is feasible only under climatic conditions of high heat and low humidity.

Drying of food involves complete removal of water under controlled conditions in such a way that the food is not altered and results in minimum changes by the drying process. Dried foods contain moisture to the extent of 1-5 per cent, and they have storage stability at room temperature of a year or longer. On reconstitution with water, dried foods are very close to and virtually indistinguishable from the original foods used in their preparation. Removal of moisture |gpm a solid with minimum change in food material is not an easy problem. Removal of only a part of water of foods, perhaps 1/3 to 2/3 of the water as in the preparation of syrups, evaporated milk, tomato paste, condensed soups, etc., is not considered as drying. Partial removal of water is known as concentration.

Advantages of Drying : Micro-organisms require water for growth and when they are growing on food they get water from food. If water is removed from food, the multiplication of micro-organisms will stop. The highest water contents at which microbial spoilage does not occur in the case of traditional dried foods are: dehydrated whole egg, 10-11 per cent; wheat flour, 13-15 per cent; dehydrated fat-free meat, 15 per cent; dehydrated vegetables, 14-20 per cent; and dehydrated fruits, 18-25 per cent. Drying of foods, thus, is primarily carried out to preserve food by controlling, micro-organisms. Partial drying as in concentration will be less effective than total drying in food preservation. However, concentration is quite sufficient to arrest the growth and multiplication of micro-organisms in some foods.

Drying, in addition to preservation, helps decrease the weight and bulk of food, e.g., 237 ml of orange juice on dehydration yields just 28 g of solids. In some cases the drying process may be chosen to retain the original shape and size. However, in such a case the volume may not be affected but there is reduction in weight. Drying thus results in great economy in storage, packaging and transport of food. Drying also results in the production of convenience foods, such as instant coffee, instant rice, etc. In these cases, cooking steps are completed before the products are dried.

Drying Rate : The amount of water removed from a given weight of material during a given time interval is called the drying rate. The most important stages in dehydration are penetration of heat into the product and removal of moisture out of the product. Various factors contribute to these two stages. A large surface area of the food to be dehydrated provides more surface area for contact witn the heating medium and for moisture to escape. Therefore, generally foods are divided into small pieces of thin layers for dehydration. This also helps reduce the distances heat must travel to reach the centre of the food and the moisture should travel to reach the sjurface to escape. Also, the greater the temperature differences between the heating medium and the food to be dried, greater is the drying rate. For any given temperature, the rate of water removal from the food is greater in vacuum than under atmospheric pressure. When the heating medium is air, it gets saturated with the moisture from the water driven from the food and this slows down subsequent moisture removal. Air in motion sweeps away moist air from the drying food surface. Thus, air velocity is also a factor that determines the drying rate.

When food is dried in air, the drier the air, the more rapid is the rate of drying. Moist air absorbs and holds less moisture than if it were dry. Dryness also determines the extent to which a food can be dried. Dried foods are hygroscopic. Each food has its own equilibrium relative humidity; i.e., the humidity at a given temperature where food neither loses moisture to the atmosphere nor picks up moisture from the atmosphere. Below this atmosphere-humidity level food cannot be further dried. For example, potato at 100°C and 46 per cent relative humidity level can be dried to 4 per cent moisture. If we wish to dry it down to

2 per cent moisture at the same temperature in air, then the relative humidity of air should be 15 per cent. Thus, the equilibrium relative humidity data of a food are important both from the point of view of its drying and storage.

There is a relationship between evaporation and temperature in drying. As water evaporates from the food it results in the cooling of the food surface. This is due to the latent heat of phase change from liquid to gas. There are several important consequences of this phenomenon in food drying. Regardless of the drying temperature or heating surface, the temperature of the food will not be higher than a particular temperature as long as water is evaporating rapidly. Thus, in a spray drier the incoming air may be at 204°C and the exit air at 121°C, but the food particle while drying may be at no more than about 71°C. As the moisture content of food decreases and evaporation slows down the particles rise in temperature. When there is no water, the incoming air and the exit air will have the same temperature (204°C). As foods are heat-sensitive, they are to be removed from the drier before this high temperature is reached.

There is also a time and temperature relationship in food preservation by drying. As food constituents are heat-sensitive, a high temperature for a short time does less damage to food than a low temperature for a long time. Also, when foods are dried they do not lose water at a constant rate all the way down to dryness. At the beginning of drying, and for some time thereafter, water generally evaporates from the food at a rather constant rate and then leaves with a falling-rate period of dryness. For example, 90 per cent of water from carrot dice can be removed in four hours and the removal of the remaining 10 per cent requires another four hours.

Thus, varying conditions, such as temperature, humidity, air velocity, direction of the air, thickness of the food and others affect the drying of food. Removal of water below 2 per cent without damage to the product is exceedingly difficult.

More than the physical factors, some of the properties of food components and the changes they undergo during drying determine the drying rate. Most foods are not homogeneous at the molecular level. For example, a piece of meat will have lean and fat interlaced or marbled together.

Therefore when a piece of meat is dried it will give up water at different rates in the regions of fat and lean. The drying rate in such a case can be increased by orienting the meat portion relative to the source of heat such that moisture escapes in a line parallel to the layers of fat rather than having to pass through them.

When sugar and low-molecular-weight substances are present in foods, they elevate the boiling point of water and thus affect the drying rate. Also, during drying, concentration of solutes become greater which slows down drying. The escape of water from food depends upon the condition in which it is present. Free water easily evaporates. Water loosely held by force of adsorption to food solids evaporates slowly. Removal of water which enters into colloidal gels, such as when starch, pectin or other gums are present, is more difficult. It is more difficult to remove chemically bound water as in hydrates of salts. The cells of blanched or cooked foods are more permeable to moisture and dry more easily than their fresh counterparts, provided cooking does not cause excessive toughening or shrinking.

In many cases, foods are pre-treated before drying with a view to make the structure more porous so as to facilitate transfer of moisture and thereby speed the drying rate. Porous sponge-like structures are excellent insulating bodies, and generally slow down the rate of heat transfer into the food. The net effect of food porosity on drying rate thus depends on whether the effect of porosity is greater on speeding the escape of moisture from food or slowing of heating transfer rate. Apart from its effects on the drying rate, food porosity has the advantages of quick solubility on reconstitution, but suffers from the disadvantages of increased bulk and shorter storage stability.

Changes during Drying : Drying brings about changes in the final product quality. One of the most obvious changes during drying of cellular as well as noncellular foods is shrinkage. The type and extent of shrinkage depend upon the rate of drying. For example, on the slow drying of a vegetable dice, first there is surface shrinkage. With continued drying, water is removed from deeper layers and finally from the centre causing continuous shrinkage towards the centre with a concave appearance and the product is dense. With quick high-temperature drying of food the surface becomes dry and rigid long before the centre dries out. Thus, when the centre dries and shrinks it pulls away from the rigid surface layer causing internal splits, voids and honeycomb effects and the product is less dense. Such a product absorbs water, reconstitutes quicker, more closely resembles the original material and is thus favoured by consumers.

With foods that contain dissolved sugar and other solutes in high concentration, drying can result in the shrinkage and sealing off of the surface pores and cracks. This results in trapping much of the remaining water with the food and drying rate dropping off severely. Dried food pieces may also contain voids, cracks and pores of various diameters. The shrinking and pore clogging by the solutes is known as core hardening. Gradual drying with low surface temperature can minimize core hardening.

Some foods which lack structure and are rich in sugar and other materials soften when heated at the elevated temperature of drying. Even after all the water has been removed the foods will be in a thermoplastic tacky condition, giving an impression that they still contain moisture; they stick to the drier. However, on cooling, the thermoplastic solids harden into crystalline or amorphous glass form. In this more brittle condition they can be easily removed from the drier.

In addition to physical changes described above, drying can bring about a range of chemical changes. These contribute to the quality of both the final product and the reconstituted food in terms of colour, flavour, texture, viscosity, nutritional value and storage stability. Complete prevention of these changes is virtually impossible. They can be minimized by appropriate technology.

Methods of Drying : Methods used for food preservation by drying should produce maximum drying rate with minimum product damage and economic drying costs. A number of drying methods are available; some are particularly suited for liquids, others for solid foods or mixtures containing food pieces. The common drier types used for liquid and solid foods may be categorized as the air-convection drier, drum or roller drier and vacuum drier. In the air-convection method, hot air supplies the heat for evaporation. If liquid, the food may be sprayed or poured into pans or on belts. Drum or roller driers are limited to be used with liquid foods, puree and mashes that can be applied as thin films. Vacuum driers are employed to lower the temperature of drying. Freeze driers are vacuum driers where, at an extremely low temperature, water vapour directly forms ice without going through the liquid state. The above division of driers is not rigid since many driers are combinations, e.g., a drum drier can be operated in vacuum or by blowing high-velocity heated air.

Air-convection Driers : There are some common aspects of the different types of air-convection driers. They all have an insulated enclosure, a means of circulating air through the enclosure and a means of heating this air. They also have means of supporting foods to be dried and devices to collect dried food.

Air may be heated directly or indirectly. In the former method, air is in direct contact with combustion gases. In indirect heating, the air is heated in contact with a hot surface, which is heated by a convenient method. A direct heating method may contaminate the food product which is not the case with indirect heating.

The simplest type of air-convection drier is the kiln drier. In this case there is direct heating of air. This kind of drier does not generally reduce moisture to below 10 per cent. A step more advanced drier is the cabinet drier. Food loaded in trays or pans in thin layers are placed in the cabinet and air heated by an indirect method is blown across food trays. This method is used for small-scale operations. Foods commonly dried by this method are fruits and vegetables. The drying time is of the order of 10-20 hours. For larger operations a tunnel drier is used. Wet food carts are moved through the tunnel on a continuous belt. Drying air is blown in a direction opposite to the movement of food carts (counter-current principle). The conveyer belt itself in some cases may form a trough (belt trough drier). The belt is usually of metal mesh and heated air is blown through the mesh. Another type of air-convection drier is the fluidized bed drier. In this case, heated air is blown up through food particles with just enough force to suspend the particle in a gentle boiling motion.

The most important kind of air-convection drier is the spray drier. More food is dehydrated by using this drier than all other kinds of driers put together. Spray drying is limited to liquids, low-viscosity pastes or purees. Food in the form of a fine spray or mist is introduced into a tower or chamber along with heated air. The small droplets make intimate contact with hot air, blast off their moisture, become small particles and drop to the bottom of the tower from where they are removed. Drying takes place in a matter of seconds. The air temperature will be 204°C but the food particles never reach a temperature above 82°C as evaporation cools the food. This method of dehydration can produce a high-quality product even with heat-sensitive materials like milk, eggs and coffee.

Drum or Roller Drier : Liquid foods, purees and mashes are dried by this method. The food to be dried is applied, as a continuous thin layer, on to the surface of a revolving drum or between a pair of drums moving in opposite directions generally heated by steam. The dried thin layer of food on the drum is scraped by a scraper blade positioned at a point on the drum. Some foods when dry are sticky and cannot be scraped off from the drum when hot. Such a sticky food becomes brittle when cold, which facilitates scraping. Providing a cold zone on a drum thus helps the drying of such foods. The drum temperature may be kept above 100°C by using steam under pressure. Generally, the drum is kept at 150°C when a film of food 1.6 mm in thickness gets dried in one minute or less. For heat resistant food products, drum drying is one of the least expensive dehydration methods. Drum-dried foods generally will have a somewhat more "cooked" character than the same material spray-dried.

Vacuum Driers : This method of drying of foods is expensive but gives high-quality foods. The drying system consists of a vacuum chamber that can withstand external air pressure and contains shelves or other supports to hold food. This kind of vacuum drier is for batch-type operation. For continuous operation a belt drier is used. The shelves are heated electrically or by circulating a heated fluid. The food gets heated by conduction and also by radiated heat from shelves above and below. The drying chamber is evacuated by a suitable device maintained outside the vacuum chamber. The water that evaporates from the food is suitably condensed. The temperature of the food and the rate of water removal are controlled by controlling the degree of vacuum and the intensity of heat output. Liquid foods dehydrated by vacuum drying have a puffed structure and are easily dissolved in water. Because of the low temperature used, there is minimun flavour change and other kinds of heat damage in this method of drying.

Freeze-drying is used to dehydrate sensitive high-quality liquid foods such as coffee and juices, and also solids of high value like strawberries, shrimps, etc., having delicate flavour, colour and taxtural attributes which cannot be preserved by any other drying method. In freeze-drying, water evaporates from ice without passing through the liquid stage, i.e., water from ice directly becomes water vapour. This happens at a temperature of 0°C or below, and at a low pressure of 4.7 mm of mercury or less. Frozen food is dried by keeping in a vacuum chamber maintained at a pressure of 0.1 to 2 mm of mercury and maintaining the temperature of the chamber just below the melting point of ice. Under such conditions water from the frozen food evaporates at the maximum rate. Since the frozen food remains rigid the evaporation of water leaves voids behind it, resulting in a porous sponge-like dried material. After the food is dried the vacuum is broken with inert nitrogen gas and packed under nitrogen. If the vacuum is broken by admitting air the dried product absorbs the air into its pores resulting in impaired storage stability.

Foam : Drying (puff dry) at atmospheric pressure can be employed to dehydrate foods and obtain products with qualities approaching vacuum-dried ones. This method of drying is very economical compared to vacuum-drying method and can be applied to liquid foods and purees which can be pre-foamed before drying. As foaming exposes an enormous surface area for quick moisture escape, drying of foams can be rapid at atmospheric pressure at a reduced temperature. With foods that do not whip readily, some whipping agents (vegetable proteins, gums, monoglycerides) are added prior to being whipped. Stable foams are cast in thin layers into trays or belts and dried by various heating schemes.

Concentration

Foods are concentrated for the same reasons that they are dried—preservation and reduction in weight and bulk. Nearly all liquid foods are first concentrated before drying because of the technical and economical advantages of such processing. Many foods are better recognized as concentrates than dried ones; examples are fruit-juice concentrates, canned soups, condensed milk, etc.

Concentration may not be effective in all cases as a means of food preservation. The levels of water in most concentrated foods are sufficient for microbial growth. Concentrated non-acid fruit juice and vegetable purees undergo spoilage unless they are further processed. On the other hand, concentrated sugar syrups, sauces and jellies are relatively free from spoilage. The solutions of sugar and salt dissolved in the remaining water give concentrates which exert high osmotic pressure and draw water from the microbial cells or prevent normal diffusion of water into the cells and thus prevent microbial contamination. Solutions containing 70 per cent of sugar or 18-25 per cent salt prevent the growth of all micro-organisms.

Methods of Concentration : As in food drying, one of the simplest methods of concentration is by utilizing solar energy. Salt has been manufactured by the concentration of sea water by this method from the earliest times.

Kettle Evaporators : A simple method of concentration is by the use of open kettles and pans, which may be heated by direct flame or steam. High temperature and long concentration times damage most foods. However, kettle or pan concentration is used in the manufacture of syrups as high heat is desirable to produce the colour from caramalized sugar and develop typical flavour.

Flash Evaporation : Purees are concentrated by flash evaporation. Superheated steam (150°C) is injected into the food pumped into a vertical tubular steam-jacketed evaporator where boiling occurs. The boiling mix then enters a separator from which the concentrated food is drained off.

Film Evaporators : Foods are also concentrated using thin film evaporators. In this case, food is pumped into a vertical cylinder which has a rotating element that spreads the food into a thin layer on the cylindrical wall. The cylinder wall is usually heated by steam. Water quickly flashes from the thin food layer and the concentrated food is simultaneously wiped from the cylinder wall. The product temperature may reach 83°C but since the concentrated food will be in contact with the heated cylinder for less than a minute, the damage is minimal.

Vacuum Evaporators : Heat-sensitive liquid foods are commonly concentrated at low temperatures in vacuum evaporators. Evaporation systems can be made that operate many times more effectively than single-effect evaporation. Several vacuumized vessels in series constitute multiple effect evaporators. In this process, the first evaporator under vacuum is heated with steam. The water vapour boiled off from the food is sent to the next evaporator kept at a higher vacuum than the first. The water vapour acts as a heat source to evaporate food in the second evaporator. The water vapour from the second can next be passed to a third evaporator having a higher vacuum than the second and so on. Grape juice and tomato juice are concentrated in this way. This method results in energy conservation.

Freeze Concentration : Concentration by freezing has been used to concentrate fruit juice. When liquid food is frozen, not all the water is converted into ice at the same time. Before the food freezes, the initially formed ice crystals are separated. By repeating this process several times on the concentrated unfrozen food a high percentage of water can be removed. The disadvantage of this method is the unavoidable entrainment loss.

Ultrafiltration and Reverse Osmosis : Another method of concentration of liquid food is by ultrafiltration and reverse osmosis. The process consists of pumping liquid foods at a high pressure against selective membranes that allow water molecules to pass through them while retaining macromble-cules, salts, sugar and other organic molecules. Membranes used in ultrafiltration are "less light" and may allow small molecules to pass through them under moderate pressure while in reverse osmosis the membranes are "tighter" and permeability does not allow even these molecules to pass through. In osmosis, there is the movement of water through membranes from a region of lower concentration to a region of higher concentration. In reverse osmosis this is reversed; under pressure there is flow of water through the membranes from a region of higher concentration to that of a lower.

The concentration of foods results in cooked flavour and darkening of colour. Concentration also causes changes in organoleptic and nutritional properties of foods. Some foods cannot be concentrated beyond a certain point. When foods containing sugar are concentrated sugar crystallizes out as concentration increases. Concentration also causes an increase in the level of salts and minerals which result in the precipitation of protein. This is the cause of gel formation of evaporated milk after a few weeks' or months' storage.

Fermentation

The methods of food preservation so far studied, such as application of heat, cold, removal of water and other methods used, have the common objective of decreasing the number of micro-organisms in food or holding them in check against further multiplication. In food preservation by fermentation, in contrast, multiplicatioin of micro-organisms and their metabolic activities are encouraged. However, the organisms that are encouraged to grow and multiply are the select groups whose metabolic products help food preservation.

Natural fermentations have played a vital role in the preservation of foods from early times. Fruit juices exposed to air underwent natural fermentation and acquired an alcoholic flavour. Milk on standing became slightly acidic. These changes were therefore used as a means of preservation of otherwise perishable foods. At the same time the changes in the texture and taste of fermented foods were found desirable. These are the principal reasons for the continued use of fermentation in food processing and preservation. The list of foods produced by fermentation is extremely long and includes the following: cheese, curd, butter, all alcoholic beverages, pickles, sauerkraut, vinegar, bread, idli, soya sauce, coffee, tea and cocoa.

The term fermentation means the breakdown of carbohydrate material by micro-organisms (or enzymes) under anaerobic conditions. In common usage, the term fermentation refers to both the anaerobic and aerobic breakdowns of carbohydrates and carbohydrate-like materials. Thus the conversion of lactose to lactic acid by *Streptococcus lactis* which takes place under anaerobic conditions and conversion of ethyl alcohol to acetic acid by the bacteria *Acetobacter aceti* under aerobic conditions are both referred to as fermentation. The term is used in a still broader and less precise manner to describe fermented foods.

In the fermentation of foods, a complex mixture of carbohydrates, proteins, fats, etc., undergo modifications simultaneously under the action of a variety of micro-organisms and enzymes present. Thus, the carbohydrates and carbohydrate like materials undergo fermentation, proteinaceous material undergo proteolysis or "putrefactive" breakdown and lipids "lipolytic" breakdown. The nature and extent of these changes depend upon the food, types of micro-organisms present and conditions affecting their growth and metabolic pattern.

The preservative effect of fermentation is caused by the chemicals excreted by the micro-organisms. The principal chemicals involved are acids (especially lactic acid) and alcohol. These inhibit the growth of common pathogenic organisms in foods. The toxin producing *Clostridium botulinum,* for example, cannot grow at pH values below 4.6.

Benefits of Fermentation : In addition to contributing to preservation, fermentation of foods has additional benefits. Fermentation produces flavour and textural changes and fermented foods are actually more nutritious than their unfermented counterparts. Microorganisms, in addition to breaking down complex compounds, synthesize several vitamins and other growth factors. In fact, the industrial production of some vitamins is largely by fermentation processes. The digestible carbohydrates and proteins of grains and seeds are enclosed in cellulosic and hemicellulosic structures which are indigestible materials. Fermentation, especially by certain molds, breaks down the indigestible protective coating as they are rich in cellulose-splitting enzymes. The altered structure of the cells makes permeability of digestive juices easy. An additional advantage of such splitting of cellulose, hemicellulose and related materials is that such materials are converted into simpler sugars and sugar derivatives which increase the nutritional value of foods.

Microbial : Activities in Foods Microbial flora associated with foods have a broad complement of enzymes and, as already stated, bring about fermentative, proteolytic and lipolytic changes among others. Proteolytic organisms break down proteins and other nitrogenous compounds resulting in putrid and rotten odour and flavour. Lipolytic organisms hydrolyze lipids giving rise to free fatty acids resulting in rancidity. These changes are un desirable in foods. On the other hand, fermentative organisms converting carbohydrates and related compounds to alcohols, acids and carbon dioxide are not offensive to food tastes. When the concentration of their fermentative products increases, they control the growth of organisms of proteolytic and lipolytic types. However, fermentation of food is complex and only one type of change to the total exclusion of other changes is impossible. Thus, to obtain a product of desired quality, controlled fermentation becomes necessary.

Control of Fermentation in Foods : The factors that influence the growth and metabolic activities of micro-organisms in food fermentation are the acidity, levels of alcohol, use of starters and levels of oxygen and salts.

Acid : Acids when present in food either as natural constituents, added or formed by fermentation, exert an inhibitory effect on harmful micro-organisms. However, the preservative effect of acid is lost if oxygen is available and surface molds grow which result in the fermentation of the acids. This happens during the ripening of cheddar cheese and constitutes a defect. Some yeasts tolerate moderately high acidity and produce ammonia from the breakdown of protein. This results in the neutralization of the acid present and permits the subsequent growth of proteolytic and lipolytic bacteria as happens in the ripening of some types of cheese.

These types of changes also occur when raw milk is allowed to ferment. Raw milk contains many types of organisms. First, *Streptococcus lactis* grows producing lactic acid and its growth is inhibited when the acid concentration reaches a particular level. *Lactobacillus* bacteria which are still more acid resistant then grow and produce more acid until the new level becomes inhibitory to their growth. This results in milk clotting and curd formation. In the high-acid environment, acid resistant yeasts and molds become active. The molds oxidize acid and the yeast produces alkaline end products. These result in a decrease of the acid level flavouring the growth of proteolytic and lipolytic spoilage bacteria resulting in an off-odour and gassy condition in the curd.

Alcohol : Alcohol is also a preservative depending upon its concentration. Yeast converts sugar to alcohol but it cannot tolerate alcohol concentration of over 12 per cent. When the alcohol content is below this level, as in beer, pasteurization of the food becomes necessary to prevent spoilage.

Use of Starters : When a particular type of micro-organisms is present in large numbers and is multiplying at a good rate, it keeps down the growth of other micro-organisms. This is the reason why in curd making or wine making a part from the previous batch of curd or wine is added to the fresh milk or grape juice. However, in commercial food fermentation, pure cultures are used as starters to obtain products of desired quality.

Temperature : Temperature has an effect on all microbial reactions and hence has to be controlled. In mixed fermentations, as in foods, control of temperature is all the more necessary as different organisms have different temperature sensitivity. For example, in the production of sauerkraut three major types of organisms which grow well at different temperatures, are involved in fermentation. In sauerkraut fermentation, therefore, an initial low temperature (about 21°C), which then is increased somewhat in the later stages of fermentation, is employed.

Oxygen : The level of oxygen determines the extent of fermentation of some foods. Thus providing or removal of air or oxygen is used to encourage or inhibit a particular micro-organism. Also, an organism may have different oxygen requirements for growth than it has for fermentation activity. For example, bakers'yeast (S. *cerevisiae)* and wine yeast (S. *ellipsoideus)* both grow well and produce greater cell masses under aerobic conditions, but they ferment sugar more rapidly under anaerobic condition. Thus, for production of bakers' yeast, the yeast is grown under the aerobic condition by bubbling air through the fermenting medium. In vinegar production there are two steps; the first step involves conversion of sugary substances to alcohol and the second the conversion of alcohol to acetic acid. Alcohol production is an anaerobic process and its conversion to acetic acid is an oxidative fermentation. Thus, in vinegar production, initially fermentation should be anaerobic and this should be followed by generous supply of air.

Salt : Salt can also be used for controlling food fermentation. Lactic acid producing micro-organisms used in the fermentation of pickles, sauerkraut, etc., are tolerant to salt solutions of the order of 10-18 per cent. Many proteolytic and other spoilage organisms that can infest lactic bacteria are not tolerant to salt above 2.5 per cent. Similarly, salt added to cheese curd controls proteolytic organisms during the long ripening periods.

Radiation : Preservation of food by ionizing radiations is a recently developed method but has not yet gained general acceptance. As is well known, the electromagnetic radiations suppress the growth of most micro-organisms. The possibilities of employing nuclear radiation to sterilize food have been extensively studied since World War II. The harmful effects on the human body from radiations from nuclear explosions have given rise to suspicion in the minds of many people about the safety of the use of irradiated foods. Much work has been done on the safety and wholesomeness of irradiated products but more careful investigations are required before allowing the irradiated food to be used on a large scale.

Kinds of Ionizing Radiations : There are several kinds of radiant energy emitted from different sources which differ in wavelength, frequency, penetrating power and in the various effects they have upon biological systems. Irradiation of foods is carried out by exposing them to high-energy radiations which penetrate them and bring about changes within them. The principal radiations used in food irradiation are gamma rays (wavelengths <2Å) emitted from excited radioactive elements ^{60}CO) and accelerated negatively charged particles, electrons (β-particles), which are emitted from a hot cathode. Gamma rays are very similar to x-rays, except that they have much greater penetrating power. An electron beam can be accelerated to very high speeds and increased energies so that it can penetrate foods, by passing it through electronic devices.

Ultraviolet radiations are also employed in preservation; but they have a very low degree of penetration and are employed to inactivate micro-organisms on the surface of food and to treat air, water and the surface of food processing equipment to reduce the number of micro-organisms.

Measurement of Radiation : Ionizing radiations are measured in terms of rads (and kilorad or megarad). A rad is 10 μJ of energy absorbed by 1 g of material. The radiation effects are related to dose by the relation:

$$n = n_o \exp(-D/D_o)$$

where $\bar{n}$ = the number of live organisms following irradiation; n_0 = initial number of organisms; D=dose radiation received (rads), and D_o = a constant depending on type of organism and environmental factors.

Different organisms are sensitive to irradiation to different extent as indicated below:

10^{3-4}—10^7 rads —micro-organisms are killed

10^3 —10^5 rads —insects are killed

10^3 —10^4 rads —sprouting of potatoes, onions, carrots, etc., are inhibited

10^2 —10^3 rads —dose is lethal for humans.

In the case of micro-organisms, the approximate sterilizing dose is: bacterial endospores, 3.0×10^6 rads; yeasts and fungi, -5.0×10^4 rads. There are, however, some micro organisms with exceptional resistance to irradiations; for example, *Micrococcus radiodurans* is resistant up to 55 times greater dosage than gram-negative organisms like *Escherichia coli.*

Mode of Action of Radiations : When gamma rays and electron beam pass through foods, there are collisions between ionizing radiations and food particles at the atomic and molecular levels, resulting in the production of ion pairs and free radicals. The reactions of these products among themselves and with other molecules result in physical and chemical phenomena inactivating micro-organisms in foods. Thus, radiation of foods qan be considered to be a means of achieving "cold sterilization" of food—a food is freed of micro-organisms without the need for high temperatures.

Water is a ubiquitous ingredient in foods. Of all the reactions brought about by ionizing radiations, the one with water is the most important in producing foods free of spoilage micro-organisms or pathogens or containing a greatly diminished content of spoilage organisms. Ionizing radiations split water to produce hydrated electrons (e^-_{aq}), highly reactive hydrogen (H) and hydroxyl (.OH) radicals, excited water (H_2O) and ionized water molecules (H_2O). Interactions between these products, or these products and other components of food containing oxygen result in the formation of highly reactive species such as hydrogen peroxide.

$$\cdot OH + OH \rightarrow H_2O_2$$

$$H + O_2 \rightarrow HO_2$$

$$HO_2 + HO_2 \rightarrow H_2O_2 + O_2$$

Hydrogen peroxide is a strong oxidizing agent and a toxicant to micro-organisms.

Uses of Radiations Ionizing radiations may be used for sterilization of foods in hermetically sealed packs, reduction in the size of the spoilage flora on perishable foods, elimination of pathogens in foods, control of infestation in stored cereals, prevention of sprouting of potatoes, onions, etc. and retardation of the development of pickled mushrooms. The destruction of the growing point causing tissue darkening of the sprouting areas of vegetables such as potatoes by radiations, eliminates the risk of sprouting during storage.

Irradiation does not very much affect the nutritional properties of foods. The destruction of various amounts of nutrients are of the same degree as in heat processing. Ionizing radiations can also hydrolyze and modify proteins, starch and cellulose. Thus, irradiation can help to improve nutritive value of certain plant materials. Significant levels of toxic or carcinogenic substances are not produced in foods irradiated with sufficient dose of radiations. At appropriate dose of radiations, sterilized or pasteurized foods, are safe from microbial standpoint.

Irradiation of foods can also result in certain undesirable effects. Ionizing radiation, in excessive doses, can alter the structure of organic and biochemical compounds in food resulting in food damage. Degradation of carbohydrates may result in loss of texture and colour. Protein degradation results in undesirable changes in colour and odour and brings about liquefaction. Egg-white proteins, on irradiation, become thin and watery. Irradiation of fats results in the development of off-flavour and off-odour and the loss of the natural antioxidants. Foods irradiated with large doses of radiation might themselves become radioactive and prove harmful when consumed.

In the irradiation of foods for preservation, the control of the radiation process is very necessary. The radiation dose must be carefully controlled to destroy micro-organisms and inactivate many food enzymes. It should be sufficient to destroy the pathogenic and spoilage causing organisms. Apart from the intensity of radiation, the amount of radiation absorbed and the length of time of radiation are to be controlled. The longer the food is in the radiation path, the more it will absorb. Radiation energy must be provided in such a manner that it reaches every particle of food to ensure adequate killing of all micro-organisms.

As already stated, the use of ionizing radiations for food preservation has been adopted very slowly. This is largely due to the unacceptable flavour of some foods irradiated to sterilization stage. Also, the fear that radioactivity might be induced in a food has come in the way of its extended use. However, recent reappraisal by the WHO and the Internatinal Atomic Energy Authority has resulted in the recommendation that irradiation dose up to 1M rad is not hazardous.

The disinfection of grains, the preservation, the prevention of sprouting of potatoes and other vegetables are of great economic value. In less developed countries lacking refrigeration facilities, losses from insects and spoilage of food account for more than half the total food production. In such cases radiation of foods will be of great significance. This requires radiation facilities at a cost that developing countries can afford.

19

Preserving Agents

The great bulk of food is comprised of chemicals such as carbohydrates, fats, proteins, vitamins, minerals, water, etc. Besides the natural components of food stuffs, additional chemicals may be incorporated, either directly or indirectly during the growing, storage or processing of food.

Food Additives

A food additive is defined as a substance or mixture of substances, other than a base foodstuff, which is present in a food as a result of any aspect of production, processing, storage or packing. This definition includes both intentional and unintentional additives. The unintentional additives, which are not added to achieve an effect in the food but which may accidentally enter into foods as a result of their use in agricultural production, raising animals, food processing or packing, are not additives in the technical sense of the term, but they are food contaminants.

An expert committee on Food Additives made up of representatives of FAO and WHO has defined food additives as non-nutritive substances added intentionally to food, generally in small quantities, to improve its appearance, flavour, texture or storage properties. This definition excludes substances added primarily for their nutritive value, such as vitamins and minerals.

A broad definition of food additive is any substance the intended use of which results, directly or indirectly, in its becoming a component of or otherwise affecting the characteristics of any food and which is safe under the condition of its use. Any substance present in food, either by intentional addition or an unintentional contaminant, has its effects on the safety of food.

The Requirement

For centuries, man has recognised the effects of food additives and has used whatever was available—marigold for colour, wood ashes for leavening, the lining of calves stomach for cheese making, etc. They were used for effects without knowing the changes they brought about. As long as the ingredient did not make one sick immediately it was alright to use it. Today, thousands of compounds are used as food additives, whose chemical identity and structure are known. They can be obtained in a very high state of purity and, when used, bring about the desired effect in foods.

The use of food additives is imperative in the complex and integrated society in which we live. The areas of food production are separated from the areas of consumption. Additives have provided protection against food spoilage during storage, transportation, distribution or processing. Also, with the present degree of urbanization, it would be impossible to maintain food distribution without the processing and packing with which many additives are involved.

A number of factors have led to the demand for foods with built-in preparation—"convenience" foods. A can of vegetable soup is a convenient food, since various vegetables have been cut, blended, supplemented with spices and so on. It just requires warming up before use. There is a great demand nowadays for "instant", heat and serve, and "ready-to-cook" convenient foods.

These foods make up about 60 per cent of the food that Americans buy. Such foods result in saving considerable amounts of time and effort in food preparation at home, restaurants, etc. The convenience food revolution would not have been possible without food additives.

Additives permit the variety of foods that we deem desirable and which certainly are objectively important in maintaining good nutrition. Vitamins and minerals are important, among other things, for good health. Many of these chemical additives can be manufactured so that foods can be "fortified" or "enriched". Potassium iodide, for instance, added to common salt can eliminate goitre, enriched rice or bread with B-complex vitamins can eliminate pellagra and adding vitamin D to cow milk prevents rickets.

Many foods, particularly those with high moisture contents, do not keep well. All foods are subject to microbial attack. Fats or oily foods become rancid, particularly when exposed to humid air. The conservation of the quality of foods against agents causing such deterioration of foods requires the addition of preservatives. Additives are also used to colour foods, add flavour, impart firmness and retard or hasten chemical reaction in food.

There is then the need for the use of food additives to maintain the nutritional quality of food, to enhance stability with resulting reduction in waste, to make food more attractive and to provide efficient aids in processing, packing and transport. The amount of additives used should be kept to a minimum; it should conform to a standard of purity and be safe. On the other hand, food additives must not be used to disguise faulty processing and handling techniques, to deceive the customers, or if it reduces the food's nutritive value, or when the desired effect can be achieved by good manufacturing practices that are economically feasible.

Over 3000 different chemical compounds are used as food additives. They are categorized into different groups. A few types of additives are indicated below.

Antioxidants : An antioxidant is a substance added to fats and fat-containing substances to retard oxidation and thereby prolong their wholesomeness, palatability and, sometimes, keeping time. An antioxidant should not contribute an objectionable odour, flavour or colour to the fat or to the food in which it is present. It should be effective in low concentrations and be fat soluble. Also, it should not have harmful physiological effect.

Some antioxidants used in foods are butylated hydroxyanisole (BHA), butylated hydroxytoluene (BHT), propyl gallate (PG) and tertiarybutyl hydroquinone (TBHQ), which are all phenolic substances. Thiodipropionic acid and dilauryl thiodipropionate are also used as food antioxidants. Naturally occurring substances that act as antioxidants are the tocopherols. The tocopherols act as biological antioxidants in plant and animal tissues, but they are rarely used as additives because they are more expensive than synthetic antioxidants.

Antioxidants function by interrupting the free radical chain mechanism involved in lipid oxidation. They are effective in small concentrations (0.01-0.02 per cent). Mixed antioxidants sometimes act synergistically. The presence of metallic ions, particularly copper and iron, promotes lipid oxidation through a catalytic action. Acidic compounds, like citric acid, complex with iron and thus, when present along with phenolic antioxidants, enhance the latter's activity.

Browning of cut fruits and vegetables is due to enzymic oxidation of phenolic substances. Antioxidants prevent this discolouration. Ascorbic acid is used as an antioxidant in this case. Acids, such as citric and phosphoric, increase the effectiveness of ascorbic acid in preventing browning.

Chelating Agents : Chelating agents or sequestrants are compounds that form complexes with metal ions. Many metals exist in food in a naturally chelated form, such as, magnesium in chlorophylls, iron in ferritin and haemoglobin, and copper, zinc and magnesium in enzymes. When metallic ions are released due to hydrolytic or other degradative reactions, they are free to participate in reactions that lead to discolouration, oxidative rancidity, turbidity, and flavour changes in foods. Addition of chelating agents results in the complexing of these metal ions and thereby the stabilization of foods.

Compounds containing two or more functional groups, such as hydroxyl, sulphydryl, carboxyl, phosphate, etc., chelate with metals under favourable conditions. Citric acid and its derivatives, phosphates and salts of ethylene-diamine tetraacetic acid (EDTA) are the most popular chelating agents used in foods.

Chelating agents are not antioxidants; they serve as scavengers of metals which catalyze oxidation. They, however, are antioxidant synergists. Citric acid and its esters in propylene glycol solution are effective synergists in lipid systems.

Polyphosphates and EDTA are used as chelating agents in canned seafoods. Seafoods contain substantial amounts of magnesium ions which sometimes react with ammonium phosphate with the formation of glossy crystals (struvite). Iron, copper and zinc containing seafoods react with sulphides that lead to product discolouration. These reactions are prevented by the addition of chelating agents.

Citric and phosphoric acids are used as acidulants in soft drink beverages. These chelate with metals which otherwise promote the oxidation of flavour compounds and catalyze discolouration reactions. Chelating agents also stabilize fermented malt beverages by complexing with copper, which otherwise catalyzes the oxidation of phenolic substances which subsequently interact with proteins to form haziness or turbidity.

Colouring Agents : These include colour stabilizers, colour fixatives, colour retention agents, etc. They consist of synthetic colours, synthesized colours that also occur naturally and other colours from natural sources. Even though colours add nothing to the nutritive value of foods, without certain colours most consumers will not buy or eat some foods. Thus, colours are frequently added to restore the natural ones lost in food processing or to give the preparations the natural colour we expect.

Originally, many colour additives were natural pigments or

dyes. For example, spinach juice or grass, marigold flower, and cochineal were used to obtain green, yellow and red colour respectively. This gave place to synthetic dyes obtained from coal tar. Synthetic colours generally excel in colouring power, colour uniformity, colour stability and cost. Further, in many cases, natural colouring materials do not exist for a desired hue. Carbonated beverages, gelatin dessert, candies and bakery goods are some foods that are coloured with coal tar dyes. As a number of coal tar compounds have been shown to be potent carcinogens, the use of coaltar dyes as food additives is restricted. Many countries have severely restricted the number of coal tar dyes for use in foods, while some other countries have completely banned their use. Food colours used also include some inorganic materials such as iron oxide to give redness and titanium dioxide to intensify whiteness.

A number of natural food colours extracted from seeds, flowers, insects and foods are also used as food additives. One of the best known and most widespread red pigment is bixin, derived from the seed coat of *Bixa orel-lana,* the lipstick pod plant of South American origin. Bixin is not considered to be carcinogenic. The major use of this plant on a worldwide basis, however, is for the annatto dye, a yellow to red colouring material extracted from the orange-red pulp of the seeds. Annatto has been used as colouring matter in butter, cheese, margarine and other foods. Another yellow colour, a carotene derived from carrot, is used in margarine. Saffron has both flavouring and colouring properties and has been used for colouring foods. Turmeric is a spice that gives the characteristic colour of curries and some meat products and salad dressings. A natural red colour, cochineal (or carnum) obtained by extraction from the female insect *(Coccus cacti),* grape skin extract and caramel, and the brown colour obtained from burnt sugar, are some natural colours that are used as food additives.

Curing Agents : These are additives to preserve (cure) meats, give them desirable colour and flavour, discourage growth of micro-organisms and prevent toxin formation.

Sodium nitrite has been used for centuries as a preservative and colour stabilizer in meat and fish products. The nitrite, when added to meat, gets converted to nitric oxide which combines with myoglobin to form nitric oxide myoglobin (nitrosylmyoglobin) which is a heat-stable pigment. The curing also contributes flavour to the meat. In addition, nitrite curing inhibits the growth of *Clostridium* and *Streptococcus,* and also lowers the temperature required to kill C. *botulinum.*

It has been discovered that cooking nitrite cured meat products results in the formation of small amounts of N-nitrosamines, which are potent carcinogens. The nitrosamines are formed by the reaction of secondary and tertiary amines, through the following type of reaction.

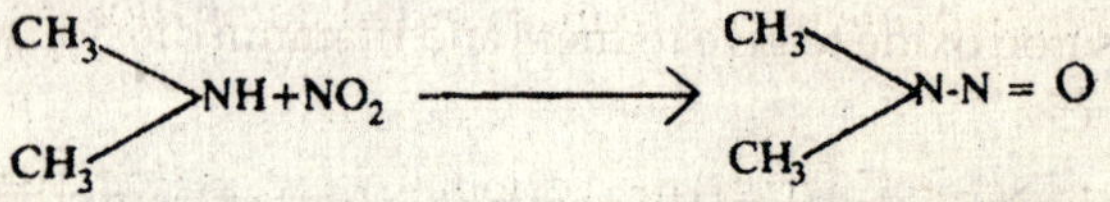

$$(CH_3)_2NH + NO_2 \longrightarrow (CH_3)_2N\text{-}N=O$$

Dimethylamine → **N-Nitrosodimethylamine**

Nitrosation may also take place in foods during storage or processing, and nitrosamines may be ingested as such. There is some evidence that nitrosamines are formed under the strong acid conditions in the human stomach, when nitrite cured meats are ingested.

In recent years, use of nitrite for curing has become controversial. Although the levels are low, the production of carcinogens during food manufacture or preparation cannot be ignored. As the derivation of nitrosamines is due to NO^-_2 in meat, a reduction in the concentration of the curing agent used helps alleviate the problem. However, the reduction in the concentration of NO^-_2 enhances the risk of food poisoning due to *Clostridium botulinum.* Recent results have shown diminished concentrations of nitrite can be used in the presence of another preservative that acts synergistically. In the presence of isoascorbate even very dilute concentrations of nitrite significantly decrease spoilage and toxin production.

Other agents used for curing meat are ascorbates and several phosphates. Ascorbate and isoascorbate react with nitrite to give nitric oxide and thereby accelerate the rate of formation of nitrosylmyoglobin. They also stabilize colour and flavour. They inhibit the formation of nitrosamines. Through chelating iron, they may contribute also to the antimicrobial stability of cured meats.

Polyphosphates, such as sodium tripolyphosphate ($Na_5P_3O_{10}$) and sodium hexametaphosphate $(NaPO_3)_n$ where $n = 10$ to 15, are used in meat curing. These compounds, through enhancing water retention, aid tenderness, juiciness and flavour of cured meats. They also influence texture and, by chelating metal ions, act as antioxidants. The latter property also contributes to the antimicrobial properties of cured meats.

Emulsions : Emulsifiers are a group of substances used to obtain a stable mixture of liquids that otherwise would not mix or would separate quickly. They also stabilize gas-in-liquid and gas-in-solid mixtures. They are widely used in dairy and confectionery products to disperse tiny globules of an oil or fatty liquid in water. Emulsifying agents are also added to margarine, salad dressings and shortenings. Peanut butter contains up to 10 per cent emulsifiers.

One of the most widely used emulsifiers is lecithin which is found in milk, egg and soyabean. Lecithin keeps, in milk, the butterfat and water phases more or less uniform. Commercial vegetable lecithin is obtained principally from soyabean. Lecithin is employed in the preparation of cocoa butter and chocolate candy. The texture and keeping qualities of bread and other fermented baking products are improved by the use of lecithin. Lecithin is a more effective emulsifying agent in combination with monoglyceryl stearate and ascorbic acid. A number of mono- and diglycerides and their derivatives are good emulsifying agents. In these cases, the ester groups make the molecule fat-soluble, while the alcohol group lends water solubility to another portion of the molecule. As a result, the molecule can serve as a bridge to keep fat molecules suspended in water.

In addition to these natural emulsifiers, there are a number of synthetic ones. These include propylene glycol monostearate, sorbitan monostearate and polysorbates.

Flavours and Flavour Enhancers : Flavouring additives are the ingredients, both naturally occurring and added, which give the characteristic flavour to almost all the foods in our diet. Flavour enhancers are not flavours themselves but they amplify the flavours of other substances through a synergistic effect. Flavour and flavour enhancers constitute the largest class of food additives. These are about 2,100 approved natural and synthetic flavours of which more than 1,600 are synthetic ones.

Natural flavour substances, such as spices, herbs, roots, essences and essential oils have been used in the past as flavour additives. The flavours of such materials are not uniform. They vary with the season and area of production. In addition, the natural flavours are in short supply and the amount of flavour substances in them is very tiny. It would take about a tonne of many spices to produce 1 g of the flavour substances and in some cases only 0.1 g could be extracted. Natural food flavours are thus being replaced by synthetic flavour materials.

The agents responsible for flavour are esters, aldehydes, ketones, alcohols and ethers. These substances are easily synthesized and can be easily substituted for natural ones. Typical of the synthetic flavour additives are amyl acetate for banana, methyl anthranilate for grapes, ethyl butyrate for pineapple, etc. Generally, most synthetic flavours are mixtures of a number of different substances. For example, one imitation cherry flavour contains fifteen different esters, alcohols and aldehydes.

One of the best known, most widely used and somewhat controversial flavour enhancers is monosodium grutamate (MSG), the sodium salt of the naturally occurring amino acid glutamic acid. This is added to over 10,000 different processed foods. This has been in use in Chinese and Japanese cooking for centuries, and was extracted from seaweeds and soyabean. About 65 years ago, a Japanese named Ikeda discovered that the flavouring from these is the MSG and that it has an attractive meat-like flavour. MSG is now manufactured on a large scale all over the world, and especially in Japan.

MSG is generally recognized as safe. However, it was reported some time back that MSG injected to young mice resulted in brain damage. Also, some individuals experience symptoms often comparable to those of heart attack, when served with food containing large amounts of MSG. The matter has now been thoroughly investigated and it has been concluded that there is no risk in its use. However, MSG which was being added to baby foods is now discontinued, as its benefits to babies are dubious.

Yeast extract has the same flavour enhancing property as MSG. It is found that, in this case, the flavour enhancing substances are the ribo-nucleotides. These are ten times more powerful than MSG.

Flour Improvers : These are bleaching and maturing agents; usually, they both bleach and "mature" the flour. These are important in the flour milling and bread-baking industries. Freshly milled flour has a yellowish tint and yields a weak dough that produces poor bread. Both the colour and baking properties improve by storing the flour for several months before making bread.

During storage, atmospheric oxygen oxidizes the carotenoid pigments responsible for the colour of the flour, converting them to colourless compounds. They also oxidize some of the proteins which form dough to give the latter increased strength and elasticity. These improvements can be obtained more rapidly with the use of chemical agents.

Chemical agents used as flour improvers are oxidizing agents, which may participate in bleaching only, in both bleaching and dough improvement, or in dough improvement only. The agent that is used only for flour bleaching is benzoyl peroxide $(C_6H_5CO)_2O_2$. This does not influence the quality of dough. Materials used both for bleaching and improving are chlorine gas, (Cl_2); Chlorine dioxide, (ClO_2); nitrosyl chloride, (NOCl); and nitrogen di-and tetroxides, (NO_2 and N_2O_4). Oxidizing agents used only for dough improvement are potassium bromate, $(KBrO_3)$; potassium iodate, (KIO_3), calcium iodate, $[(Ca(IO_3)_2]$ and calcium peroxide, (CaO_2).

Benzoyl peroxide oxidation takes several hours. The gaseous agents used for bleaching and improvement act immediately upon contact with flour. Oxidizing agents used for dough improvement only remain inactive until yeast fermentation lowers the pH of the dough sufficiently to activate them. As a result of late action they cause increase of loaf volume, improved loaf symmetry and improved crumb and texture characteristics. The dough improving oxidizing agents oxidize sulphydryl groups (-SH) in the procems of gluten to yield an increased number of intermolecular disulphide bonds (-S-S-), resulting in a tougher, drier, more extensible dough that gives rise to improved characteristics in finished products.

Humecants and Anticaking Agents : Humecants are moisture retention agents. Their functions in foods include control of viscosity and texture, bulking, retention of moisture, reduction of water activity, control of crystallization and improvement or retention of softness. They also help improve the rehydration of dehydrated food and solubilization of flavour compounds.

Polyhydroxy alcohols are water soluble, hygroscopic materials which exhibit moderate viscosities at high concentrations in water and are used as humecants in foods. Some of them are propylene glycol ($CH_3.CHOH.CH_2OH$), glycerol, and sorbitol and mannitol [CH_2OH $(CHOH)_4OH_2OH$]. Polyhydric alcohols are sugar derivatives and most of them, except propylene glycol, occur naturally.

Anticaking agents help prevent particles from adhering to each other and turning into a solid chunk during damp weather. The help free flowing of salts and other powders. These materials function by readily absorbing excess moisture, by coating particles to impart a degree of water repellency, and/or by imparting an insoluble particulate diluent to the mixture. Calcium silicate (Ca SiO_3 X H_2O) can absorb liquids in amounts two and a half times its weight and still remain free flowing. In addition to absorbing water, some anticaking agents effectively absorb oils and other non-polar organic compounds.

Calcium silicate is used to prevent caking in baking powder, table salt and other foods and food ingredients. Because it can absorb oils, calcium silicate is a useful anticaking agent in complex powdered mixes and certain spices which contain free essential oils. Calcium and magnesium salts of long-chain fatty acids (e.g., calcium stearate) are used as conditioning agents for dehydrated vegetable products, salt and other food ingredients in powdered form. Other anticaking agents used in food industry are sodium silicoaluminate, tricalcium phosphate, magnesium silicate and magnesium carbonate.

Leavening Agents : Leavening agents produce light fluffy baked goods. Originally, yeast was used almost exclusively to leaven baked products. It is still an important leavening agent in bread making. When yeast is used, ammonium salts are added to dough to provide a ready source of nitrogen for yeast growth. Phosphate salts (sodium phosphate, calcium phosphate) are added to aid in control of pH.

To make light cakes, biscuits, waffles, muffins, and many other baked products, chemical leavening agents are used. Baking powders generate carbon dioxide for leavening purposes.

Nutrient Supplements : Nutrient supplements restore values lost in processing or storage, or ensure higher nutritional value than what nature may have provided. When foods are processed, there may be loss of some nutrients and additives may be added to restore the original value. For example, to produce white flour, wheat is milled in such a way as to remove the brown coloured part of the grain which is rich in vitamins and minerals. To restore the nutritive value, thiamine, nicotinic acid, iron and calcium, are added to the flour. Similarly, vitamin C is added to canned citrus fruits to make up the loss of the vitamin during processing.

When manufactured foods are used as substitutes for natural ones, nutrients are to be added to the former to ensure that their nutritional value is at least equal to the natural product. For example, margarine is used as a substitute for butter on account of its cheapness. To ensure that the nutritional status of those who use margarine does not suffer addition of vitamins A and D to it, at least equal to that of the natural product, is necessary.

Some foods are to be fortified by adding specified nutrients in excess of what nature provides. Milk, for instance, which is a nutritious food is low in vitamin D content. Addition of this vitamin to milk has helped some countries to reduce the incidence of rickets. Similarly, cereals, baby foods and fruit juices are fortified with vitamins to improve the nutritional benefits. Some proteins of foods are deficient in essential amino acids and such foods are fortified with lysine and methionine. Similarly, foods are fortified with essential fatty acids, if they are deficient in them.

Iodine deficiency causes goitre. Sea foods are a source of iodine and where these do not form part of the diet, goitre may be endemic. Iodine in the form of potassium iodide added to common salt in controlled amount (iodized salt) is a safeguard against this disease. Similarly, fluorine in small quantities in food and water is required for normal tooth development. When there is this deficiency, controlled addition of fluoride to drinking water ensures effective protection against dental decay.

Non-nutritive Sweeteners : In many ways sucrose is an ideal sweetener; it is colourless, soluble in water and has a "pure" taste, not mixed with overtones of bitterness or saltiness. But it is rich in calories. The diabetics and overweights who must restrict their intake of sugar must have an alternative to sucrose. Thus, synthetic non-nutritive sweeteners having less than two per cent of the calorific value of sucrose for equivalent unit of sweetening capacity came into use.

The first synthetic sweetening agent used was saccharin (sodium ortho benzenesulphonamide or the calcium salt), which is about 300 times sweeter than sucrose in concentrations up to the equivalent of a 10 per cent sucrose solution.

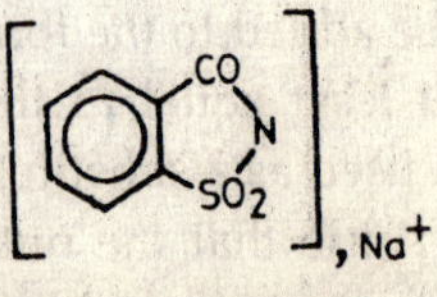

CO N SO_2 , Na^+

Sodium saccharin

Use of saccharin often leaves a bitter and unpleasant after-taste. Attempts to find better substitutes resulted in the accidental discovery of cyclamates (sodium and calcium salts of cyclamic acid—cydohexane sulpha-mate), which are about 30 times sweeter than sucrose but have little of the after-taste of saccharine. So, cyclamates were widely used as sweetening agents in the manufacture of soft drinks, other low-calories liquid foods and dietetic forms of foods. However, the use of cyclamates has been banned after high dosages were found to produce bladder cancer in rats, probably from the formation of cyclohexylamine, a known carcinogen.

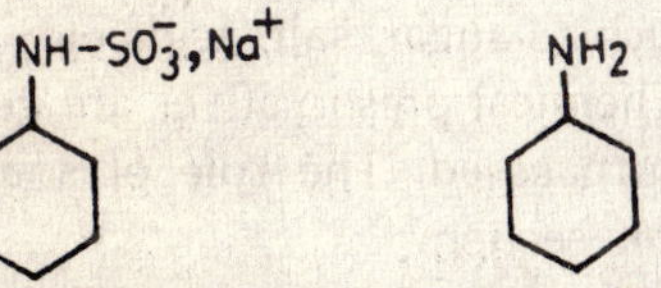

$NH-SO_3^-, Na^+$ NH_2

Sodium cyclamate **Cyclohexylamine**

Newer non-nutritive sweetening agents, ranging in sweetness from 10 to 3,000 times of sucrose have been discovered. Among them is glycyrrhiza acid, obtained from the roots of a European leguminous plant *Glycyrrhiza glabra* (licorice). The sweet taste of glycyrrhizic acid is detectable at one-fiftieth the threshold taste level of sucrose. It is used in tobacco products, confectioneries and beverages. Neohespiridine dihydrochalcone isolated from citrus peels is about 1,000-2,000 times as sweet as sucrose.

The tropical African fruits, kutemfe and serendipity berry, contain low-calorie sweeteners. Kutemfe contains two proteins thaumatin I and II. On a molar basis these substances are about 10^5 times as sweet as sucrose. The protein substance, monellin, obtained from serendipity berries, is as sweet as the sweeteners from kutemfe. But these substances are unstable to heat and lose their sweetness at pH 2 at room temperature.

A potentially useful low-calorie sweetener is the diester of L-aspartic acid and L-phenylalanine. The methyl ester of L-aspartyl-L-phenylalanine, is reported to be 100-200 times sweeter than sucrose, with taste characteristics very similar to those of sucrose.

pH Control Agents : These include acids, alkalis and buffers. They not only control the pH of foods but also affect a number of food properties such as flavour, texture, cooking qualities, etc.

Preservatives : A preservative is defined as any substance which is capable of inhibiting, retarding or arresting the growth of micro-organisms, of any deterioration of food due to micro-organisms, or of masking the evidence of any such deterioration. It is estimated that nearly 1/5 of the world's food is lost by microbial spoilage. Chemical preservatives interfere with cell membrane of micro-organisms, their enzymes or their genetic mechanisms. The compounds used as preservatives include natural preservatives such as sugar, salt, acids etc., as well as synthetic preservatives. Chemical preservatives are generally added after the foods are processed. The role of some preservatives is considered in this section.

Sodium Chloride : This has been used as a food preservative from early times. Salt stops the growth of micro-organisms and interferes with the action of proteolytic enzymes. Salt also causes food dehydration by drawing out water from the tissue cells. Salt is employed to control microbial population in foods, such as butter, cheese, cabbage, olives, cucumbers, meats, fish and bread. The amount of salt added determines the extent of protection afforded to the food. The term "brine" is used to denote the percentage of NaCl in the water phase of a food. In the preservative action of NaCl there is synefgistic action with other intrinsic factors such as pH, or extrinsic factors such as temperature, partial pressure of oxygen, etc.

Sugar : Sugar aids in the preservation of products in which it is used. The high osmotic pressure of sugar creates conditions that are unfavourable for the growth and reproduction of most species of bacteria, yeasts and molds. The preservative action of moderate strength of sugars can be improved if invertase is used to increase the concentration of glucose relative to sucrose. Foods in which sugars aid preservation include syrups and confectionery products, fondant fillings in chocolate, honey, jams, jellies, marmalades, conserves, and fruits such as dates, sultanas and currants.

Sulphur Dioxide : Sulphur dioxide has been used in foods for long as a general preservative. It is used in the treatment of fruits and vegetables before and after dehydration to extend the storage life of fresh grapes, prevent the growth of undesirable micro-organisms during wine making and in the manufacture of fruit juices. Sulphur dioxide is also the most useful agent for the prevention of browning reactions in dried fruits. Most cut fruits are treated with sulphur dioxide to prevent enzymic browning.

Forms in which sulphur dioxide is employed as a preservative include the gas (SO_2), the sodium or potassium bisulphites ($NaHSO_3$ or $KHSO_3$), sulphites (Na_2SO_3 or K_2SO_3), and metabisulphite ($Na_2S_2O_5$; or $K_2S_2O_5$). In aqueous solutions, sulphur dioxide and the sulphite salts form sulphurous acid (H_2SO_3) and ions of bisulphite (HSO^-_3) and sulphite(SO^{2-}_3). At low pH values (lower than 4.5), the undissociated sulphurous acid predominates and inhibits the growth of yeasts and molds. At high values, the $HSO^{2\prime}$ion is effective against bacteria but not against yeast. The sulphurous acid antimicrobial activity may be due to the reaction of bisulphite with acetaldehyde in the cell, the reduction of essential disulphide linkages in enzymes and the formation of bisulphite addition compounds which interfere with respiration.

One of the defects of use of sulphur dioxide is it leaves an unmistakable taste in the mouth. It also causes the breakdown of vitamin B-l, so that foods containing sulphur dioxide may not be good sources of this vitamin.

Sorbic Acid : Straight chain monocarboxylic acids and α-unsaturated fatty acid analogues have antimicrobial activity. Sorbic acid (CH_3-CH=CH-CH=CH-COOH) and its sodium and potassium salts inhibit molds and yeasts, in foods such as cheese, baked products, fruit juices, wines and pickles. The antimycotic action of sorbic acid is due to the inability of molds to metabolize the conjugated unsaturated structure.

Acetic Acid : Acetic acid (CH_3COOH) in the form of vinegar (4 per cent acetic acid) has been used to preserve pickled vegetables from antiquity. Acetates of sodium, potassium and calcium are used in bread and other baked goods to prevent ropiness and the growth of molds, but they do not interfere with yeasts. The acid is also used in foods, such as catsup, mayonnaise and pickles, primarily for flavour, but these products also benefit from the concurrent antimicrobial action. The antimicrobial activity of acetic acid increases as the pH decreases.

Propionic Add : Propionic acid ($CH_3.CH_2.COOH$) and its sodium and calcium salts exert antimicrobial activity against molds and some bacteria. The acid finds extensive use in the bakery field, where it not only inhibits molds effectively but is also active against the ropy bread organism

Bacillus Mesentericus : The toxicity of propionic acid to molds and certain bacteria is related to the inability of the organisms to metabolize the three-carbon unit.

Benzoic Acid : Benzoic acid is widely used as an antimicrobial agent. Its sodium salt is more soluble in water than the free acid and hence it is generally used. However, once in the product some of sodium benzoate is converted to the acid form. The undissociated acid is the form with anti-microbial activity. The acid is most active against yeasts and bacteria, and least active against molds. It exhibits optimum activity in the pH range 2.5-4.0 and thus is well suited for use in acid foods, such as fruit juices, carbonated beverages, pickles and sauerkraut.

Parabens : These are alkyl esters of p-hydroxybenzoic acid. The methyl, ethyl, propyl and heptyl esters are generally used. These are effective inhibitors of molds and yeasts, but are relatively ineffective against bacteria. They are active at pH 7 and higher and have little effect on flavour.

Epoxides : Epoxides are cyclic ethers that destroy all forms of micro-organisms including spores and even viruses. The epoxides used as preservatives are ethylene oxide and propylene oxide.

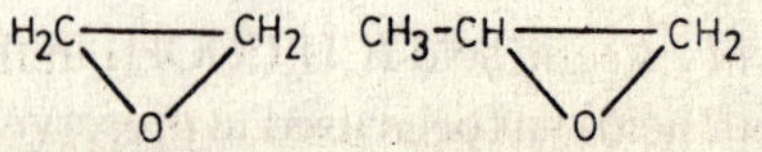

H_2C——CH_2 (bridged by O) CH_3–CH——CH_2 (bridged by O)

Ethylene oxide **Propylene oxide**

In order to achieve intimate contact with micro-organisms the epoxides are used in the gaseous form and, after adequate exposure, the residual epoxide is removed by flushing and evacuation. Their use is limited to dry items, such as nuts and spices. Spices often contain a high microbial load and they cannot be sterilized by heat because of the instability to heat of volatile flavour compounds. Thus, treatment with epoxides is a suitable method of reducing microbial load of spices.

Antibiotics : Antibiotics are antimicrobial agents produced naturally by a variety of micro-organisms. Antibiotics are of great chemotherapeutic value in controlling pathogenic micro-organisms in living animals. Their use in food preservation could lead to the development of resistant strains of organisms, thus making their medicinal use ineffective. Therefore, the use of antibiotics as food preservatives is not permitted in certain countries, while some countries allow the limited use of a relatively few antibiotics. These include nisin, pimaracin, chlorotetracycline (aureomycin) and oxytetracycline (terramycin).

Nisin is used to control the growth of sporeforming bacteria of dairy products, such as cheese and condensed milk. Nisin is nontoxic to human beings and does not lead to cross-resistance with medical antibiotics. Pimaracin is an antifungal substance and used to control the growth of fungi in cheese and sausages. Its toxicity in human beings is low and it is active in low concentrations of 10-100 parts per minion. Chlorotetracycline and oxytetracycline are used to control the growth of bacteria in fish and poultry. The residual antibiotics are destroyed by usual cooking methods.

Diethyl Pyrocarbonate : Diethyl pyrocarbonate

$$(H_5C_2O-\overset{\overset{\displaystyle O}{\|}}{C}-O\overset{\overset{\displaystyle O}{\|}}{C}-OCl_2H_5)$$

is used as an antimicrobial food additive for fruit juices, wines and carbonated beverages. It acts as a "cold sterilizing" agent for aqueous solutions. Its advantage is that following its action it is readily hydrolyzed to ethanol and carbon dioxide. It is active in low concentrations (120-300 parts per million). In concentrated solutions, it is an irritant. It is likely to react with ammonia, which is ubiquitous in plant and animal tissues, forming urethane (ethyl carbamate, $C_2H_5-O-\overset{\overset{\displaystyle O}{\|}}{C}-NH_2$) a carcinogen. Because of this, it is of limited use today. Dimethyl pyrocarbbnate, a lower member of this group of compounds, may be widely used in future as a cold sterilizing agent.

Stabilizers and Thickeners : These compounds function to improve and stabilize the texture of foods, inhibit crystallization (sugar, ice), stabilize emulsions and foams, reduce the stickiness of icings on baked products and encapsulate flavours. Substances used as stabilizers and thickeners are polysaccharides, such as gum arabic, guar gum, carrageenan, agar-agar, alginic acids, starch and its derivatives, carboxymethylcelluloses and pectin. Gelatin is one noncarbohydrate material used extensively for this purpose. Stabilizers and thickeners are hydro-philic and are dispersed in solution as colloids. These swell in hot or even cold water and help thicken food. Gravies, pie fillings, cake toppings, chocolate milk drinks, jellies, puddings and salad dressings are some among the many foods that contain stabilizers and thickeners.

Other Additives : There are a number of food additives that provide functions other than those indicated above. Clarifying agents like bentonite, gelatin, synthetic resins (polyamides and polyvinylpyrrolidone) are used to remove haziness or sediments and oxidative deterioration products in fruit juices, beers and wines. Enzymes are added to bring about desirable changes; rennin for producing curd and cheese, papain for tenderizing meat and pectinase for clarifying beverages. Firming agents like aluminium sulphates and calcium salts are used to keep the tissues of fruits and vegetables crisp. Freezing agents like liquid nitrogen and dichlorofluoromethane, which are extremely volatile and rapidly evaporate at ordinary temperatures, are used to chill foods. Solvents like alcohol, propylene glycol and glycerine are used to dissolve suspended flavours, colours and many other ingredients. Packing gases, such as inert gases, are added to packets of instant foods to prevent oxidative and many other changes.

The use of additives, as well as their numbers, is increasing with years. Use of additives has helped not only to produce more food but also to protect what is produced until it is harvested, processed, marketed, bought and eaten. Use of additives has made it possible to feed an increased population and in a better way than before. In the advanced countries of the world, the use of food additives has resulted in an increase in the number of food items available from about 900 in 1941 to 7,500 in 1975.

Sugar and salt, together with other nutritive sweeteners, corn syrup and dextrose, account for about 90 per cent of 1,800 intentional additives consumed. There are some fifty five additives which are moderately used, half of these are used as leavening agents or to control pH. Use of all other additives amounts to about 10 g per person per year. The consumption of several flavours and micronutrients may be less than 0.01 mg per person per year.

Role of Additives

Although most food additives are apparently harmless, the rapidly increasing number and types of chemicals added to our food has increased concern regarding their harmfulness. Their use has provoked many emotional responses from consumers. There are those who strongly believe that essentially all chemicals in foods are bad and we should eat only natural foods. There are others who feel that there is nothing to worry about food additives since there is no absolute proof that any chemical has harmed a human being. It thus becomes necessary to consider if food additives are safe and how to protect the consumer about unsafe additives.

There are many types of food hazards. Millions of people die every year due to microbiological hazards in the form of food-borne infections caused by unsatisfactory handling practices. There is the nutritional hazard due to sub-optimal intake of several key nutrients, due to poverty, ignorance, indifference and misinformation. Then, there are the environmental pollutants due to pollution in water. Some natural foods contain toxic substances (natural toxicants). They cause harm when consumed in sufficient quantity. Pesticides applied to food crops result in pesticide residues in food, and this is a hazard. Finally, there is the hazard of the food additives. Of all food hazards, microbiological and nutritional hazards are far greater than others; but are widely ignored. The hazards from food additives and others are remote and small; yet they receive the most attention of consumers, administrators and others.

The presence of synthetic additives does not necessarily mean that a food is harmful and the fact that a food is completely "natural" is no guarantee of its safety. Eating halibut liver can cause vitamin-A poisoning. Cabbage, lettuce, spinach, tea and a number of other foods contain very small amounts of benzopyrene, a known carcinogenic chemical. Lima beans, sweet potato and tapioca contain compounds which give deadly hydrogen cyanide in the human intestine. Some vegetables (cabbage, cauliflower, turnip brussel sprouts, etc.) can cause goitre in some susceptible individuals. Spinach and rhubarb have high oxalic acid content which can precipitate kidney stones. On the other hand, many synthetic food additives, such as vitamins, citric acid, etc., are identical to safe chemicals found in natural foods. So it is not a question of natural versus synthetic additives. The issue is the need and safety of the additive. The need for food additives has already been discussed at the beginning of this chapter and tests for the safety of food additives are to be considered now.

Evaluation of Safety : In the evaluation of safety of additives it has to be proved that harmful effects have not occurred with the addition of the chemicals. As it is difficult to carry out toxicity studies with human beings, animal experiments are carried out. The simplest way to express toxicity is by the value LD_{50}, i.e., the dosage (lethal dosage) necessary to kill 50 per cent of a population of test animals under precisely stated conditions. The four following types of toxicity studies are employed.

1. Acute toxicity, or single dose experiment
2. Subacute toxicity (daily ingestion for days or weeks)
3. Chronic toxicity (daily ingestion for weeks to months)

4. Studies of carcinogenicity, mutagenicity, teratogenicity and reproduction.

Acute Toxicity Tests : In acute toxicity studies, groups of animals (two species) are given a wide range of single doses of the additives orally or by injection into the blood stream. The LD_{50} values in a specified period of time (24 hours, 7 days) and abnormalities seen on autopsy may provide clues to the inherent toxicity of the additive.

Subacute Toxicity Tests : In a subacute toxicity test, two or more species of animals (usually rats and dogs) are used. The duration of test is 90 days. The study is made at different dose levels. They vary from near zero to those sufficiently high to produce some type of adverse effect, after the study has continued for several days. Regular evaluation of the state of health of the animals is made and the physiological and biological tests are carried out. Complete autopsy and histological examination of all organ systems of these animals given high doses of additives are carried out. These studies help determine the acceptable daily intake, in milligrams per kilogram of the body weight, allowed for human being.

Chronic Toxicity Tests : Chronic toxicity tests are conducted in a manner similar to the subacute test but the duration of the test extends for 1 to 2 years. The number of animals used at each dose and the number of dose level will be more than in the subacute test. Additives are administered at 10 to 100 times human allowable levels calculated from subacute tests. This type of test also helps determine the carcinogenicity (cancer causing) and mutagenicity (heritable changes in genetic material) of the additive. Long-term tests also help study the effect of additives on the permanent structural or functional changes induced in embryo (teratogenicity) and in reproduction, i.e., male or female fertility, litter size, litter weight and number of the surviving young.

An additive which according to the above evaluation procedure is not harmful is considered safe in some countries and permitted as a food additive. The control of additives in foods is being gradually improved and tightened and testing procedures are becoming more rigorous in different economically advanced countries of the world. The laws regulating the use the additives differ in different countries. In order to try to formulate food standards on an international basis, the FAO and WHO have set up a permanent commission designated as Codex Alimentarius, to develop international and regional food standards, which include standards of food additives and contaminants, with the hope of improving food standards all over the world. The proposals of the Codex Alimentarius is highly valuable to developing nations which as yet have few standards of their own.

Limitations of Tests : Tests for safety do not solve all the problems associated with the use of food additives. Results of animal experiments, though very useful, have their own limitations. Not all biological species respond in the same way to the same compound. Further, metabolic pathways of several animals are not identical to those of man. This raises the question of which results with animals are really applicable to human beings? In addition, a chemical that has been thoroughly tested and found to be harmless may react synergistically with another chemical to produce harmful (or beneficial) effects greater than with each of the chemicals used. It is financially and scientifically not feasible to test for all synergistic reactions with the many thousands, even millions, of the natural and synthetic chemicals. Then there is the question of what is to be done when the test for safety reveals a low order of risk or leaves doubts about toxicity.

Safety Versus Hazards : The benefits involved in the use of food additives are many, such as increased shelf-life, quality, nutritive value and economic saving. Even if there is some risk involved in the use of a food additive it becomes necessary to accept it if the benefits are sufficiently great. The benefit of saccharin as a sweetener, in the absence of an alternative, to diabetics and obese persons outweighs the risks. Nitrite used for meat preservation also prevents the growth of the micro-organism *Clostridium botulinum.* The banning of the use of nitrite for its suspected adverse effect greatly increases the toxic effects of the microbes in meat. There is no such thing as an absolute safety in food additives. Even common salt, which is essential for life in small amounts, can probably kill a person if taken at one time in large quantity. Similarly, metals like copper, chromium and zinc are essential for life in trace amounts. These can also be toxic and mortal if ingested in large amounts. The toxic effects observed with some food additives are at levels far higher than are present in food. Factors like age, sex, weight and nutritional status, are also to be taken into consideration in considering the hazards of an additive. Fortunately, our bodies possess a multitude of mechanisms for dealing safely with small amounts of toxic substances from any source. Thus, from a rational standpoint, the use of additives in foods should be accepted when they serve some useful purpose. As one cannot live in modern society without them, we must ensure that their use is controlled so as to gain benefits while eliminating hazards and abuses.

Unintentional Additives

The unintentional incorporation of chemicals into food is as widespread as intentional addition and may present health hazards. The sources of contamination are radioactive fallout, thousands of chemicals used in agricultural production, animal food additives and accidental contaminants during food processing.

Radioactive Fallout : Radioactive fallout through nuclear explosions is a serious modern problem. Nuclear explosions inject into the stratosphere as well as into the atmosphere considerable amounts of smaller particles called fission products. These contain unstable atoms, called radio-isotopes, which spontaneously break down emitting radiations and particles that are highly injurious to living tissues. The fission products finally reach the ground through rain, snow or wind. This is known as fallout. The fallout matter reaches man directly in drinking water, fruits and vegetables or indirectly through animals, which eat contaminated feed or graze on contaminated pastures.

Many of the fission-produced radioisotopes have half-lives

(length of time that has to elapse before the amount of radioactivity measured has dropped to half the original value) of less than one day. Some have a half-life of a few days (8 days for ^{131}iodine) while others are radioactive for many years. The half-life of ^{90}strontium is 28 years and that of ^{137}cesium is 30 years. Even ^{131}iodine, with a half-life of only 8 days, is hazardous for the normal functioning of thyroid. ^{90}Strontium is considered to be the most hazardous radioactive isotope. It is closely related to calcium and the body treats both strontium and calcium in exactly the same way. ^{90}Strontium induces bone cancer and leukaemia. ^{137}Cesium passes through the human body quickly but it emits radiations which, through blood, reach all tissues and can be a potential genetic danger.

Agricultural Contaminants : Chemicals in the form of insecticides, fungicides, herbicides (in general biocides), growth promoting substances and protectants, etc., are extensively used in large numbers in agricultural production. Without mem much food would be lost. Commercial production of some crops would be impossible if chemicals are not used. It is estimated that 23 per cent of the commercial cabbage crop and 37 per cent of the potato crop would be lost if chemicals were not used. Small quantities of chemical residues often remain in such crops.

The residues of the pesticide DDT has been observed in small amounts in soil, water, vegetables and animal tissues in all parts of the world. From these sources, the pesticide residues reach man. The widespread use of this chemical as an insecticide has contaminated even the air we breathe. The presence of pesticide and other residues in food is a serious international problem. WHO has attempted to control the extent of contamination by prescribing the limits for the amount of many pesticides that may be present in foods. Some countries have banned the use of chemicals like DDT.

Animal Food Additives : The use of some antibiotics as food additives has been considered in Subsection 29.15.11. They are also used as plant and animal additives. In some countries (particularly the USA), about 80 per cent of animal feed it treated with small quantities of antibiotics for enhancing growth, improved feed utilization and the checking of intestinal flora of animals. This has helped to produce less expensive meat and poultry. In all the cases where antibiotics have been used residues may remain in meat. As already indicated, the presence of antibiotics in foods may result in the development of strains resistant to antibiotic drugs.

The synthetic female hormone, diethylstilbesterol (DES), is used on chicken, cattle, sheep as implants and as a daily additive to the feed. This helps the conversion of foodstuffs into meat more efficiently in such animals. On an average the growth is one-fourth faster than in untreated animals; and the increase is more in muscle than fat. Residues of DES when present in food are potential cancer hazards.

Contamination of food in any way is bad. Just as in the case of food additives, food contamination must be considered in the light of any benefits that ensue. Use of pesticides is hazardous; but without pesticides much food would be lost. Some type of packing may result in contamination but the protection of food requiring long-distance transport from dirt and infection requires packing. Again, contamination of any type in very small quantities may not be harmful and in many cases the reported hazard has not been proved conclusively.

Aspects and Prospects

Man's basic drive is for food to satisfy his hunger. Food is intimately woven into the physical, economic, psychological, intellectual and social life of man. It is a part of his culture and is filled with many different meanings and symbolism for all individuals at various ages and stages of their maturity.

Agricultural produce, such as cereals, pulses, fruits and vegetables, and reared animals for slaughter, milk, eggs, etc., are foods or food raw materials. When consumed, foods undergo digestive and other changes to supply the body its requirements. After production and before consumption, foods are subjected to numerous adverse physical, chemical, microbial or parasitic factors which may cause their spoilage or cause disease when consumed. To prevent these and prepare food for immediate or future use requires processing, preservation and storage. Food for consumption should have the proper appearance, colour, juiciness, texture, odour and taste. During the past few decades great advances have been made in the study of the whole field of the properties, preservation and processing of raw food and of the behaviour of finished food products.

There is a tremendous growth of world population. In spite

of increased food production there is a danger of shortfall in supply. Consequently, there must be greater and more efficient utilization of the existing food sources and development of entirely new ones. Also, artificial foods, which have been controlled with respect to the attributes of eating quality, nutritional content and ease of assimilation, have to be developed to meet the requirements of man.

Great Source

Food is a more basic need of man than shelter and clothing. It provides adequately for the body's growth, maintenance, repair and reproduction. Food furnishes the body with the energy required for all human activities—it provides materials required for the building and renewal of body tissues and the substances that act to regulate body processes. An individual food, such as milk, may fulfil all these functions or, as in the case of sugar, any one function. However, all the above functions of food must be served by the diet.

All through history food has played important roles besides that of nutrition. Wars have been fought for food. People have been known to steal, rob and kill for it. Explorers have searched the world for new foods. Sciences have been built on food and food related discoveries have been rewarded. Fortunes have been made and lost in foodstuffs. Food has helped in creating history!

Food is also a Source of Power : People have been made to starve for submission. Wars have been won by blockading food supplies to the enemy. Power of food may be exerted in society and in the family, through its use as a reward or punishment. A child may be sent to bed without food because of bad behaviour or may be given something special as a reward for some in order to maintain the body in good health. Most foods fulfil more than one function as they are complex mixtures of a number of chemical substances.

Nutrients Foods are composed of dozens or even hundreds of different kinds of substances—the nutrients which when consumed in adequate amounts, fulfil all the functions of the body. Six general classes or kinds of nutrients found in all foods are carbohydrates, fats, proteins, vitamins, minerals and water.

Carbohydrates make up the bulk of our diet. They are our chief source of energy. About 70 per cent of the energy requirements for all body functions is obtained from carbohydrates. Energy is produced by the oxidation or 'internal burning' (cellular respiration) of carbohydrates in the animal cells using oxygen. Carbohydrates also help in the utilization of proteins and fats. Carbohydrates when consumed in excess are converted into fats (some glycogen also) to be used when needed.

The main sources of carbohydrates in the diet are starch and sugar. The sources of the former are mainly cereal grains (wheat, rice, etc.) or tubers (potato, sweet potato, cassova) and those of the latter are sugarcane and fruits.

Fats or lipids are the most concentrated form of energy in the food. They furnish more than twice the number of calories per gram furnished by carbohydrates or proteins. When compared to carbohydrates, fats contain a less percentage of oxygen and more of hydrogen, and consequently on oxidation yield more energy. Generally about 30 per cent of human energy requirements are met by fats. When excess energy is supplied to the body, it is stored as fat.

Fats are abundant in both plant and animal materials. In plants they may be confined to the cytoplasmic membrane or may also be present as reserve material. The fat content of fruits (except avacado and olive) is poor. Fat up to about 15 per cent is present in the germ of cereals. Nuts, such as groundnuts, are rich sources of fats. Butter from milk is an important source of fat. The adipose tissue of animals consists mainly of fats.

Proteins are the major source of building material for the body. They play an important role as structural constituents of cellular membranes and function in the maintenance and repair of body tissues. Proteins also function as biocatalysts. The food value of the protein depends upon the nature and content of its amino acids, which are its structural units. The excess of protein not required for building may be used as a source of ene gy.

Proteins are found in both animal and plant tissues. Meat, fish, poultry, eggs, milk and cheese are good sources of protein foods from animal sources. Pulses and cereals contain considerable amounts of storage proteins. Soyabean contains over 40per cent protein on dry weight basis. Nuts and seeds are also good sources of proteins. Starchy vegetables contain up to 2 per cent protein. Other vegetables and fruits are poor sources of proteins.

Vitamins are "accessory nutrients". They are required for the proper utilization of the bulk food of the diet—carbohydrates, fats and proteins, and for the maintenance of good health. Vitamins together with minerals are involved in small quantities in the regulation of body processes. They are constituents of enzymes, which function as catalysts for many biological reactions within the body.

Vitamins are found in plant and animal tissues. Their content in plant tissues varies widely depending upon the growing condition, stage of maturity, handling, processing and storage. They are not uniformly distributed in plant tissues. Vegetables and fruits are good sources of vitamins. Wheat is an excellent source of B vitamins, but the bran and germ, containing the bulk of these nutrients, are usually removed during processing. Since vitamins are simple organic substances they are easily synthesized and the synthetic vitamins are added to enrich or supplement those found in food products.

Minerals also act as catalysts for many biological reactions within the body. Their other functions include the building of bones and other structural parts of the body, muscular contraction, transmission of messages through the nervous system, and the digestion and utilization of nutrients in food. Some minerals like calcium, phosphorus, iron, magnesium and sulphur are required in large quantities, while others like zinc, copper, iodine, manganese, cobalt, etc. are required in small quantities.

Minerals are found in foods from animal and plant sources.

The mineral content of plant foods varies depending upon the mineral elements present in the medium of cultivation. The distribution of a particular mineral element varies in different tissues. Minerals, as vitamins, are added to food to enrich it.

Water is second only to oxygen in importance for the body. It is an ideal medium for transporting dissolved nutrients and wastes throughout the body.

Apart from the consumption of water as such, body needs of water are supplied by the foods we consume. Some foods contain a high percentage of water. Apart from this, oxidation of carbohydrates, fats and proteins in the body yields water.

Value of Food

In addition to the above nutrients foods contain enzymes which function as catalysts in chemical reaction, colouring material and flavour compounds achievement. Food is now being used as an experience of revolt against "the establishment".

Food is a source of security. An infant learns security from the way his mother feeds him. His behavioural patterns will be influenced by the extent to which he feels secure as regards his food supply. Similarly a growing child gains confidence and a feeling of belonging when he knows there is food in the house and he will be fed. People feel reasonably secure when they have enough food stored up to take care of them during periods of scarcity. Familiar foods give a sense of security when one has to eat away from home.

Food is a status symbol. The well-to-do eat foods the common man cannot afford, even though they may not be nutritious. It is prestigious to use polished white rice instead of brown rice which protects one against beriberi. The same is true of white flour and white bread which have replaced "black bread". The status factor associated with certain foods used by the so-called upper class makes others prefer them, to easily available, less expensive and often more nutritious foods. We serve certain foods for family meals and different foods when we have guests.

Food is a symbol of hospitality and friendship throughout the world. We express our hospitality to a guest through an offer of food or a drink. In times of disaster or sorrow we take food to the affected persons. In our country offering a cup of coffee or tea is a symbol of friendship.

Food is an outlet for emotion. As a relief from tension one may eat or overeat. For some people loneliness and boredom are relieved by continuous nibbling at food. Anger and frustration may turn one against food. Specific foods are associated with unhappy experiences. Foods consumed by some people are unacceptable and even revolting for others. Such concepts have no rhyme or reason, nor are they related to nutritive value; they are just emotional reactions.

Thus, for an average man, food is much more than a substance supplying nutrients for health. It is the sum of his culture and traditions, emotional outlet, gratification of pleasure and a relief from stress, a means of communication, security, status—all of these interwoven in the fabric of life and unconsciously expressed in food likes and dislikes. The psychological and emotional reaction to food do not yield easily to reasoning or scientific facts about nutrition.

Food Intake and its Regulations : All animals must eat to live and all have mechanisms that direct them to take food. In almost every case some control is exerted over the amount and kind of food that is taken. When hungry the animal responds by locating and ingesting foods and eating stops when hunger is satisfied.

Hunger, Appetite and Satiety : Hunger is usually an unpleasant sensation that compels a person to seek food and eat it, it is a physiological, condition which is associated with the contraction of the stomach. The contractions are forceful and occur for a period and then die away as the stomach passes into a resting stage. Hunger conditions that subside without eating will reappear later with greater intensity. In addition to stomach contractions resulting in tenseness, rumbling and a feeling of emptiness, a hungry person may experience certain general sensations, e.g. weakness, irritability, occasional headache or even nausea.

Appetite in most people is a pleasant sensation that causes a person to desire and anticipate food. An appetite can be for a certain kind of food. Appetite also has physiological components but is basically a psychological state. It is less easily localized than hunger, and is usually felt in the mouth or palate. It appears to depend more on the odour and memory of pleasant food. Appetite is clearly distinct from hunger, as a person may express a desire for some food at the end of dinner when he is comfortably replete.

Satiety is the sensation accompanying the satisfaction of the desire for food that comes after eating. It is not just the opposite of hunger and has far fewer sensations. While hunger, builds up slowly, satiety occurs rapidly. Absence of the desire for food, when it is needed, is an abnormal condition and is known as Anorexia.

Regulation of Hunger : Hypothalamus is a small portion of the brain located at its base near the brain stem. This has been identified as the area which evokes the sensation of hunger and satiety. In the central portion of the hypothalamus (the ventromedial hypothalamus), the destruction of a small area causes animals to eat voraciously and become obese, because of destruction of the satiety centre. Again, the destruction of a small centre in the side region of the hypothalamus (the lateral hypothalamus) results in the opposite effect, that is, the animals refuse to eat because of the destruction of feeding centre and become anorexic. A stimulation of the satiety centre causes organisms to stop eating and that of the feeding centre causes them to eat.

The satiety and the feeding centres of the hypothalamus are connected by nerve fibres. When stimulated, the satiety centre sends signals to the feeding centre to inhibit feeding activity. That is, the feeding centre controls the feeding behaviour and satiety centre regulates it.

A number of factors stimulate the satiety centre so that it can regulate the feeding centre. There are sensory, metabolic and hormonal influences controlling the food intake.

Sensory Influences : Stomach contraction results in hunger. But hunger contraction is not the only feature of food intake regulation, as hunger contraction continues even when the main nerve to the stomach is severed. However, there are stretch and chemo receptors in the gastro-intestinal system that record the distensions of the stomach and the presence of food after a meal, which relay information to the brain resulting in short-term regulation.

Several other stimuli involved in the gastro-intestinal system contribute to the sensation of eating. Sensory stimuli coming from the taste, smell and texture of food are relayed to the cortex of the brain, which are then transmitted to the satiety centre in the hypothalamus which results in signals to stop or to continue eating. Further, some psychological factors also have an influence on this centre.

Metabolic Factors : There are glucose receptors in the satiety centre which are receptive to glucose utilization. When food is taken, blood sugar level increases and the rate of utilization of glucose in the tissues rises. Then the receptors are stimulated, and the satiety centre signals responses to stop eating. Some hours after eating, the blood glucose level falls resulting in a low utilization rate. The satiety centre then stops sending signals to the feeding centre. This mechanism of food intake regulation is known as glucostatic regulation.

The regulation of food intake over a long-term is regulated by the amount of fat stored in the adipose tissues (lipostatic regulation). According to this theory precise information on the fat stores is relayed from the adipose tissues to the nervous control centre. If the stores are filled, signals are given to stop eating and when the fat level is reduced, eating continues till the satiety centre is activated. The manner in which the information on the fat content of adipose tissue is transmitted is not clear.

The plasma concentration of amino acid patterns produced by the diet have an effect on the amount of food intake. Since many brain neuro-transmitters are affected by the supply of amino acids, it is definitely possible that the feeding behaviour could also be so influenced (aminostatic regulation).

Hormonal Centre : A number of hormones, such as insulin, glucogen, etc. which are involved directly or indirectly in the regulation of the utilization of glucose which can be sensed by the hypothalamus glucose receptors, regulate the intake of food.

Various Patterns

Man eats what his forefathers ate, if possible, and what his environment offers. A young child does not form fixed food habits, but is patterned by adults, who eat certain foods and not others. The foods which his father does not like and which his mother therefore does not serve, do not become familiar to the child and would not be eaten by him. The environment—the physical, psychological and social setting, which relates to the culture of a group—also determines the food patterns.

Historical : Some of our knowledge of what early man ate comes from archeological studies of cave drawings of food getting and preparation activities. Other evidence of what primitive people ate includes the study of remnants of discarded food found by archeologists in mounds, pits, bogs, lake beds and tombs. The remnants of human faces (coproliter) also tell the story of early human food. From such remains of prehistoric man a picture of the food eaten by him has been reconstituted with some degree of certainty from the study of anthropologists and other scientists.

Primitive men lived as hunters and gatherers. They collected their food from wild animals and plants. They depended upon fruits, nuts, roots and other plant foods, meat from animals and fish catch in seas, lakes and rivers. They were forced to spend their days and nights in search of food. They roamed from place to place to correspond to the changing season, the coming and going of various fruits and leaves or the migration and movement of game animals. They lived this way till about 10,000 years ago in a few places and 5000 years ago inmost of the world.

Gradually, food gatherers learned to domesticate plants and

animals. They were no longer roaming about eating what was available. They settled down, built shelters and raised plants and animals to provide food. Plant domestication began in China about 10,000 B.C. followed by India, the eastern Mediterranean area and Africa. The first crops to be grown were wheat and barley from wild grasses. Simultaneously, livestock were domesticated. Cows were domesticated first and then sheep and goats. Milk was probably the first food to be extracted from animals. In the early stages, food production did not develop beyond an inefficient subsistence level and small farming communities developed around the areas of farming. The development of agricultural skills over the last two centuries and consequent supply of a sufficient amount of food, its preservation and storage, resulted in the emergence of cities and urban civilization.

One of the first great changes which occurred in man's food pattern must have been when he learnt to use fire to cook. It is not known when he first used fire for this purpose. Man eats most of his food cooked and this is one of the many characteristics which separate him from other animals. The type and amount of fuel available determines the pattern of food of a society. In areas where fuel is scarce, quick cooking foods are prepared. The use of chapatis, thin unleavened bread, and stew-like mixtures has developed in our country, and in other parts of Asia and Africa because their preparation requires meagre equipment and little fire.

Many changes took place in food patterns prior to middle ages. As man moved from one place to another, he found new foods growing in his new settlement. Since he usually carried the seeds of foods grown where he lived to his new place of residence, there was a migration of foods. Thus, sugar went from India to other parts of the world. Sweet oranges from China and sour ones from India went to Europe with the early overland traders. The dispersion of foods indigenous to one country into another has always increased the variety of man's diet from ancient times. Today, with the rapid means of communication, the differences in the diets of different countries are becoming less marked.

Effect of Population

Population Growth : The population of the entire world when agriculture or settled cultivation was started over 10,000 years ago was about 15 million. The estimate of the world population about 2000 years ago was 250 million. This was doubled in 1650. Since then there has been a threatening increase in the population growth reaching a billion in 1830,2 billion in 1940 and 4.42 billion in 1980, with more than half of the world population living in Asia. The regions of fastest population growth are Africa and South and Central America, although the world's largest growth and largest absolute increase are in South Asia. It is estimated that at the turn of the century the world population will be 6.13 billion and 90 per cent of this would be in developing countries. At present the world population is increasing by about 80 million per year.

The population of India at the time of partition of the country (1947) which was about 350 million jumped to 683 million in 1981 and is expected to exceed one billion in 2001. Now, the annual addition to the population of India is over 15 million.

The world is already facing hunger. According to recent (1985) Food and Agricultural Organization (FAO) report, abnormal food shortages have been reported in 30 countries of Africa, Asia and Latin America. The present growth rate of the world population tends to further aggravate the food situation. Also, about one-third of humanity consumes two-thirds of the world's food supply. About one quarter of the people in developing countries are undernourished. India is one of the countries which suffers from undernourishment on a vast scale.

The people of developing countries consume food corresponding to 1800-2000 kilocalories (Kcal) per day (Indian consumption is 1969 kilo-calories) . The consumption in developed countries is in the range of 3000-3500 Kcal. A utilization of under 2000 Kcal per person per day can be definitely said to be on the low side. Within any country, the distribution of food is very much in favour of the better-off people.

In developing countries, the inadequacies of food are not only in the quantity of food, but also in its quality, leading to malnutrition as well as undernutrition. The diet of people in these countries is unbalanced, because the bulk of their diet consist mainly of cereals—rice, maize, millet and starchy root. Over 80 per cent of their calories are derived from these food sources. The lack of variety in their food and particularly the shortage of protective foods leads to deficiency diseases. Protein-calorie malnutrition, particularly among children, is extremely common in these countries. In 1975, in Africa, Asia and Latin America, 20.9 million out of 34.6 million children of the age group 1-4 suffered from protein-calorie malnutrition.

Food Production : From 1950 to 1971 there was an unprecedented growth in world food production. Yields on existing crop land were raised dramatically by energy intensive agriculture. The introduction of high yielding wheat and rice strains in parts of Asia and Africa resulted in a large increase in yield and this is referred to as the "Green Revolution". During this period the world grain production increased from 631 million tonnes to 1237 million tonnes; resulting in an increase in grain availability per head, per year from 251 to 330 kg.

Even after 1971, there has been a gradual increase in the world grain production. It stood at 1432 million tonnes in 1980 as against 1237 million tonnes in 1971. But the output per head barely kept pace with population growth. During this period the availability of grain per head per year came down from 330 to 324 kg.

The position in developing countries was even worse. There was a decline in their total grain production. These countries face a widening food gap between their production and consumption. Their food import needs to be increased dramatically. The total food import of developing countries in 1984 was of the order of 100 million tonnes.

In India, the progress in agricultural production during the last 35 years has been very impressive. There has been a consistent upward trend in foodgrain production except during the years marked by acute weather aberrations. The foodgrain production has risen from 51 million tonnes in 1950-51 to a record production of 151.5 million tonnes in 1983-84 and further increases are anticipated in the coming years. Our requirement in 2000 A. D. is of the order of about 190 million tonnes.

The increase in agricultural production during the last three decades is a result of the increase in the application of science and technology in agriculture. Great strides have been made in agricultural research, education and extension. However, we cannot be complacent and ignore major problems concerned with food production. Farm management efficiency has to be improved. Input factors like water, seeds and fertilizers are to be increased. The diminishing size of an average land-holding and its adverse effect on the net income of the farmer has to be avoided. The consistent damage to the ecosystem, whose maintenance is essential for sustained agricultural advance should be prevented. Our dry farming has to be improved.

Future Prospects

The shooting population growth, rising energy costs, doubts about the adequacy of agricultural resource base, disproportionate share of available food by the well-to-do, lagging behind of new agricultural knowledge and unfavourable weather conditions have given rise to pessimism about the ability of the earth to feed its people. This assessment is also explicit or implicit in the reports of a number of international institutions concerned with world food production and demand.

It appears as though one need not be frightened about the world food situation. Actually, hunger is not new; it is as old as history. The world lives from hand to mouth, never more than one crop away from hunger. Actually, the world food problem is diminishing. The average life-span is lengthening even in the poorest countries. The life expectancy at birth is now said to be 58 years, which was 42 years in 1960. The child death rate is dropping. In the low-income countries the death rate among children in the age group 1-4 declined from 30 per thousand in 1960 to 20 in 1978. These recently born children were getting the food and health care that increased their survival rate by 14 per cent in eighteen years.

There is a decline in birth-rate. In low-income countries, the birth rate in 1960 was 48 per thousand; by 1978 it had fallen to 39. The decline in birth rate has decreased the world population growth rate from 2.0 per cent to 1.8 per cent.

The average food production in developing countries has crept upwards though it is not ahead of population growth. More land could be brought under cultivation though such development would require enormous investment and much time. There is great scope for increasing food production in the developing countries; the yield per hectare in some of them is less than half of what it is in developed countries. The poorer countries are arranging for proper distribution of available food through fair-price shops and food-for-work programmes.

The discoveries in agriculture are not lagging behind. International research has resulted in the production of high-yielding varieties of wheat and rice which has helped increase the world food supply. The number of agricultural research institutions with good financial resources is increasing. It may be hoped that the work in such institutions will result in technological breakthroughs in fields, such as gene-splicing, textured vegetable proteins, nitrogen fixation from non-leguminous crops, salt tolerant crops, wild crosses of plants and animals, improved photosynthesis, long-range weather forecasting or computer-aided agriculture management.

Food products are being used for non-food purposes, e.g., because of fuel scarcity, some countries are using petrol mixed with alcohol. If this is practised on a world scale, produce from 5 per cent of farmland would be required for this purpose. We can ill afford this when hunger is threatening the world.

A large amount of vegetable material like grasses are available. They are not eaten because they consist largely of cellulose which man is unable to digest. Proteins are extracted from grasses and other vegetable matter. Such protein concentrates are not used as foods now as they lack both taste and smell. But they could be used as foods after improved processing.

After the oils are extracted from nuts, a residue rich in proteins is left. This residue at present is mostly used as animal food or fertilizer. It is estimated that the amount of protein contained in such oilseed residues is sufficient to provide twice the world's deficit of protein. Oilseed cake can be processed and used as food. It is already being used to a certain extent in some poor countries. This could be expanded.

New foods can be obtained in future. We are now mostly depending on foods derived from plants grown on land. Unicellular organisms, such as yeasts, algae and fungi may be cultivated on liquids. These are rich sources of high-quality proteins and could be developed as food. New foods may also be developed by chemical synthesis.

Thus, it should be possible to have sufficient food for future generations if we make the needed investment to develop and distribute new agricultural knowledge, the developed countries share their knowledge and experience with the less developed ones and the developing countries are diligent enough to improve their agriculture and reduce the rate of growth of their population number. Action should also be taken to prevent the conversion of a high share of our food into non-food products, and to develop food from non-traditional sources. Scientific and technological improvements will help meet the food needs of the future.

Bibliography

Ainaduraj, S.G.: *A Review of Research on Spices and Cashewnuts in India*, ICAR, New Delhi,

Andrews, S.: *Food and Beverage Science*, Tata McGraw Hill, Publishing Co. Ltd., New Delhi, 1980.

Ansell, G.B., J,N. Hawthrone and R.M.C. Dawson : *Functions of Phospholipids*, Elsevier, New York., 1973.

Arora, K.: *Theory of Cooking*, K.N. Gupta & Co., Delhi, 1982.

Aurand, L.W. and A.E. Woods : *Food Chemistry*, The AVI Publishing Co., Connecticut, 1973.

Austin, A. and A. Ram : *Studies on Chapati-Making Quality of Wheat*, Indian Council of Agricultural Research, New Delhi, 1971.

Aykrod, W.R. and J. Doughty : *Legumes in Human Nutrition*, FAO, Rome, 1973.

Bachman, W.: *Continental Confectionery*, Maclaren and Sons Ltd.London, 1955.

Banerjee, G.C.: *Poultry, Oxford and IBH Publishing Co.*, New Delhi, 1979.

Barrow, G.M.: *Physical Chemistry for Life Science*, McGraw-Hill Book Company, New York, 1992

Bennion, M.: *Introductory Foods*, Macmillan Publishing Co., New York, 1980.

Birch, G.C., A.G. Cameron, and M. Spencer : *Food Science*, Pargamon Press, New York,1984.

Birch, G.G., J.G. Prennan and K.J. Parker : *The Sensory Properties of Foods*, Applied Science Publication Ltd., London, 1977.

Bland, J.W. : *Clinical Metabolism of Body Water and Electrolytes*, U.B. Saunders Company, Philadelphia, 1962.

Board, R.G.: *A Modern Introduction to Food Microbiology*, Blackwell Scientific Publications, Oxford, 1983.

Borgstrom, G.: *Fish as Food*, Academic Press, New York, 1962.

Borgstrom, G.: *Principles of Food Science*, The Macmillan Co., London, 1971.

Briggs, G.M. and D.H. Calloway : *Nutrition and Physical Fitness*, W.B. Saunders Co., Philadelphia, 1979.

Cambell, A.M., M.P. Penfield, and R.M. Griswold : *Experimental Study of Foods*, Houghton, 1990.

Cesaerani, V. and R. Kinton : *Practical Cookery*, Edward Arnold, London, 1981.

Chandy, M.: *Fishes*, National Book Trust, India, 1970.

Chang, R.: *Physical Chemistry with Application to Biological System*, Collier Macmillan, International Edition, 1977.

Charalambons, G., and G. Inglett : *The Quality of Foods and Beverages: Chemistry and Technology*, Academic Press, New York, 1981.

Charley, H.: *Food Science*, John Wiley and Sons Inc., New York. 1982.

Cherry, J.P.: *Protein Functionality in Foods*, American Chemical Society, Washington D.C., 1981.

Chichester, C.O. : *The Chemistry of Plant Pigments*, Academic Press, New York, 1972.

Choudhury, B. : *Vegetables*, National Book Trust, New Delhi, 1977.

Clydesale, F. : *Food Science and Nutrition*, Prentice-Hall, Inc., New Jersey, 1979.

Copson, D. A.: *Microwave Heating*, The AVI Publishing Co. Inc., Connecticut, 1975.

Davidson, E.A.: *Carbohydrate Chemistry*, Holt, New York, 1967.

Desrosier, N.C.: *Food Preservation*, The AVI Publishing Co. Inc., Connecticut, 1970.

Dick, D.A.T. : *Cell Water*, Butterworth, Washington, 1966.

Dickerson, R.E. and I. Geiss : *Proteins: Structure, Function and Evolution*, Menlo Park, California, 1983.

Duckworth, R.B.: *Fruits and Vegetables*, Ptrgamon Press, New York, 1966.

Dyke, S .F.: *The Chemistry of Vitamins*, Interscience Publishers Inc., New York, 1965.

Eckles, C.H., W.B. Combs and H. Macy : *Milk and Milk Products*, Tata McGraw-Hill, Bombay, 1980.

Eisenberg, D. and H. Kauzmann : *The Structure and Properties of Water*, Clarendon, Oxford, 1969.

Eley, G.: *Wild Fruits and Nuts*, E.P. Publishing Ltd., Yorkshire, 1976.

Farrington, D. and A.A. Roberts : *Physical Chemistry*, John Wiley & Sons Inc., New York, 1962.

Fennema, O.R.: *Food Chemistry*, Marcell Dekker Inc., New York, 1976.

Fersht, A. : *Enzyme Structure and Mechanism*, W.H. Freeman & Co., 1977.

Forrest, J.C., E.D. Aberle, H.B. Hedrick, M.D. Judge and R.A Merkel : *Principles of Meat Science*, W.H. Freeman and Co., San Francisco, 1975.

Furia, T.E.: *Hand Book of Food Additives*, C.R.C. Press, T.C. Ohio, 1977.

Goodwin, T.W: *The Biochemistry of Carotenoids*, Academic Press, New York, 1980-84.

Gould, R.F. : *Flavour Chemistry*, American Chemical Society, Washington, D.C., 1966.

Gould, W. A.: *Food Quality Assurance*, The AVI Publishing Co. Inc., Connecticut, 1977.

Greenstein, J.P. and M. Winitz : *Chemistry of Amino Acids*, John Wiley & Sons, New York, 1961.

Gunstone, F.D.: *An Introduction to the Chemistry and Biochemistry of Fatty Acids and their Glycerides*, Chapman and Hall, London, 1967.

Gurr, M.E. and A.T. James : *Lipid Biochemistry—An Introduction*, Cornell, Ithaca, New York, 1975.

Gyorgy, P. and W.N. Pearson : *The Vitamin*, Academic Press Inc., New York, 1967.

Hall, C.W.: *Dictionery of Drying*, Marcel Dekker, Inc., New York, 1979.

Harrison, S.G., G.B. Masefield and M. Wallis: *The Oxford Book of Food Plants*, Oxford University Press, London, 1975.

Hascherneyer, R. and A.H. Haschemeyer : *Proteins: A Guide to Study of Physical and Chemical Methods*, John Wiley & Sons, New York, 1973.

Hilditch, T.P. and P.N. Williams: *The Chemical Constitution of Natural Fats*, Chapman and Hall, London, 1964.

Hobbs,B.C. : *Food Microbiology*, Arnold-Heine Mann, New Delhi, 1982.

Holman, R.T. : *The Progress in the Chemistry of Fats and other Lipids*, Pergamon Press, New York, 1971.

Howes, F.N.: *Nuts*, Fabers and Fabers Ltd., London, 1948.

Hudson, B.J.F. : *Development in Food Proteins*, Applied Science Publisher, London, 1982.

Hunt, P. : *Fruit and Vegetables*, Ward Lock Ltd., London, 1972.

Jacob, M.B. : *Chemistry and Technology of Foods*, Interscience Publishers Inc., New York, 1951.

Jasscler, D.K. and M.A. Joslyn : *Fruit and Vegetables Juice*, The AVI Publishing Co. Inc., Connecticut, 1971.

Jull, M.A.: *Poultry Husbandry*, Tata McGraw-Hill Publishing Co. Ltd., New Delhi, 1977.

Juuka, W.R. and H.M. Pancoast, *Hand Book of Sugars*, The AVI Publishing Co. Inc., Connecticut, 1973.

Kacharoo, P.: *Pulse Crops of India*, ICAR, New Delhi, 1970.

Kadans, J.M.: *Encyclopedia of Fruits, Vegetables, Nuts and Seeds*, Parker Publishing Co. Inc., New York, 1973.

Katyal, S.L. : *Vegetable Growing in India*, Oxford and IBH Publishing Co., New Delhi, 1977.

Kent, N.L.: *Technology of Cereals*, Pergamon Press, New York, 1978.

Krause, M.V. and L.K. Mahann: *Food Nutrition and Diet Therapy*, W.B. Saunders Co., Philadelphia, 1979.

Lal, G., G.S. Siddappa and G.L. Tandon : *Preservation of Fruits and Vegetables*, Indian Council of Agricultural Research, New Delhi, 1960.

Lennarz, W.J. : *The Biochemistry of Glycoproteins and Proteoglycans*, Plenum, New York, 1980.

Less, R. and E.B. Jackson : *Sugar Confectionery and Chocolate Manufacture*, Leonard Hill Books, An Intertext Publisher, Burks, 1973.

Levie, A. : *The Meat Hand book*, The AVI Publishing Co. Inc., Connecticut, 1967.

Lloydryall, A. and W.T. Pendzer: *Handling Transportation and Storage of Fruits and Vegetables: Fruits and Peanuts*, The AVI Publishing Co. Inc., Connecticut, 1974.

MacGregor, E. A. and C.T. Greenwood : *Polymers in Nature*, John Wiley & Sons, New York,

Mackinney, G. and A.C. Little : *Colour of Foods*, The AVI Publishing Company, Connecticut, 1972.

Malik, R.K. and K.C. Dhingra : *Up-to-date Confectionery Industries*, Small Industry Research Institute, New Delhi, 1976.

Marks, J., A : *Guide to the Vitamins: Their Role in Health and Disease*, University Park Press, Baltimore, 1975.

Marton, I.D. and A.J.Macbod : *Food Flavours*, Elesvier Scientific Publishing Co., New York, 1982.

Mate, S. A.: *Cereal as Foods and Feeds*, The AVI Publishing Co. Inc., Connecticut, 1959.

—: *Cereal Sciences*, The AVI Publishing Co. Inc., Connecticut, 1969.

—: *Cookie and Craker Technology*, The AVI Publishing Co. Inc., Connecticut, 1978.

—: *Bakery Technology and Engineering*, The AVI Publishing Co. Inc., Connecticut, 1972.

—: *Cereal Technology*, The AVI Publishing Co. Inc., Connecticut, 1970.

Mcwilliams, M.: *Food Fundamentals*, John Wiley & Sons Inc., New York, 1979.

Mellor, J. D.: *Fundamentals of Freete-Drying*, Academic Press, London, 1978.

Meyer, L.H. : *Food Chemistry*, Reinhold Publishing Corporation, New York, 1961.

Michael Eskin, N.A. : *Plant Pigments, Flavours and Textures*, Academic Presss, New York, 1979.

Murthy, R.B.: *Breeding Procedures in Pearl Millet*, ICAR, New Delhi, 1977.

Nagy, S., P.E. Shaw and M.K. Veldhnis : *Citrus Science and Technology*, The AVI Publishing Co. Inc., Connecticut, 1977.

Nath, P. : *Vegetables for the Tropical Region*, Indian Council of Agricultural Research, New Delhi, 1976.

Palmer, T.: *Understanding Enzymes*, John Wiley & Sons, New York, 1981.

Pamela, V.P. : *Directory of Wines and Spirits*, North Wood Publication, London, 1974.

Parry, J.W. : *Spices*, Chemical Publishing Co. Inc., New York, 1969.

Paul, P.C. and H.H. Palmer: *Food Theory and Application*, John Wiley.& Sons Inc., New York, 1972.

Peckham, G.G. and J.H. Freeland-Graves : *Foundations of Food Preparation*, Macmillan Publishing Co. Inc., New York, 1979.

Peterson, M.S. and A.H. Johnson : *Encyclopedia of Food Science,* The AVI Publishing Co. Inc., Connecticut, 1978.

Peterson, M.S. and D.K. Tressler : *Food Technology the World Over,* The AVI Publishing Co. Inc., Connecticut, 1963.

Pigman, W.W. and D. Horton : *The Carbohydrates: Chemistry and Biochemistry, Plants,* C.S.I.R, New Delhi, 1969.

Potter,N.M. : *Food Science,*The AVI Publishing Co. Inc., Connecticut, 1978.

Prasad, A.S. and D. Oberleas : *Trace Elements in Health and Disease,* Academic Press, New York, 1976.

Puruthi, J.S.: *Spices and Condiments,* National Book Trust of India, New Delhi, 1976.

Ranganna, K.S. and K.T. Achaya : *Indian Dairy Products,* Asia Publishing House, Bangalore, 1974.

Ranganna, S. : *Manual of Analysis of Fruit and Vegetable Products,* Tata McGraw-Hill Publishing Co. Ltd., New Delhi, 1984.

Roberts, D.V. : *Enzyme Kinetics,* Cambridge University Press, 1977.

Rogers, C.A.C.: *Profitable Poultry Keeping in India and the East,* Treasure House of Books, Bombay, 1966.

Rudolph Ballentine: *Diet and Nutrition,* The Himalayan International Institution, Honesdale, Pennsylvania, USA, 1979.

Runeckles, V.C. : *Recent Advances in Phytochemistry,* Academic Press, New York, 1972.

Schapira, J.: *The Book of Coffee and Tea,* St. Martin's Press, New York, 1975.

Schultz, G.E. and R.H. Schirmer : *Principles of Protein Structure,* Springer-Verlage, New York, 1979.

Sebrell, W.H. (Jr.) and R.S. Harris : *The Vitamins,* Academic Press Inc., New York, 1967.

Simms, A.E. : *Fish and Shellfish,* Virtue and Company Limited, London, 1973.

Singh, B., : *Races of Maize,* ICAR, New Delhi, 1975.

Smartt, J.: *Tropical Pulses*, Longman Group Ltd., London, 1976.

Sri Aurobindo : *The Upanishads,* Sri Aurobindo Ashram, Pondicherry, 1977.

Stadlmare, W.J. and. O.Y. Cotterill : *Egg Science and Technology,* The AVI Publishing Co. Inc., Connecticut, 1973.

Stumbo,C.R. : *Thermobacteriology in Food Processing,* Academic Press, Inc., New York,

Sultan, W. J.: *Modem Pastry Cheff,* The AVI Publishing Co. Inc., Connecticut, 1977.

Swern, D, : *Bailey's Industrial Oil and Fat Products,* Interscience Publishers Division, John Wiley & Sons, New York, 1964.

Tandon, H.P.: *Egg and its Care,* Ministry of Agriculture, Govt. of India, New Delhi, 1973.

Thangam, P.E.: *Modern Cookery for Teaching and Trade,* Orient Longmans Ltd., Bombay, 1983.

Thankamma, J.: *Food Adulteration,* S.G. Wasani, New Delhi, 1976.

Underwood, E.J: *Trace Elements in Human and Animal Nutrition,* Academic Press, New York, 1977.

Warner, J.N.: *Principles of Dairy Processing,* Wiley Eastern Ltd., New Delhi, 1976.

Weiss.T. J.: *Food Oils and their Uses,* The AVI Publishing Inc., Connecticut, 1970.

Whistler, R.L. and J.N. BeMiller : *Industrial Gums,* Academic Press, New York, 1972.

Whitaker, J.R. : *Principles of Enzymology for Food Science,* Marcel Dekker Inc., New York, 1977.

Whiteley, P.P. : *Biscuit Manufacture,* Elsevier Publishing Co. Ltd., London, 1971.

Williams, A, : *Bread Making,* Hutchinson, Benhan, London, 1975.

Williams, J., R. E. Eakin, E. Beersteeker, (Jr.) and W. Shine : *The Biochemistry of Vitamins,* Reinhold, New York, 1950.